Praise for the 3-Day Solution Plan

"The Solution Plan is the whole package! I not only lost weight but also feel healthier and happier. The Solution is just what I needed, physically and mentally."

—Annie, *Prescott, Arizona*

"After a lifetime of searching, I have found a solution for my overeating! Thank you!"

—Kathryn, *Vancouver, B.C.*

"Finally, a plan which eliminated my cravings. I even passed on chocolate, without regrets! Thank you! Thank you!"

—Lee, *Huntsville, Oregon*

"I feel this is my solution to permanent weight control. It focuses on the real reasons I'm overeating and a detailed plan to combat it."

—Jackie, *Los Angeles*

"Thank you for a great way to jump-start not only a diet but a new way of life."

—Janice, *Knoxville, Tennessee*

"The Solution helped me be a 'mindful' eater rather than an 'unconscious' eater. It's what I needed."

—Laurie, *Nashua, New Hampshire*

"I've tried Weight Watchers (twice!), South Beach, and diet pills. This is the first plan I ever tried that made me believe I could solve my weight problem once and for all!"

—Joanna, *Philadelphia*

"My drive to overeat decreased a lot. I lost about four pounds over the three days. Sometimes I still wanted a cookie, but I didn't eat it!"

—Frank, *Cincinnati*

"The best I have felt in years."

—Selma, *Seattle*

"By the end of the third day, I had lost six pounds—and that's without doing the plan perfectly!"

—Diane, *Cincinnati*

"It really does turn off the drive to overeat! No more fruitless attempts to 'control myself.' I felt like I was enjoying food for the first time."

—Jennifer, *Eugene, Oregon*

"I have been binge-free for the entire past week for the first time in years."

—Carol, *Austin*

"I used the 12-step approach for years, but this is far more powerful. The drive to overeat is gone."

—Dave, *Detroit*

"By the middle of the third day, I felt physically as if there was an aura of well-being surrounding me and a glow of health I haven't felt in many years. Thanks!"

—Christine, *Oklahoma City*

"Wow! I want to share this experience with everyone I care about! Finally, something that teaches me how to *keep* the weight off!"

—Sharon, *Boston*

"In three days, I felt healthier and more at peace with myself and the world."

—Lisa, *Cincinnati*

"It was so easy to follow and so rewarding that I didn't want it to end! This is how I want to experience *every day* of my life!"

—Jeanette, *Denver*

"My husband and I did it together. In my thirtysome years of marriage, we have never felt as close and intimate, plus we both lost weight. Thank you!"

—Christine, *Richmond, Virginia*

"What a way to live each day!"

—Jason, *Cleveland*

"Most of us know 'it's not about the food,' but that doesn't help us discover and change what it's really about. Finally, a program that allows us to fix what's really been going on."

—Judy, *Phoenix*

"Even though I kept second-guessing myself, I was amazed at how fast my body responded. Not to mention the body-soul connection. Thank you!!!"

—Jane, *Mountain View, California*

"What a great feeling to awaken to a spring in my step and my thoughts turning to what creative things I could do for the day . . . instead of what I was going to have for breakfast!"

—Kathy, *San Diego*

"I didn't have any sugar cravings. I had so much energy. I knew clearly that I wanted a lot more of this!"

—Ken, *Gainesville, Florida*

"Wow! I feel free, light, and I have such energy! I want to have this be my life."

—Chris, *Austin*

"I felt so energized on this plan, and I'm balanced for the first time in years. The drive to overeat was turned off in three days. . . . And I lost five pounds!"

—Christine, *Oklahoma City*

"Using this plan, I was less likely to overeat. It really works!"

—Matt, *Springfield, Illinois*

"It felt very comforting to be on the three-day plan. I felt a sense of emotional structure that is usually missing from my day-to-day life."

—Barbara, *Sonoma, California*

"I found out that my emotions controlled my eating more than I thought! Once I made the connection, I felt free to eat responsibly! It was liberating!"

—Val, *Comox, B.C.*

"I found a peace in those three days that grows stronger as I continue to use the tools."

—Angelica, *Walla Walla, Washington*

"The three-day plan is three days of fun and energy—and I lost six pounds!"

—Jennifer, *Eugene, Oregon*

"I was the happiest I have been in years during these three days! This plan really works!"

—Cara, *Ontario, Canada*

"This is *not* a diet. This plan goes to the heart of *why* we overeat. I felt cared for and guided into my own wisdom!"

—Jacqueline, *Kansas City, Missouri*

"I couldn't believe that I didn't crave chocolate for the entire three days! That's a miracle!"

—Lee, *Ontario, Canada*

"It feels like a light has been turned on inside my body. I have more energy and vitality than ever!"

—Lyssette, *Los Angeles*

"Thanks for helping me discover the power of real feelings!"

—Ron, *Eugene, Oregon*

"I was amazed at how confident I felt after just three days. The drive to overeat just vanished!"

—Emily, *Long Beach, California*

"Who knew losing weight could feel so good and be such fun?"

—Karen, *Providence, Rhode Island*

"What a wonderfully creative program! Just what I needed to lift my spirits and lose some weight!"

—JoAnn, *San Diego*

"I lost four pounds in three days. Taking some time for myself was such a great idea—long overdue!"

—Doug, *San Mateo, California*

"The plan freed me from focusing on food, what to eat, when to eat, and put the focus on where I feel it needed to be—on the why."

—Deidre, *Westwood, New York*

"I've finally found what I've been looking for my entire life: the power to stop overeating!"

—Ann, *Salem, Massachusetts*

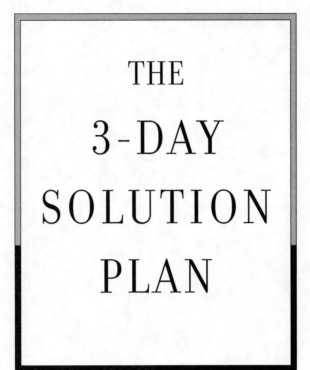

THE
3-DAY
SOLUTION
PLAN

ALSO BY LAUREL MELLIN

The Pathway

The Solution

The Shapedown Program

THE
3-DAY
SOLUTION
PLAN

*Jump-Start Lasting Weight Loss
by Turning Off the Drive to Overeat*

Laurel Mellin, M.A., R.D.

A Solution® Method Book

BALLANTINE BOOKS
New York

The information in this book is provided for general reference and educational purposes only and is not intended to address, diagnose, or treat any medical or psychological condition. If you have or suspect you may have a medical or mental health condition, or if you are taking any medication, use dietary supplements, consume three or more alcoholic beverages daily, use recreational, prescription, or over-the-counter drugs or have a history of addictive behaviors or dependencies, you must be supervised by a knowledgeable physician who is fully aware of your condition and medical history. Always consult with your doctor before embarking on any exercise or dietary regimen or altering an established dietary or exercise plan, particularly if you are pregnant or breastfeeding or have any other medical or mental condition. Do not combine this plan with any other plan except under appropriate medical supervision.

Published in the United States by Ballantine Books, an imprint of The Random House Publishing Group, a division of Random House, Inc., New York.

Ballantine and colophon are registered trademarks of Random House, Inc.
The Solution® and the nurturing and limits symbols are registered trademarks used under license by The Institute for Health Solutions, a non-profit organization.

Library of Congress Cataloging-in-Publication Data

Mellin, Laurel.
The 3-day solution method : jump-start lasting weight loss by turning off the drive to overeat / Laurel Mellin.
p. cm.
"A solution method book."
ISBN 1-4000-6377-9 (alk. paper)
1. Weight loss—Psychological aspects. 2. Appetite.
3. Compulsive eating. I. Title: Three-day solution method. II. Title.

RM222.2.M4513 2005
619.2'5—dc22   2004061590

Printed in the United States of America

Ballantine Books website address: www.ballantinebooks.com

2 4 6 8 9 7 5 3 1

First Edition

Text design by Nicola Ferguson

FOR MY FAMILY

Mackey and Papa, Haley, Joe and John,
Steve and Viv, Sarah, Lisa, and Michael

Contents

Introduction

WHEN I WAS twelve years old, devouring three cinnamon rolls
for my after-school snack and worrying incessantly about the size of
my thighs, my mother put me on a diet. I gained five pounds immediately.

Dieting made me hungrier!

That experience fueled my interest in nutrition. Enough so that
when a physician erroneously told me in my early twenties that I
couldn't have kids, I turned to find my life's purpose in promoting
health through good nutrition. Plus, I thought that knowing more
about nutrition might just solve my own struggles with food and
weight. So I went to graduate school in nutrition science, but even
after that experience, my own issues with food didn't magically disappear. Part of me was still that little girl who craved cinnamon
rolls and had terrible things to say about her thighs. Knowledge was
clearly not the answer.

As fate would have it, a position in adolescent medicine on the
faculty at UCSF enabled me to train in other disciplines and gave
me the clinical experience and intellectual nourishment to reflect
on the true roots of weight and eating problems. Many people—
Charlie Irwin, Carl Greenberg, Vilia Frost, Susan Johnson, Marion
Nestle, Marna Cohen, Mary Crittenden, and many others—guided
my learning. I applied these ideas to treating adolescent obesity and
developed The Shapedown Program, which launched in 1979. At
the time, the program was not all that different from most family-
based diet, exercise, and behavioral programs. The results were

similar, too. There were always one or two star pupils in every group, but how did the rest do? Not all that well. I knew that there was a missing link in weight control but I didn't know what it was.

Then one day, seven stories below ground level in the UCSF medical library, I found a largely overlooked research paper published in 1940. Hilde Bruch, M.D., a Baylor College of Medicine professor, conducted a study that showed that, other than genetics, parental indulgence and deprivation were at the root of children's weight problems. The repeated contact with an indulging or depriving environment did not meet the children's needs, and their appetites ramped up. Later, emerging neuroscience showed that repeated contact with an indulging or depriving environment also wired children's brains to tend to indulge and/or deprive themselves. In a culture in which food is glorified, tantalizing, and abundant, it made sense that that pattern of deprivation and indulgence would be expressed in eating. Even if they didn't overeat as children, they would be primed to go to excess with food or another external solution later on in life.

Bruch's findings were consistent with psychological development and family systems theories. Indulgence and deprivation are two sides of the same coin, and they both have the same source: not enough skill in self-nurturing and effective limit setting. If we can't nurture ourselves, how can we nurture our children? If we can't set limits with ourselves, how can we set limits with our kids? Not enough nurturing leads to deprivation and not enough limits lead to indulgence. Both indulgence and deprivation block development and fan the flames of emotional appetites. Excesses are passed from one generation to the next not just by genetics or modeling of the behavior, but by a parent's unconscious transmission to their young of the tendency to indulge and deprive.

Bruch's findings were in harmony with what we saw in our clinic. Parents had plenty of love for their children. They felt the *emotion* of love, but they struggled with having the *skill* to nurture and set limits with their kids, particularly given all the stresses of modern life. The good news was that this missing link was something that could be *taught*! It was something as concrete as skills, not something genetic but learned. Moreover, if insufficient nurturing and limit setting blocked development, then pumping up those tools could facilitate development. If we could teach the skills, the level, we now know, rewires the elusive feeling brain, and the drive to go to excess could possibly fade. Those urges and cravings for cookies, candy, and chips—and even cigarettes, alcohol, pill popping, spending, and overworking—could subside. And because changes in the feeling brain tend to persist, maybe these changes could even be lasting.

Immediately, my colleagues and I began teaching the skills to parents and children in our clinic, and then watched with amazement. The simple act of pumping up these developmental skills changed nearly everything! It was as if these children had been freed. They could so readily connect with themselves and others that they didn't need the extra food. They lost weight without rigid dieting. They ate less because they wanted less. They felt like getting off the couch and going out to play.

These twenty-five years of teaching these skills have gone rather quickly. I've raised my three children and been through my share of ups and downs. Despite some daunting and humorous challenges, there has been an astonishing amount of grace, for the method has continued to develop and evolve.

The first program, Shapedown, was revised so that it is now based on this interweaving of developmental skills mastery and healthy lifestyles. It is provided in 1,000 hospitals and clinics nationwide (for a list of providers see www.shapedown.com). With a new developmental skills approach, the results showed great improvement compared to the old program that involved diet, exercise, and cognitive-behavioral treatment. In fact, parents who watched their children participate in this program said, "We want more of these skills, too. Why isn't there a program for us?"

The program for adults, The Solution, began in 1991 and was first developed for weight loss. However, our research showed that those using the method saw improvement in the whole range of common excessive appetites. Their moods tended to improve: depression decreased 50 percent in the first 12 weeks of training and the participants' relationships and spiritual lives blossomed. The feeling brain is the seat of excessive appetites, emotional balance, relationship intimacy, and spiritual connection, so our results made a lot of sense. If the long-term use of the method rewired the neural networks in the feeling brain, these broad-spectrum changes would naturally follow.

We began to stop thinking about simple weight loss or even lasting weight loss and turned our sights to something more: a Solution, that is, freedom from the whole range of common excesses and a life abundant in the rewards of maturity, such as balance, self-acceptance, sanctuary, vibrancy, intimacy . . . and joy! Since that time, this paradigm shift from the narrow focus on one excess to concentrating on the roots of the excesses has made more and more sense. After all, the obesity epidemic was fueled, in part, by the tremendous success of the anti-tobacco initiative. Many people stopped smoking and started overeating! Reducing health care expenditure and maximizing personal health and happiness takes going to the roots of problems rather than just chasing symptoms.

The first person I saw reach a Solution was ten years old, a little girl with curly dark hair and dancing brown eyes. After about 10 weeks of using the method, her mother said to me, "I don't know what's going on, but this child is a different person. She's happy! She doesn't even *want* the extra food. It's like . . . her weight and food are not even issues in her life." That was a time when I still didn't have *my own* Solution!

How to explain this rapid change? The brains of children are like little sponges: they soak in these skills and transform so quickly! The same transformation happens for adults but it takes longer to achieve, typically through 18 months of training. So if you want a quick fix, this is not the right program for you. However, those who are committed to rewiring their feeling brain to naturally favor a life of balance and freedom from external solutions, typically say that it is a godsend. Although these changes can occur through many means, one usually has to forge a path for oneself, with all the attendant missteps and strife. This method offers a clear and certain pathway for those who want to use it.

A non-profit organization, the Institute for Health Solutions, now disseminates Solution training and provides professional certification in the clinical use of the method. We learned early on that being a psychologist, family therapist, physician, or dietitian did not provide enough training for us to administer the method effectively. Most health professionals don't have a Solution in their own lives, just the way I didn't when I started doing this work. We can't teach skills to others that we don't have ourselves! More training—personal and clinical—is essential, and a professional training program, now accredited by the American Psychological Association and other professional organizations, is available to licensed health professionals.

Every year, we continue to learn more about the method. In the late 1990s we began to understand that the magical changes we were seeing—in almost all the participants—reflected the power of the method to retrain the elusive feeling brain. Only in the last few years have we really appreciated the immense power of a fulfilling, vibrant lifestyle in turning off the drive to go to excess. Doubtless, there will be more to learn. Our priority now is to bring the method to more people who are at highest risk and to children, in order to decrease the risk of the legacy of external solutions from being transmitted generation to generation. Children have always been a major focus, as well as parents and grandparents who can pass the skills along to the young.

Although the program for adults was initially used by women, that has changed. There are now many men who come into training, and many couples, too. While our original focus was on solving weight problems, that has changed as well. In recent years, numerous people have challenged us: "Do I have to develop a weight problem to be eligible to get these skills?" they asked. The book *The Pathway* opened the door to the use of the method in combating excess and reaping life's rewards. It is a perfect companion to this book and essential reading for those who use the method.

It's taken a long time to develop the method and to get the word out about it; however, the timing has been perfect in its own way. We have learned more not only about the mechanism through which the method works, but how to make mastering these skills and reaching a Solution easier, safer, and quicker. Our complete Solution course ("The Solution Kits") doesn't just tell you what you should do and hopes that you do it. Rather, it gently and effectively guides you through the process, giving you just what you need at each point of the journey. It offers a predictable pathway to rewiring the feeling brain and, within the limits of genetics and circumstance, appears for many people to end weight problems and other excesses for good. This book is an introduction to that course.

Counting all the books and workbooks written for the Institute and Shapedown, this is my thirty-fourth book! Yet it's the *first one* that has offered a plain and simple plan for beginning to experience the power of the method. Sometimes the best things come last.

The 3-Day Solution Plan will offer you an easy, effective way to use the method to appreciate the power you have to turn off your drive to overeat. It will also enable you to jump-start the journey that leads to having a Solution in your own life. However, the most important immediate benefit of using this plan may not be the weight you lose (typically three pounds in three days), or even the introduction to this method. It may well be a feeling you have on the third day of the plan: a sense of being complete, a moment in which you know that on the day that you were born, you had all the inherent strength, goodness, and wisdom you would ever need to be free of common excesses, to live life to the fullest, and to do what you came to Earth to do.

All you required were the tools to access it.

—Laurel Mellin
San Anselmo, California
October 20, 2004

Part 1

JUMP-START

LASTING

WEIGHT LOSS

1

Three Days That Will
Change Your Life

DIETS DON'T WORK for one reason: we can't stay on them.

We can't stay on them because the drive to overeat is very powerful. When we really want that luscious dessert, that second plate of pasta, or that late night snack, we're going to get it. The drive to overeat is *that* strong!

Sure, we can force ourselves to stick with a diet for a day, a week, or a year. In fact, we can be absolutely *perfect* at dieting, but sooner or later we'll relent and go back to overeating. We gain all that weight back and more.

It's so frustrating, so discouraging, and such a waste of energy!

The solution to weight problems is to *stop* dieting. The real solution is to start setting our sights on something more powerful. Diets never worked for me or for the people in our groups at the university. However, something else has worked, and that is focusing on one thing: *turning off the drive to overeat.*

In this book, I'll guide you through a three-day plan so that you can experiment with turning off the drive to overeat. You can watch your appetite fade, your energy increase, and your body let go of fat rather than storing it. Better yet, by the third day you will experience a new sense of clarity and vibrancy, or what we call "life above the line."

You can do this. You can do *anything* for three days! And these three days could just change your life.

The whole premise of traditional weight programs is that if we just knew what to do, we could do it! We could turn away from that candy bar when we hit a low in the late afternoon and resist those salty, crunchy chips while watching television. Traditional weight programs are based on knowledge, insight, planning, and decision-making—all of which are processed primarily by the thinking brain.

Unfortunately, there is no significant relationship between what is processed by the thinking brain and the most primitive human drives, including the drive to eat! The drive to overeat resides in the feeling brain. As long as our feeling brain is hardwired to trigger us to overeat, we'll overeat! Our desire for food is not rational. It's emotional! We eat when we're very high, very low, or emotionally numb, that is, lost in our thoughts, analyzing everything, and cut off from our feelings.

This method, The Solution, equips us with the skills we need to rewire our feeling brain to turnoff the drive to overeat. It maps out a healthy lifestyle that satisfies us in ways that food never could. The combination of tools and lifestyle can bring lasting weight loss without rigid dieting or weight-loss drugs. It can offer us a true solution.

You can jump-start using the method with this 3-Day Solution Plan, and, if you're anything like the people I've worked with, you'll want to incorporate The Solution into your life. Also, if you prefer to move straight to using the plan, without knowing the particulars about why this method works, you can do that quite easily. Just read the series of brief chapters in part 1 of the book, Jump Start Lasting Weight Loss, then skip to part 3, The 3-Day Solution Plan, and begin experiencing three days that will change your life!

For Just Three Days . . .

Here's how it works. For three days, you jump in and use this plan. It's an adventure! During these three days, you will use the powerful mental tools of the method, and you will create a healthy, satisfying lifestyle. You will eat delicious food, exercise daily, and take time for love, work, play, and rest. There are step-by-step plans, and no guesswork is involved. The method is so powerful that you don't have to do this plan perfectly for it to have an astonishing effect on your weight and your life. With these three days, you will:

- *Acquire tools to turn off the drive to overeat.* When you are in the kitchen, wondering whether you should reach for ice cream, cookies, or leftover spaghetti, you can reach instead for these tools and stop wanting *any* of them.
- *Lose up to 6 pounds without dieting.* In testing this plan,[1] many people lost about 3 pounds in three days, but some lost more—all without dieting.
- *Enjoy 3 days of personal vibrancy.* Modern life makes us feel pulled in all directions. For three days, you will live in an especially rewarding way, and by the third day, you will have a renewed sense of clarity, vibrancy, and peace.

If you would like to, after three days, you can continue to use the plan in a less intensive form to complete two weeks of using the method. At that time, you may have what you want from the method, but if you want more, there is an active, warm Solution community online and a complete Solution course that takes you step-by-step to finding a Solution—that is, rewiring your feeling brain to the point that you have lasting weight loss, freedom from other common excesses, and an abundance of life's richest rewards.

In many areas of the country, there are Solution providers who give coaching, lead groups, and conduct weekend retreats based on the method. In fact, this 3-Day Solution Plan was inspired by our Solution retreats, in which, in just three days of intensive Solution work, people see tremendous progress toward reaching their solution. This plan brings you many of those same experiences in the comfort of your own home.

The Three-Day Plan

One thing you will *not* do on this plan is diet. You will use our new 1-2-3 Eating system, in which no foods are forbidden. You can either use the preselected menus for the three days or select from many alternate menus. The foods are easy to prepare and very delicious.

You will also exercise, but you probably won't go to the gym, unless you want to. Instead, you will exercise daily by doing something that you love, like walking with a friend, playing sports, rocking out to music, or going for a bike ride. You'll also take time for love, work, play, and rest.

One thing you will not do on this plan is diet.

Most important, you'll use the powerful tools of the method to begin to retrain your feeling brain so that your inner life spontaneously favors a state of clarity, vibrancy, and peace. Food will become . . . just food! You'll enjoy it, but you'll be perfectly capable of pushing away from the table. You'll *eat* less because you'll *want* less.

In our testing of the plan, some people said they were afraid they wouldn't do it perfectly. *You don't have to do it perfectly.* You simply need to jump in and do it. If you do your best to follow the plan, wonderful things will happen!

Others feared that the method would turn their lives upside down. Many people who have used the method over time say, "The Solution changed my life." This method can transform your life in a spectacularly wonderful way. However, after these three days, you may decide to make *no changes* at all. Or you may prefer to take small steps, keeping your pace of change completely within your personal comfort zone.

On each of the three days, you will use the skills to begin both to retrain the feeling brain and to put into practice a satisfying and healthful lifestyle. Based on our testing of the plan, this is what you're likely to experience on each of the three days:

Day 1: Detox

This is the first day of experiencing a new life. Most people feel a sense of adventure at the idea of using these skills and adopting a vibrant lifestyle to turn off the drive to overeat. It's a time of detoxing from too much sugar, fat, salt, and calories. For some, it feels as if they are detoxing and cleansing. Others are emotionally attached to the food and find themselves grieving the loss of overeating for comfort and fear that they will not be able to stay on the plan. However, most people think that this is just what they most need to do and are proud that they have started the plan.

On this first day, you will use the skill of checking in, asking yourself how you feel and what you need, and begin to experience the power of the method. In a sense, this is the most challenging day of the plan, as you are setting into place both the lifestyle changes and the habit of checking in with yourself. Using the skills and squeezing in all the elements of the day will keep you busy, however, the overriding feelings you're likely to have are hope and pride.

Day 2: Connection

You can do anything for one day, but for two days? That's more challenging. So the plan for the second day is full of ways to make this easier and gratify, satisfy, and please you. In fact, the goal in planning the day was for you to feel so satisfied and vibrant that you wouldn't even notice that you are taking in less food. So the lifestyle part of the program emphasizes finding pleasure in your body, with physical activity and sensual activities on your own or with a partner.

> *After three days, you will feel so vibrant and alive that you will want more days like these.*

In terms of the mental part of the plan, you will continue to use the skill of checking in but will also add a second skill, emotional housecleaning. This is an easy but extremely effective skill, one that flushes out our feelings, literally cleaning house inside. When you use it, within a few minutes, you will feel emotionally lighter and less likely to have an urge to eat. The overriding feeling of the day: happy!

This is a highly pleasurable day!

Day 3: Vibrancy

Day 3 is when all your effort and focus will pay off. By today, you may feel so vibrant and healthy and so free from the drive to overeat that you will amaze yourself. Even if your weight is very high or you have a long-standing attachment to overeating, your drive will begin to fade, and you will see that you have more power to push away from the table and get off the couch.

On this day, you will use the most powerful skill of the three basic tools: doing cycles. Because you have used the first two skills on days 1 and 2 of the plan, using this skill will be far easier and more effective. This is the skill that has the most potent effect on turning off the drive to overeat and rewiring your feeling brain. You will also experience more emotional connection on this third day, and that experience will further turn off your drive to overeat.

After three days, you will feel so vibrant and alive that you will probably want more days like these. If you do, you can transition into using the second phase of the plan and move toward a life of lasting weight loss.

The first step, however, is to focus on these three days.

2

Retraining Your
Feeling Brain

PLEASE RECALL A time recently when your mind turned to food. You weren't hungry, but you definitely wanted something to eat. Perhaps you were restless, upset, or bored, and you knew that you *should* be dieting—but the food was calling to you.

Chances are that you were in a state we call "below the line." The more moments of the day that we spend below the line, the more our appetites will ramp up.

Every moment of every day, we are in one of two states: above the line or below the line. The Solution Method gives us the tools to stay above the line more of the time, where the drive to overeat naturally fades. We check in with ourselves often, and if we're below the line, we reach for the tools of the method and move ourselves above the line. It's as simple as that!

> *Every moment of every day,*
> *we're either above the line or below.*

When our feeling brain is overloaded or out of balance, lots of things change. That's because the feeling brain, the limbic system, is the center of many fundamental aspects of our lives. It's the seat of emotional balance, relationship intimacy, spiritual connection, and all those red-hot drives to go to excess, including overeating. When we're below the line, a cascade of changes in neurochemicals and hormones follow. Each imbalance leads to another and taken together, these changes can foster weight gain. The first law of thermodynamics still applies and calories do count. However, the fallout from life below the line triggers cravings and urges to eat more and exercise less. It encourages our bodies to store those extra calories rather than release them.

Are You Above or Below the Line?

In Solution groups, the first questions new participants often ask are "What's below the line?" and "How do I know I'm below the line?" The signs are unique to each individual, and you'll develop an awareness of your own particular signs that you're below the line. I know I am when I start wanting food, when I start worrying about everyone else's problems and forget to deal with my own, or when I feel numb or depressed. You'll develop an awareness of your own signposts as you use the 3-Day Solution Plan. But here are some clues to watch for:

Appetites Ramp Up

When we're above the line, the drive to overeat is low, as are other urges and cravings. We don't care about the extra food, don't think about our weight that much, as we are too busy living active, vibrant lives. When we're below the line, we have cravings and urges to eat that we know have nothing whatsoever to do with body hunger. We may think far too much about food and obsess about our weight, or, on the other hand, we may be unaware of our bodies. We don't feel fat even though our weight may pose serious medical risks.

Our appetites for the other common external solutions may ramp up, too. An external solution is anything that we do to excess because we are disconnected from ourselves and the present moment. We can't soothe and comfort ourselves from within, so we do the logical thing. We reach outside ourselves for soothing and comforting.

In the 3-Day Solution Plan, there are no judgments about external solutions, and even after you have a Solution in your life, you will probably still use them now and then. But you won't judge yourself for it. Plus you don't turn to external solutions that often or for that long.

When we're below the line, our appetites ramp up.

Common external solutions besides overeating are: smoking, drinking, overworking, overspending, using unneeded prescription drugs ("pill popping") or recreational drugs, and the softer excesses such as people pleasing, rescuing others, thinking too much, and isolating. The drives for these common external solutions fade when we're above the line.

We're High, Low, or Numb

Emotionally, when we're above the line, the feelings can be positive or negative and can be intense or mild. They are balanced feelings, such as angry, grateful, sad, happy, afraid, secure, guilty, and proud. One of the things that sets these feelings apart is that they don't spin us out of control. They lead us to our true need rather than our want. They don't stay stuck for hours or days. We feel them, and then they fade and we are open to feeling the next feeling.

When we're above the line, our appetites fade.

When we're below the line, the feelings can again be positive or negative, but we're either very high or very low. In this state, balanced feelings turn into something else: sadness becomes depression, anger becomes hostility, and fear turns to panic. Simple guilt—a beneficial feeling that leads to learning and change— turns into debilitating shame. Pure happiness becomes such elation that we forget to eat reasonably or pay our light bills. These feelings tend to stay stuck and can last hours, days, or years. They also tend to come with other clues that we are below the line. For example, we can be intensely sad and cry, whereas when the sadness turns to depression, we become passive and withdrawn. When we're intensely angry and above the line, we may stand up for ourselves in an assertive way, but when we're below the line, the anger turns into hostility and we become aggressive.

When we're above the line, we are present in the current moment, experiencing what is occurring in our lives. When we're below the line, the current moment escapes us. We're consumed by the past or obsessed about the future. In fact, we're likely to be so wrapped up in our thoughts or moods that we are not aware of our bodies. We feel like walking heads, as if our bodies were just vehicles to carry our thoughts around all day!

Some people who are below the line emotionally aren't high or low. They're emotionally numb. They are aware of thoughts but not feelings. The thoughts tend to be repetitive and even obsessive. Those thoughts may exhibit conventional intelligence, but they lack emotional intelligence. Basic to our survival is having ongoing access to our emotions because feelings are more accurate than thoughts in pointing us to our needs. Meeting our true "above-the-line" needs rather than our "below-the-line" wants is the key to turning off the drive to overeat.

Feelings are more accurate in pointing us to our needs because of the very nature of the feeling brain. It's the central clearinghouse for everything that is going on in our lives: feelings, thoughts, memories, sensory input, body signals—everything! It collects, processes, and prioritizes that information, then coordinates a response to it by sending messages to other parts of the brain and to the body, in order to keep us in a state of balance. With all this chaos of information flooding into the feeling brain, it distills a feeling to motivate us to meet our most important needs. When we miss out on those feelings, we cannot move forward with our day with enough sensitivity toward ourselves to avoid having excessive appetites.

The solution to weight problems is to spend more moments of the day above the line.

Also, when we're below the line, feelings clump up and form what we call "smoke screens." Perhaps we feel confused, stressed, miserable, or upset. These smoke screens are clusters of feelings and thoughts. Because we can't sort them out, we can't recognize what they are. If we can't recognize our feelings, we can't know what we need.

Corrections Weaken

Other clues to our emotional state involve spirituality and relationships. When we're above the line, we feel spiritually connected, if that is our belief. When we're below the line, we feel lost, empty, or disconnected, or we tend to use religion in unhealthy ways. In our relationships when we are above the line, we are assertive, rather than passive or aggressive. When we are below the line, instead of being intimate with others, we merge with them, to lose ourselves in others. Perhaps we're rescuers or people pleasers or simply find ourselves so wrapped up in the feelings and needs of *others* that we have no idea how *we* feel or what *we* need!

Or we can go in the other direction. We can "cut and run" emotionally, trying to distance ourselves or being so cut off from our feelings that we can't empathize with others. When we're below the line, we can find ourselves in control struggles, persecute others, or seek revenge!

Life below the line is not pretty! Nor is it rewarding. But that's not a problem, because with the Solution tools, we can pop ourselves above the line. I say "pop" because when you use the third skill you will learn during the 3-Day Solution Plan, doing cycles, the shift inside is so profound that it feels like a sudden burst. When you use these skills consistently, at some point, you will find that a wave of relaxation and peace—and warm energy—flows through your body. It's the effect of your feeling brain flipping the switch from life below the line to life above the line.

Rewiring the Feeling Brain

The feeling brain is just one of our three brains, which interact in a tangle of electrical and chemical exchanges involving a hundred billion cells:

- *The thinking brain* is the part of us that stores our conventional intelligence. It's what enables us to memorize the Gettysburg Address or to remember that $a^2 + b^2 = c^2$ is the Pythagorean theorem.
- *The brain stem* monitors our basic bodily functions, such as heart rate and blood pressure.
- *The feeling brain* is our emotional intelligence. It's the seat of emotional balance, relationship intimacy, and spiritual connection, as well as those red-hot passions and

pleasure drives, including overeating and the central clearinghouse of input from the external environment and the internal milieu.

Most treatments for weight problems target the thinking brain. The thinking brain processes knowledge, insight, planning, and deciding. When we read diet books and acquire knowledge, see a therapist to gain insight into why we overeat, plan what we will eat the next day, or make a personal resolution to lose weight, we are using our thinking brain.

> *To pop yourself above the line when*
> *you are below, use these skills. They work!*

Unfortunately, there is no significant relationship between what is processed by the thinking brain and primitive drives such as the drive to overeat. That's why you can have both a Ph.D. in nutrition and an eating disorder. *Knowing* what to do is not enough. Even if you force yourself to have positive thoughts, those thoughts can be blown away like a speck of dust in a sandstorm when the passions and cravings of the feeling brain say otherwise. In a face-off between reason and passion, passion usually wins. The pathway to lasting weight loss is to change the feeling brain.

Imagine that, moment to moment, information is flooding into the central clearinghouse of your brain, your feeling brain, through your senses, thoughts, emotional memories, and bodily processes. All that flows through in any given moment reflects all that is going on and has gone on in your life: environmental stresses, major life events, trauma and abuse, genes, development, experience, and health behaviors. All at once!

> *You eat less because you want less.*
> *You do not have to go on a rigid diet.*

Sometimes life is easy, and there isn't much activity in the feeling brain. Other times we're completely overloaded. If the sum total of what pours into the feeling brain at any given moment is more than our brain can effectively process, the brain perceives stress and we begin to go below the line. When we go below the line, the brain draws upon all that it has at its disposal. Sometimes this requires the brain to temporarily change how it digests information in order to prevent damage and enable itself to regain balance. This is a process that occurs in many different organs and is called allostatis, or an allostatic response[1]. All this is done in an effort to return the body to balance, to homeostasis, to life above the line.

If the stresses from the body or the environment are frequent or so extreme that the brain can't process them properly, the changes that were temporary allostatic protective responses in the neural networks of the brain become fixed! Lifting weights leads to the body expecting this to be a new state and increasing muscle mass; repeated increases in blood pressure lead to the cardiovascular system creating a new higher set point for blood pressure.

In a similar way, frequent or extreme stress can put into place a new emotional set point that is below the line. We become neurologically prone to depression, disappointment, or anxiety, which amounts to an enduring tendency that is called our allostatic load. In other words, we pay a neurological price when our upsets find no resolution, or our losses are not fully grieved, or when life presents us with such a rapid-fire series of stresses that we don't have time between upsets to recover.

With a high allostatic load, we more easily and more often find ourselves in that emotional state in which the drive to overeat ramps up and we reach for an external solution to our distress: a bag of chips or a candy bar. What's more, those neural networks in the feeling brain, that new emotional set point, causes us to interpret information more negatively. That further adds to our allostatic load and stokes the fires of our excessive appetites. We reach for food to activate the "feel good" neurotransmitters in our brain and alleviate our pain. Unfortunately, overeating fails to cure the cause of our upset, so our problems don't disappear. In fact, they mount. Overeating also reinforces this new state of reaching for external solutions rather than dealing more effectively with the everyday challenges of life. This pattern becomes more hardwired in the neural circuits of our brain, so we reach for external solutions in response to stress rather than for soothing and comforting from within. If our allostatic load is high, we are also apt to have more health problems. For example, all that stress and all those candy bars lead to more artherosclerotic plaque and increased insulin levels in the blood, which stimulates the appetite. As problems pile up, we're more likely to establish a new homeostasis below the line, in which we are dependent upon various external solutions—behavioral, emotional, mental, relational, and spiritual—to stay in balance. We may dabble in overeating, spending too much, languishing in self-pity, or overanalyzing everything. These external solutions serve a purpose by "propping us up" and getting us through the day. In essence, when our allostatic load is high, we may take up residence below the line.

The good news is that if we visit life below the line more often than we'd like to or have taken up residence there, we can move. We can do this by living life above the line, using the method effectively so that one synapse at a time, we change the neural networks that favor emotional imbalance.

In time, we decrease our allostatic load and trigger the allostatic response less often. Even when we do go below the line, we are not as apt to take a free fall in which those cravings and urges are overwhelming. More often, we simply dip below the line, and then pop ourselves back up above the line again, perhaps having felt depressed, disappointed, or anxious for a while, but not having felt a strong need to overeat.

So how do you stay above the line?

You do two things: decrease the pain, stress, and overload that flow into the feeling brain and retrain the feeling brain to process that pain, stress, and overload more effectively. You do this by using the two key parts of the method: Solution Skills and Mastery Living.

Solution Skills

During these three days, you will use three basic Solution Skills. These are the skills that retrain your feeling brain.

It's important to retrain our feeling brain because as long as it is hardwired to trigger us to overeat, we will gravitate toward a stalled lifestyle of unbalanced eating that makes us gain weight.

The wiring of the feeling brain is based on neural networks. Each time we experience something, nerve cells couple. They link. With repeated or emotionally charged experiences, the links strengthen into neural networks that fire in our brain unconsciously, like lightning, controlling much of what we do.

If we're raised in a responsive environment, one that is neither indulging nor depriving, our parents nurture us well and set effective limits in our lives. Their own capacity to nurture themselves and to set limits in their lives is naturally downloaded into our feeling brain by their repeated contact with us, creating neural networks that automatically favor life above the line.

Even though they loved us, if they didn't have these skills within their own feeling brains, they could not download them into ours. Love is an emotion, and this process is a reflection of skills. Even if they did download those skills into our brain, modern life is so stressful and losing weight is so challenging that we still might need more of them. Fortunately these skills are not genetic but learned, and virtually anyone can learn them.

The symbol of The Solution Method is an infinity sign in motion, with the *N* standing for nurturing and the *L* standing for limits. It symbolizes our commitment to do something our parents may not have had the skills to do: to stay with ourselves when we are upset, giving ourselves the nurturing and the limits we need until we are back in balance and have popped ourselves above the line.

*During these three days, you will cultivate
the habit of living life above the line.*

During these three days, you will begin to cultivate the habit of using these skills in your daily life. The way that our feeling brain processes daily life is unconscious and automatic. Changing it is very different from changing the thinking brain. It involves emotional learning, not conventional learning.

Emotional learning is far more challenging to change than conventional learning. We can consciously remember what happened last evening on our favorite television show, but our moment-to-moment processing of our own emotional experience is far more difficult to be aware of, let alone change. When someone insults us, or we spill coffee in our laps, or a child screams, we react sponta-

neously on an emotional level. We're not in control of those feelings! They just rise up and grab us—then saturate our being, a reflection of factors ranging from whether or not we ate breakfast
that morning or had a spat with a close friend moments before, and
the wiring of our feeling brains.

The first time you pop yourself above the line by using the skills,
it's amazing! All you did was use these skills, and your feeling brain . . .
changed! Each time you pop yourself above the line, you will create
one small change, rewiring the feeling brain one synapse at a time.
Sometimes it feels as if you're nudging yourself above the line or
slipping above the line, but regardless of how it feels, when that
switch flips and you move above the line, you are creating a new life.

The mental part, Solution Skills, and the lifestyle part, Mastery Living, work together.

I like to think in terms of parties. When we're below the line,
there's a whole party of negativity going on. We notice one guest—
perhaps the craving for a candy bar. However, because the feeling
brain is out of balance, other guests join in: numbness, obsessive
thinking, mood swings, passivity, aggression, deprivation, indulgence, merging, distancing, control struggles, rescuing others, people pleasing, persecuting, and other external solutions.

It's quite a party!

The power of the method is to get just one molecule of our
being above the line, enough to bring up a nurturing, supportive
inner voice. Just one cell, that's all it takes! And use these skills to seduce the rest of our being to come above the line. When we do that,
we accomplish two things that are of monumental importance.

First, we break up the internal party that is below the line, and
we throw a new party that is above the line. That is, we weaken the
neural networks that support life below the line and strengthen
the ones that support life above the line.

We get immediate relief and feel better, but more important,
we change the hardwiring in the brain. As we continue to pop ourselves above the line, we use the skills when our spouse won't listen,
when the dog poops in the house, when the cookies burn, when the
stock market nose-dives, when hormones rage, when solicitors keep
calling—whenever we go below the line! Each time, the networks

that favor life above the line strengthen, and those that support life below the line weaken.

At some point in your use of the method, the networks that support life above the line will become dominant over those that support life below the line. The switch flips, and instead of automatically going below the line, you will spontaneously stay above the line more of the time.

You won't have to memorize the skills. You will have one pocket reminder for each day's experience.

To get a taste of life above the line, you can't just use the skills now and then. During these three days, you will use them hourly. That might sound like a lot to accomplish, but you probably won't mind doing it, because it will make you feel better right away. Plus, you'll know that you're on the pathway to rewiring your feeling brain, and there is security and satisfaction in that.

You won't have to memorize the skills, because included in the appendix is a pocket reminder for each of the three days, to give you structure and support. You can use the skills in your mind, on paper, aloud, or on your computer—whatever works best for you. If you want extra support, you can program your watch or computer to remind you hourly to use the skills, and more support is available on our website (www.thepathway.org), including a discussion board.

These skills will fit in well with your normal daily routine. You can use them anywhere, and nobody will know. They will notice only the aftereffects: that you look vibrant, relaxed, and happy. Two of the three skills take just a couple of minutes to use. The third one, doing a cycle, takes longer—usually 10 to 20 minutes—but you use that skill only on the third day and only a couple of times.

It's just for three days. You can do *anything* for three days!

The three Solution Skills are: checking in, emotional housecleaning, and doing cycles. When you're above the line, you use checking in to stay there. When you're headed below the line or are a little below the line, you use emotional housecleaning to move solidly above the line. When you're below the line, emotional housecleaning isn't enough. You need to do a cycle to pop yourself above the line.

• *Checking in:* Most of us check our wallet, our lipstick, or our belt buckle throughout the day. This is that kind of skill, except that you are checking in with your feeling brain. You are checking to see whether you are above the line or below it. This is the skill you will learn on the first day of the plan, and you will use it hourly for all three days.

• *Emotional housecleaning:* On the second day, you will add the emotional housecleaning skill. When you check in with yourself and know you are headed below the line—starting to think too much and to go numb, or beginning to feel way high or way low—you'll use this skill to move back above the line. With this skill, you check for eight basic feelings. Four are positive feelings: grateful, happy, secure, proud. Four are negative feelings: angry, sad, afraid, guilty.

• *The cycles:* This is the skill that enables you to pop yourself above the line when you are below it. Doing cycles is so powerful because it precisely mirrors responsive parental nurturing and effective limits, the patterns that make us emotionally intelligent, more conscious, and living in the present moment. You will use this skill on the third day of the plan. It takes some practice, but the first time you feel that "pop" above the line, with all the emotional lightness and clarity that follow, it will be more than worth it.

Mastery Living

In addition to using the internal skills during these three days, you'll be living a vibrant lifestyle. Eating balances serotonin, dopamine, and endorphins. Unless your lifestyle does its part to balance those neurotransmitters, when you begin to eat less, you're going to trigger cravings and urges. The following subsections explain how each element of the plan turns off the drive to overeat in its own way.

Solution 1-2-3 Eating

At each meal, you choose at least one food from each of three groups: The Fiber Group, Healthy Fats, and The Protein Group.

1. *The Fiber Group:* This group consists of vegetables,
   fruits, and whole grains, not the ones that just look
   like whole grains, such as "brown bread," but really
   gnarly whole grains that contain lots of fiber, such as
   100 percent stone-ground whole-wheat bran or high-
   fiber whole-grain cereals. Each food in this group
   contains at least 3 grams of fiber per 100 calories.
2. *Healthy Fats:* These are foods high in monounsaturated
   fats or omega-3 fatty acids. Examples are oils such as
   olive oil and canola oil, as well as foods such as nuts,
   seeds, and avocados. All contain at least 30 percent of
   their calories from monounsaturated fats or at least
   .5 grams of omega-3 fatty acids per 100 calories.
3. *The Protein Group:* This group consists of low-fat
   sources of protein, including low-fat meats and poultry,
   fish and seafood, low-fat and nonfat dairy products, eggs
   and egg products, beans, and soybeans. Each food in
   this group provides at least 7 grams of protein per
   100 calories, no trans fats, and no more than 2 grams of
   saturated fat.

There is one more group: *White Stuff.* These foods are
not bad or wrong, but they are not the foods that
promote vibrancy and calm the appetite. This category
includes foods high in saturated fats, trans fats, refined
carbohydrates, alcohol, and caffeine.

To have a life of vibrancy and lasting weight loss, choose most
of your foods from The Solution 1-2-3 Food List (see Chapter 22).
Then, to be sure you aren't depriving yourself, check to see whether
you really need some White Stuff. *If you do, have it and enjoy every
bite without guilt.* But if you don't really need it, rather than eating
mindlessly, just skip it. With this plan, you are apt to find that you
don't often need White Stuff. But if you do, by all means have it!

This way of eating provides about 30 percent protein, 30 percent
fat, 40 percent carbohydrates with less than 10 percent saturated fat
(typically about 7 percent), no trans fats, 17 percent monounsaturated
fat, and 22 grams of fiber, all with a food intake that is high in nutri-

ent density and rich in phytochemicals. In contrast, high protein diets typically provide an average of 40 percent protein, 50 percent fat, and as little as 15 percent carbohydrates. The brain needs carbohydrates to function well! High protein diets also dish up as much as 15 percent saturated fat, with only 8 percent monounsaturated fat. Most are low in fiber and lack important vitamins, minerals, and power phytochemicals. We believe The Solution 1-2-3 Eating will nourish your body (and spirit) in ways that diets never could.

Body Work

You will exercise for one hour a day, split into two periods of activity. One will be when you first awaken in the morning, when you'll take a few minutes to stretch and enjoy your body. The other will be at any time during the day. Some people are morning exercisers, whereas others prefer late in the day or the evening. What matters isn't *when* you do it but *that* you do it.

During that hour a day, do something you love! Find a sport you enjoy, exercise with others, compete against yourself, or do something playful that you haven't done since childhood. Your body work time is not just for health but for pleasure, creativity, relaxation, and personal nourishing. Exercise increases dopamine and serotonin, and if you exercise for a long time intensely, you can increase endorphins and get "runner's high."

Meaningful Pursuits

You will spend no fewer than six hours and no more than eight hours engaged in some activity that enables you to focus on something other than yourself and brings rewards that you value. It could be a job, parenting, going to school, or doing volunteer work. Most of us work too much or not enough. Overwork leaves little time for activities that turn off the drive to overeat, and working too little deprives us of the experience of working hard, then reaping the rewards.

Working in a focused way increases dopamine. We get charged up! After being charged up, we relax and reflect on our accomplishments. Serotonin, the neurotransmitter that makes us relaxed and fulfilled, increases. We get an intrinsic reward. If we work too much, we drain dopamine, miss the serotonin reward, and feel exhausted and depleted. If we don't work hard enough, we never get that dopamine rise, which triggers the serotonin reward. Working either too hard or not hard enough creates a reward-deficiency syndrome. No wonder we want that extra cookie!

Time to Restore

During your 3-Day Solution Plan, you will reserve one hour daily for doing whatever you want to do that is truly restoring. That doesn't mean junk time—watching television or logging on to the computer. It means giving yourself precisely what you need, something that lifts you above the line and balances your neurotransmitters. Examples include taking a hot bath, playing the guitar, creating a painting, listening to music, walking in nature, reading a good book, laughing out loud at a comedy, praying or meditating, or just being completely alone and listening to the beauty of the quiet. This is one sacred hour each day to do whatever nourishes you in ways that food never could.

Intimacy Time

On each of the three days, you will take one hour for intimacy time. Connection with others is the most effective way to balance neurotransmitters and turn off the drive to overeat. There are three kinds of intimacy time: social, sexual, and emotional. On the first day, the focus is on social intimacy—being with people other than your family who give you a sense of belonging or with whom you share an interest. On the second day, you will satisfy more of your needs for sensuality or sexuality, and on the last day, your intimacy time will focus on creating more emotional intimacy with someone you care about.

These skills and this lifestyle will give you the power to move yourself above the line. When you are there, a whole cascade of changes follow that shift your body from holding on to weight to losing weight.

3

Small Changes, Great Results!

HOW CAN MAKING small changes, such as checking your feelings and taking an hour for yourself each day, trigger weight loss? How could these small changes yield such great results?

It's because they pop us above the line, and in that state, we experience a myriad of small but important changes in body, mind, behavior, and spirit that favor losing weight. They reverse the changes that our body naturally makes when it's below the line. Here's a sampling of the ways in which life below the line packs on pounds:

- Chronic stress causes increases in cortisol, the stress hormone.
- Cortisol secretion increases blood glucose, which prepares us for fight or flight.
- The stress is not physical, so the blood glucose is not used by the muscles.
- The pancreas secretes insulin to clear away the extra glucose.
- Cortisol drains our neurotransmitters, including serotonin, which relaxes and satisfies; dopamine, for energy; and endorphins, for pleasure.
- Increases in insulin and cortisol cause cravings for foods high in sugar and fat.
- Increased cortisol sends glucose to the center of the body, where it forms cortisol receptors, further increasing cortisol, decreasing serotonin in the brain, and triggering mood swings and depression.

- Increases in weight cause insulin resistance, so the pancreas secretes more insulin, which prompts more overeating and weight gain.
- Eating more dietary fat reduces our metabolism because dietary fat is metabolized efficiently and most of the calories normally lost because of digestion are conserved.
- Eating more sugar further increases insulin levels and triggers hypoglycemia, which increases tension, tiredness, depression, and anxiety.
- Diets high in fat and sugar are low in fiber. The intestines, which account for a quarter of our metabolic energy needs, shrink, and our metabolic rate slows.
- Depression can lead to decreased spontaneous movement and physical activity.
- Decreased physical activity deprives us of the mood-elevating effects of exercise, contributing to further mood problems.
- Chronic inactivity promotes decreased metabolism, decreased muscle mass, and further weight gain.
- Once weight is gained, fat begets fat, and a host of body mechanisms, such as higher levels of fat-storage enzymes and a higher weight set point, make it harder to lose.

When we stay above the line, the layers of the problem begin to fade, one by one. We step out of the toxic spiral.

- Obesity and overeating can trigger high dopamine levels, coupled with low serotonin levels, which prompt food cravings.
- Weight gain causes health problems, which add to our stress, including joint and bone problems that interfere with our exercise.
- Stress disturbs sleep. When sleep is disturbed, less growth hormone is secreted. Growth hormone boosts metabolism, and we lose out on that effect. Metabolic rate decreases.
- Sleep deprivation decreases leptin, which suppresses appetite, and increases grehlin, which amplifies hunger.

- Depression coupled with negative social attitudes toward obesity affect body image. Body image and self-image are intertwined, so both take a downturn.
- Changes in sex hormones due to stress and a more negative body image affect sexual desire and/or functioning. We feel less sexually satisfied and miss out on the serotonin boost that touching and orgasm bring.
- Stress and depression have a negative impact on relationships. We are more isolated, and we turn to television, food, and other external solutions to cope.
- Media images of delicious food affect the sensory center in our thinking brain—the orbitofrontal cortex—and make us hungrier. We develop a craving brain with imbalances of neurochemicals that motivate us to eat to prevent the pain of withdrawal.
- We go on a diet and start thinking about food. Stress, thoughts of food, and worries about weight trigger cognitive overload of our thinking brain, and impulse control declines.
- By now, food has become addictive, so we stay on the diet for a while, then return to overeating or we stay on the diet but develop another crossover external solution.
- Problems in our lives mount up, which trigger more stress.
- We're in the toxic spiral of weight gain, and we're spinning out of control!

What amazes me when I have been in the toxic spiral and when I listen to the reflections of participants in Solution groups is that we are not eating tubs of chocolate ice cream or having three cheeseburgers for dinner. The difference between maintaining weight and gaining weight is an average of 50 calories per day, or the amount of energy in half a small apple. That's all it takes!

The good news is that if small differences draw us into the toxic spiral, then small changes can draw us out of it. We don't have to focus on each aspect of the spiral. All we have to do is focus on this very moment, then the next moment, and the next, doing what we can to stay above the line. When we do, the layers of the problem begin to fade, one by one, and we step out of the toxic spiral.

Cameron's Story

Weight is not just about diet and exercise but about a spiral of changes that naturally occur when we're below the line: the domino effect! This shows up in our research as well as in the groups at the university.

For instance, Cameron, a portfolio manager, juggled raising two children, keeping together a difficult marriage, and holding down a demanding job. She had never been slender, but when her new boss doubled her workload, she had no time to go to the gym and started going to the vending machine instead. Candy bars boosted her energy in the late afternoon.

Cameron's stress triggered family stress.

The problem was not the candy but the stress! What's more, Cameron's stress triggered the domino effect. Her whole family could feel her upset. Soon her children began going below the line: her older son became more demanding, and her younger one got clingy and sullen. Her husband, Jack, had his own difficulties with a threatened layoff at work. His external solutions were television and spending, so the more stress Cameron brought into the house, the more he went below the line. One day he came home beaming. He had spent money they didn't have on a new flat-screen television for the family room. Shortly thereafter, he began seeking refuge in late-night TV.

Cameron coped by working even more and now had no time to cook. So she started bringing home takeout food and between skipping the gym and feeling bloated from all that sugary, fatty food and resentful of Jack's retreat into the family room, she lost interest in making love. Without that tenderness and gratification, both she and Jack were even grumpier.

Then Jack was notified that he would not be laid off, but he did have a new position that required traveling four days per week for the first two months. When Cameron heard that news, she felt like strangling him! How could he leave her all alone to take care of two kids *and* the house as well as her work?

Food never looked so good to Cameron—
particularly ice cream.

Jack went on his trips and Cameron went . . . to the kitchen. Food had never looked so good to her, and she developed a taste for designer ice creams, particularly those with caramel swirls or little fudge brownies.

She was definitely in survival mode, but the kids did reasonably well and she and Jack made their way through his comings and goings. However, when the two months were almost up, Cameron slipped on her pants one morning and went to button them. The waistband was too tight. She weighed herself—and found she had gained 10 pounds!

She was furious. That was it! She had gone on diets, and she knew how to lose weight: just cut out bread, cookies, and ice cream. But whenever she lost weight, she always regained it.

Instead, Cameron went to a Solution group. She jump-started her program with the 3-Day Solution Plan, then started using the courses, deepening her skills and doing more lifestyle surgery.

Lifestyle surgery was relatively easy for her. She cleaned out the kitchen, getting rid of the potato chips, the sugary cereals, and the banana bread, and she started buying more fresh fruits and vegetables and whole foods. She started walking for an hour at noon—sometimes on her own with headphones and music and sometimes with a coworker. Cameron even committed to leaving work at 6:00 p.m. no matter what.

Instead of going on a diet,
she got on the pathway to finding a Solution.

The Solution Skills were harder for her. When she checked in with herself at first, she found that she didn't know how she felt. Most of the time, she was numb. She knew how her boys felt and how Jack felt, but her mind was so full of thoughts—she analyzed everything—that she rarely took the time to figure out how she felt.

And as for her limits, Cameron was too harsh on herself, on Jack, and on her older son, and too easy on her younger son. He got away with everything! She began popping herself above the line more and more, beginning to retrain her feeling brain. In time, she began easing up on her older son and setting more limits with her younger son. The children were happier and calmer, which helped her stress level.

> *One by one, the family stresses faded.*
> *Peace, connection, and vibrancy returned.*

Rekindling intimacy with Jack took longer. He was still watching a lot of television, and Cameron was still fed up with him. But instead of getting ice cream or nagging him, she went for walks, and did cycles. As she began to stay more above the line, instead of judging him for watching television, she started feeling empathy for him. The tenderness between them started to return and their marriage began to improve.

Cameron noticed that she was losing weight. For the first time in years, she was consistently eating more sensibly. Doing so was almost effortless because she had stopped wanting the extra food.

She lost 15 pounds, and a year later, she had kept the weight off, and lost more, but more importantly, weight and food were no longer issues in her life.

She had not dieted—but she had focused on staying above the line and turning off the drive to overeat. Instead of being perfect on her diet, she had made many small but immensely important changes. . . .

4

Why Diets Don't Work

LIKE MANY PEOPLE who use this method, Cameron had dieted off and on for years. Each time she started a new diet, she hoped that this particular one would work. When it didn't, she usually blamed herself.

However, gaining back that weight wasn't her fault. It was the natural consequence of using dieting as a treatment for being overweight. There are scores of studies that show that diets do not work.[1] No matter what diet and exercise plan we use, on average, we lose weight but gain it back. Sometimes, we gain back more than we initially lost!

With the obesity epidemic on the nightly news, never have more people been dieting,[2] and never have more been overweight.[3] It makes sense that if we just know what to do—how to eat—we'll do it. It should work! But there are interconnected reasons why dieting is not the answer:

- When we're below the line, we go to extremes with any diet plan. It's all or nothing. We try to be perfect on the diet, but when we can't stand that anymore, we go off the diet and overeat anything in sight.
- When we diet and force ourselves to change what we eat without turning off our desire for the extra food, there is a backlash. Slowly, over time, we find ourselves eating just a little bit more and treating ourselves to sweets and fats slightly more often. Before long, we've stopped losing weight.

- Dieting makes us think more about our food, and those thoughts are toxic. They can overload the decision-making part of our thinking brain and shut down our impulse control. Also, thinking about food increases insulin levels, so blood sugar drops, we get hungry, and we eat more.
- Ultimately, the problem with dieting is that it doesn't go to the root of the problem, which is that we're below the line, stuck with a whole spiral of changes in our bodies and minds that fosters overeating and weight gain. Diet is only one part of that spiral.

Everyone knows someone who has dieted successfully, lost weight, and kept it off without substituting another excess. Some of them did it through lifestyle surgery, such as stopping their three-hour daily commute or leaving an unsatisfying relationship—something that so definitively lightened the overload in their feeling brain that they could cope well without overeating. Others retrained their feeling brain, some through means other than Solution training:

- Long-term psychotherapy that is not analytical but loving can give the repeated contact with warm support and effective limits that retrains the feeling brain.
- Having a loving partner can do the same. Love heals, but we usually choose partners who seem different from us but are equally below the line, and repeated contact with them inadvertently reinforces the networks that send us below the line rather than revising them.
- Support groups can offer caring and create community. However, the risk is that we'll substitute connecting with the group rather than doing the more challenging work of mastering the skills to connect with ourselves.
- Perhaps the most common way to gain these skills is through the "school of life." The lessons learned from the lumps and bumps of our daily lives can prompt us to be aware of our feelings and needs and adopt healthy limits.

Regardless of the method one uses to retrain the feeling brain, that rewiring is the key to lasting weight loss that sidesteps the replacement of overeating with another excessive behavior.

Without revising the feeling brain, weight loss is usually short-term. Right now, there is such desperation about the obesity epidemic that the focus of research and clinical treatment has turned toward drug and surgical options. So far, the results have not been encouraging.

> *Unless the feeling brain is retrained,*
> *weight loss usually doesn't last.*

Given that there are at least 200 genetic factors that can explain our tendencies to gain weight,[4] it's unlikely that there will be a magic bullet to treat obesity. Even if there is, the drive to overeat is so primitive and deep that most drugs effective enough to turn it off would be likely to affect other bodily systems in unfavorable ways or have unpleasant or serious side effects. A magic pill that turned off the drive to overeat wouldn't really offer a true solution. Except for those whose weight problem is influenced by medical conditions such as the metabolic syndrome or drugs that pack on pounds such as steroids, weight-loss drugs cover up the symptoms rather than solving the problem. Just as antidepressants do not solve the problem of depression, drugs that tinker with normal chemical functioning to promote weight loss don't cure the causes of the obesity problem.

> *A magic pill for obesity would never*
> *offer a true solution.*

When used in combination with a diet and exercise program, the currently approved weight-loss drugs offer only a modest advantage over diet and exercise alone and only do so for the short term.[5] The annual cost per person of administering these drugs is about $1,000,[6] and as soon as the prescription ends, often the lost weight is rapidly regained.[7] Gastric surgery is often a last resort for those with extreme obesity. The cost is $12,000 to $30,000 initially, based on the procedure chosen, and there can be complications and repeated surgeries, which further increase costs.[8]

Health improves as weight is lost, but excising the fat in the absence of rewiring the emotional brain leaves some feeling like "dry drunks." Their behavior has changed without having acquired the requisite internal skills to prompt that change. These are the same skills that would have enabled them to grieve the losses of the past and cope with the stresses brought on by their new body size. The original cause of the problem was not a large stomach, so the "cure" of gastric stapling or banding only masked the problem rather than solving it.

> *The trouble is that* external *nurturing and* external *limits are inherently unstable.*

On the other hand, the scientific literature shows that no matter what the weight-loss approach, it works, on average, in the short term. However, success is often based on the fact that these treatments provide *external* forms of nurturing and limits. Having the support of a counselor, sponsor, therapist, group, or drug attempts to make up for the absence of the skill to nurture from within. Gastric staples place physical limits on our eating, and diets attempt to impose boundaries when it comes to eating.

The trouble is that *external* nurturing and *external* limits are inherently unstable. You can't depend on them! Your support group can disband. Your counselor is available an hour a week. Where is your counselor when you are peering into the refrigerator and really need him or her? You can tire of that diet—eating chicken breasts and steamed broccoli gets old—and your prescription for that pill can run out. Even if it doesn't, most drugs only retain their power to aid weight loss for six months to a year. After that time, what then?

> *Weight goes down when we use external supports, then increases once they're removed.*

The reliance of weight-loss programs on external nurturing and limits is one reason that research studies on these programs all demonstrate the same results: a "V-shaped" weight change. The average weight of subjects goes down during the time that external nurturing and limits are in place. When the external nurturing and limits are removed, the weight rebounds.

If overweight didn't strongly affect our health and happiness, none of this would matter. But since it does, we need to stop hoping that the next diet will be the answer and start looking seriously at what lies at the root of the problem . . .

5

The Crossover Effect

THE DRIVE TO overeat shares its roots with those other common excesses. In Solution groups, people join in the training regardless of excess or even if they have no excesses but just want to live life above the line.

If the roots are shared, then it's easy to stop one external solution only to start another. You've probably seen it in your friends or even in yourself. You force yourself to lose weight, and after all that hard work, once it seems that the problem has finally disappeared, another one crops up:

- We stop overeating and start overspending.
- We stick to a budget but start drinking.
- We abstain from drinking and start smoking.
- We quit smoking and start eating sweets.

As people living in the modern world, we're prone to excessive behaviors, some of us more than others, but most of us tend to use one external solution or another. That's because of our genes. It's not that we have a rare defect but that our shared genes are those of our hunter-gatherer ancestors.[1] They lived in small tribes, had virtually no chronic stress, and ate whole foods, not processed foods—and even those foods were scarce.

Life today is completely the opposite. We are faced with information overload, impossible demands, constant chaos, social isolation, existential crises, and endless temptations. Our bodies respond to this life with changes in hormones and neurotransmitters that create cravings and appetites to a greater extent than our ancestors had.

> *There is a security in mastering these skills.*
> *Once we have them, we've got them for life.*

That's why, worldwide, when a country modernizes, obesity rates soar. So do other problems, such as crime, child abuse, suicide, divorce, smoking, alcoholism, depression, anxiety, and psychosomatic illnesses. It all stems from the mismatch between our hunter-gatherer genes and the stresses, isolation, and temptations of modern life.

Our tendency is to try to address one symptom at a time rather than going to their roots and addressing the cause. Forcing a change in our "bad habits," such as eating, drinking, smoking, and spending, without turning off the *drive* to go to excess is much like cutting weeds at ground level rather than pulling them out by the roots. They just grow back. Either they grow back in the same form or cross over and become other external solutions.

For example, a study published in the *New England Journal of Medicine*[2] found that those who stopped smoking were at least twice as likely to become overweight as those who had never smoked. The research concluded that one-quarter of the recent rise in obesity rates for men and one-sixth of the rise in obesity rates for women were attributable to the success of the antitobacco initiative. If we used a similar approach for the obesity epidemic now—with education, taxation, and legal actions—we might well improve obesity rates but prompt an increase in smoking or other external solutions, most likely spending, drinking, and pill popping.

> *Instead of pushing down one symptom after another,*
> *we go to the roots of the problem and end them all.*

What about the idea of not pushing down symptoms? That's the intention of The Solution Method. It's to accept our genetic tendencies, then use the method to fill in the gap between the genes we have and the genes we need in order to be free of various compulsions, addictions, and bad habits. It's to go to the roots of the problem and end the whole range of symptoms. We do that by shifting our lifestyle to something more akin to the lifestyle of our ancestors, if only slightly so. We gain the skills to move through the stresses of modern life rather than have them bore into us and trigger our reaching for food or another external solution. Plus, once we have the skills, we have them for life, so changes are apt to persist.

Then we'll be able to indulge ourselves now and then and enjoy our lives to the fullest. We won't have to worry that one wrong step will cause us to fall off the cliff and crash on the rocks of one personal excess or another. We won't fear that if we ever got thin, we'd start smoking, overspending, drinking too much, overexercising, pill popping, or overworking.

That would be a true solution.

6

Solution Method Research

THE SOLUTION METHOD was developed during the last 25 years at the University of California–San Francisco's School of Medicine, in the department of family and community medicine and pediatrics. We have much to learn about the method. However, some research has been conducted. It has shown a trend toward producing lasting weight loss and improvements in a whole range of common excesses.

A survey conducted independently by a University of Illinois– Chicago researcher evaluated program results in 155 participants who had enrolled in Solution training for at least one year and reported on the 134 who responded, an 86 percent response rate.[1]

Several studies suggest that the method turns off the drive to overeat.

Respondents were largely white women in their forties and fifties, and 43 percent had participated in Solution telegroups (audio-conferencing groups with a Solution provider), 33 percent had participated in a Solution group (an in-person group with a Solution provider), and 17 percent had completed the program through self-study Solution circles. All used the program's complete course, including at least four of the six Solution Kits.

There were significant improvements in all five of the most common excesses:

- 92 percent improved overeating.
- 88 percent improved excessive drinking.
- 83 percent improved smoking.
- 90 percent improved overspending.
- 82 percent improved excessive working.

In addition, improvements in happiness, health, personal relationships, work relationships, coping with work stress, work productivity, and physical activity were seen in the majority of participants. Since most subjects participated in the program to treat weight problems, fewer reported problems with the other excesses. Therefore, this research pertains mostly to obesity. But improvements in all of the excesses were highly significant.

A 15-month controlled clinical trial of sixty-three overweight and obese adolescents using the method was conducted in four sites in Northern California by health professionals trained in the method.[2] Participants were randomly assigned to one of two groups: a 10-week family-based program based on the method (The Shapedown Program) or a no-treatment control group. Those participating in the 10-week group lost weight during the program, then kept that weight off and had lost more by the time of a one-year follow-up. Their diet, exercise, and mood also improved. The control group made few changes and had no significant improvement in weight loss initially or in the long term.

The changes appear to continue
after the program ends.

A small group of adult subjects that participated in a Solution group at the university was followed at two years and at six years.[3] On average, participants not only lost weight and kept it off but also decreased their weight even more after the program ended. Other common excesses—smoking, excessive drinking, and overspending—decreased significantly, too. Depression dropped 50 percent in the first three months of using the method and continued to show decreases at the two-year follow-up and the six-year follow-up. Most subjects reported improved relationships and a spiritual deepening.

Although more studies are planned on the method, these initial studies are encouraging. In fact, they offer the first report in medical literature of a nonsurgical method in which weight loss continues after treatment ends. These findings resulted in *Health* magazine naming the method "One of the Top 10 Medical Advances of the Year."[4]

In the coming years, we hope to learn more about the effectiveness of bringing these skills to children, as well as to high-risk groups, and to explore the physiology associated with using the method and living life above the line.

7
Getting Started!

THE WAY YOU use this method is to begin! Just follow the 3-Day Solution Plan step-by-step. Again, if you want more detail about why the method works, that information is provided in Part 2 of the book. If you're interested in starting right away, you can skip directly to Part 3 and begin!

After three days on this plan, you will very likely feel so good and see such important results that you will be inspired to continue using the method. If you continue past these three days and the transition plan that lasts for the first two weeks, then you'll probably become involved with a Solution self-help circle, our Solution Internet support, or even a Solution group, coaching, or retreat.

Either way, you'll notice changes right away and realize that the method is infectious. When people do cycles together, the combination of using powerful skills and the warmth and closeness of community create a powerful experience. There is a sense of shared mission, that no matter what our differences, we are all committed to retraining our inner lives to naturally favor life above the line. Solution groups have sprung up around the country, for the skills are "catching"!

- A father is struggling with his two school-age kids, who are always fighting and scowling. He starts checking in with himself, using the skills, and soon, they are doing the same thing—and they are not squabbling!

- A woman joins a Solution group to take off some weight. Her husband becomes curious about it and listens to her do a cycle. She starts losing weight, and so does he. When they have an argument, they use the method together. Instead of going to bed angry, they make up first.
- One professor who uses the method attends scientific meetings all over the world and regularly sits in the lobby of her hotel with a colleague or two and does cycles. They all feel more relaxed and satisfied. Plus, they're less likely to overeat the hotel food.
- Two women are walking partners. One day, instead of complaining about her husband, children, and work, the woman who has Solution Skills asks the other woman to listen to her do a cycle. Their closeness deepens, and they both feel more invigorated by their walk.

That's why I encourage you to consider asking someone to use this plan with you. It's easier and more fun than doing it alone. However, if you prefer complete privacy and still want support, there is plenty of anonymous support from our Solution community. On our website (www.thepathway.org), there is a discussion board for 3-Day Solution Plan users, which is free to those who have a copy of this book. Also on the website, there are options for groups or personal coaching with Solution providers, health professionals trained in the method and access to Solution materials that prompt the rewiring of the feeling brain.

Despite all this community and support, this is not a program of dependency. The way you use the method is to get in, roll up your sleeves, master the skills, and rewire your feeling brain. Then, instead of spending your time in groups or coaching or with sponsors, you get on with your life.

You go fly kites, make love, and eat strawberries in bed. You follow your passions—you'll have plenty of them. Your creative energies will ramp up, too, so that you can fulfill your purpose in life and follow your spiritual path. Life below the line has stolen too much of your time. Now, you're back—so why not enjoy it!

For these three days, consider starting fresh.

As you prepare to use this plan, please be aware that it's important to stop any lingering judgments you may have about yourself due to your weight.

They are not fair to you. You've seen evidence in this book that the treatments available for weight problems are processed by the wrong part of the brain—the thinking brain instead of the feeling brain. What's more, you've seen that they target only diet and exercise, not the whole spiral of changes that trigger us to gain weight.

Apart from being unfair, that harsh, judging voice can get in the way of this work. The skills themselves are used with your own voice, so if that voice is unkind, then it's more difficult to use this method. For example, when you use the skills and ask yourself, "How do I feel?" and still have a harsh tone, the question could end up sounding not at all soothing, comforting, and empowering. It could be harmful rather than helpful.

So for these three days, consider starting fresh. Intentionally drop any nuance of harshness in your inner voice and replace it with a warmer and more supportive tone. Even if you have leftover emotional trash about how you really "should" have been smarter or better than you were, give yourself the benefit of the doubt. And consider giving the method the benefit of the doubt, too.

Even though you may have bought stacks of diet books, experimented with weight-loss drugs, or tried gastric surgery and deeply believe that nothing will work for you, consider opening your heart to the possibility that something could work for you. This method could work for you.

You don't have to do this perfectly. You simply need to begin. Just take three days and let some of the power and joy of this method come into your life.

It's only three days.

You can do *anything* for three days.

Part 2

TURNING OFF

THE DRIVE

TO OVEREAT

8

It's a Toxic World

IT USED TO be that when I ate too much, I blamed myself.

"How could I blow it again? What's wrong with me, anyway?"

That's the familiar self-bashing that goes on all over America after the holidays pass, the big meal ends, or the bag of cookies is empty.

But I didn't blow it at all! I just did what comes so very naturally when we're below the line. Instead of thinking "How could I blow it?" a more accurate response would be: "Oh, I overate. Wow. That makes perfect sense. My threshold of need must be way up today!"

At every moment of every day, each of us has a very specific and ever-changing "threshold of need" of the skills. Our threshold of need is the demand that the circumstances of life, both the external environment and the internal milieu, place on us. It can be low, moderate, high . . . or in the stratosphere.

> *"Oh, I overate. Wow. That makes perfect sense. My threshold of need must be way up today!"*

When the level of the skill we have to stay in balance, in homeostasis, is greater than the skill our threshold for need requires, we'll stay above the line. If we have less skill than what we need, we go below the line. Our threshold of need for the skills change in a moment, for that is the nature of the feeling brain. It's that sensitive, that responsive to the environment inside and out. The moment our need for the skills increases beyond our skill level—whether it's due to a critical glance from our boss, our own negative thinking, or street noise—the allostatic[1] response is triggered and we head below the line. Our body sets in motion a cascade of physiological changes in an effort to return us to balance.

That's the nature of the feeling brain, and it's so disorienting! Our threshold of need of the skills is constantly in flux. We can feel solidly above the line one moment where food is just food—not a fix. Then, something changes and, in a flash, we're below the line, where the world simply does not look the same—and neither does food. All of a sudden, our appetites soar and, no matter what, we're going to get that food.

We are still the same person. The only difference is that our threshold of need of the skills has increased!

If you will, think back to the times when your penchant for sweets or evenings spent on the couch devouring pizza led to creeping bulges around the waist. Wasn't that the year when your work-pressure mounted or your mother-in-law moved in or the time when you were in a funk for no reason you can put your finger on—*you just were.* The topography of our weight changes—or our use of the external solution of choice—seems to make more sense when you consider your threshold of need.

With all the stress, isolation, and temptations of modern life, most of us have a high threshold of need of the skills just from our current life situation. The breakneck pace of modern life is daunting, and there are fewer of the calming influences of stable, caring relationships and enduring social affiliations. Add to that the endless temptations of modern life—luscious inexpensive junk food *everywhere*—and it's no wonder obesity rates are soaring.

> *"Wasn't the year I gained all that weight the year my lover left, the dog died, and the basement kept flooding?"*

However, our threshold of need of the skills is a function of more than the immediate situation. It's a reflection of our genes, early experiences, temperament, major life events, traumas, workplace, and home and world environment, all of which can lead to increases in our allostatic loads.

Here's how it works. Say something happens that triggers us to go out of homeostasis and into allostatis, the process of maintaining the body during change. That adaptive response of rallying to this stress changes the body even though it enables us to respond to challenges presented and/or to prevent damage that would other-wise occur. It draws on all its resources and, albeit temporarily, brings the body to a new set point. For example, the allostatic re-sponse to weight lifting is the aches that are associated with the breakdown of muscle fibers. The body interprets this as a need to grow in order to respond to the new demand. Our muscles grow and we can lift those weights! However, if that weight lifting intensifies to the point that it brings about too much damage to the muscle and some damage to the joint, that wear and tear and new set point en-dures and adds to our allostatic load. The higher our allostatic load, the higher our threshold of need of the skills and the more our new homeostasis, our new norm, is apt to be below the line.

There are four common ways that allostasis can increase our al-lostatic load and make us more likely to establish a new set point that is below the line. First, we experience a rapid-fire series of stresses. Our cat dies, then we get laid off, then our car breaks down. We never really get a chance to recover and be fully, squarely, and soundly above the line. Second, for some reason our bodies do not adapt to stress. We don't just "get over it" each time we face a par-ticular stress and, in fact, each time the same stress crops up, it's as if it happens for the first time! Third, we just could be one of those people whose body simply doesn't respond effectively to stress, we don't turn on the stress response when we should, so there is no full recovery back to balance. And fourth, our physiological stress re-sponse turns on, but it doesn't turn off. Like a note stuck on the piano, we're in a chronic state of stress that leads us not above the line but drained, and we find ourselves taking up residence below the line.

Instead of being equipped with the skills to change those neural networks one synapse at a time, we're put on a diet.

One of the reasons weight problems can be so challenging—or even vexing—is because they often involve changes in our bodies and brains that are the result of our having a high allostatic load both psychologically and physiologically. Many of the factors are described later in this book (see Chapter 10, Spinning Out of Control), for example:

- Stress eating triggers central body fat accumulation and when these cells increase in size, they become resistant to insulin, thus increasing insulin in the blood, which in turn stimulates the appetite and the cortisol-induced draining of "feel good" neurotransmitters that leaves us distressed.
- We didn't learn these skills early in life because our environment was abusive or neglectful, and that abuse and neglect predisposes us to over-reacting physiologically to stressful events throughout life. The early abuse or neglect led to overfeeding or underfeeding as a child, both of which have been associated with weight problems in adulthood.
- A series of losses or changes results in our becoming fixed psychologically below the line, depressed, discouraged, and/or anxious, then we eat to feel better, but that overeating triggers weight gain, which leaves us vulnerable to health problems that further weight gain.

When we have a high allostatic load, our threshold of need of the skills may be chronically high. It may be stuck in the stratosphere and we may well be neurologically fixed at a set point that is way below the line. It feels normal to use various external solutions, not as an indulgence, but as a way to prop ourselves up and get through the day. We are apt to feel as if we're clawing our way above the line and we're always right on the edge of losing it. We are in constant survival mode not because we are wrong or bad, but because our own combination of genetics, temperament, acquired biological changes, stress, isolation, and temptation is keeping our threshold of need sky high nearly all the time.

In that situation, we need to get our threshold of need of the skills down and pump up our levels of skills so that we find ourselves above the line more often. We need to unload some of that stress, isolation, temptation, thus decreasing our allostatic load and pumping up our skills and using them over time to retrain our feeling brain one synapse at a time. Instead, we often go on a diet, take pills, or even think about gastric surgery.

We don't all have a high threshold of need of the skills. Some of us have mild weight problems, a low allostatic load, and a low ongoing threshold of need of the skills. Maybe we have an easy temperament, a body that tends to release energy rather than store it, and a natural affinity for pleasing ourselves with music, art, sports, and other noncaloric activities. We might notice a weight gain only when there seems to be a direct temporal cause, such as taking steroids, caretaking a child or parent, or going to work at an ice cream parlor. Something changed in our life and our weight increased and when that situation resolved, so did the weight problem.

Also, the threshold of need of the skills can creep up without us being fully aware that it has. Perhaps menopause begins and we put on a couple of pounds, then our last child leaves home and we put on a few more pounds, but it may not be until we sprain our ankle and have to give up brisk morning walks that we realize that we're below the line. By that time we may have increased our allostatic load considerably and may be more "fixed" below the line than we had imagined.

On the other hand, some of us may not really know how high our threshold of need of the skills is because we don't see ourselves as being below the line. Perhaps our weight doesn't bother us that much, or we're emotionally very even, so we have always thought that those extra pounds were just a matter of a few bad habits. They had no roots. Often this is because we've confused emotional imbalance with highs and lows and may not appreciate the debilitating effects of being emotionally numb, caught up in our thoughts but missing our own responsiveness and depth that feelings bring. We might say, "My life is wonderful. The only problem is this pesky weight problem that simply doesn't seem to go away." We may also be confused about our threshold of need because we're dabblers, using several external solutions. Not one of them is very noticeable. Or the external solutions we use may not be the common observable ones: smoking, drinking, pill popping, recreational drugs, overworking, or excessive exercise. They may be subtler. Perhaps our external solution is the tendency to stay stuck in a particular mood, such as self-pity, hostility, depression, or shame, or to be wedded to a childhood role that no longer works well for us, such as being the "victim," the "savior," or the "failure."

You might take a moment to think about how these external solutions apply to you. Consider the times you gained weight and how your threshold of need increased, whether it was because of stress, isolation, or temptations, and how much of a load you carry because of the repeated or long-term experiences of being below the line. Your need of the skills may have popped up or crept up—or you may have a threshold of need that is always high.

Does my threshold pop up or creep up, or is it always high?

Cameron's weight gain was caused by her threshold of need for the skills popping up when her new boss came on board and doubled her workload. With all that stress and the change in lifestyle, she couldn't connect with herself, let alone with her husband, Jack.

She was more isolated.

Her stress affected Jack and the children, too. Our feeling brains resonate with one another, so stress can literally be catching! The stress that Cameron brought into the home increased each family member's threshold of need for the skills, and each of them slipped a little bit more below the line. In that state, their emotional connections and capacity to regulate their moods based on one another's presence decreased.

Their elder son became demanding, and their younger one became sullen and needy. When he was below the line, Jack tended to distance emotionally and by using the external solution of watching television.

These changes in her children and husband further increased Cameron's isolation and stress. When a whole family goes below the line, they can easily drag one another further and further below, with each person living in his or her own private hell but acting as if everything were okay—until they can't anymore, and the screaming and use of external solutions starts.

If Cameron's family were not living in modern times, things would be apt to right themselves quite naturally. If there were nothing in the kitchen to eat but berries, milk, and corn, and nothing to do but garden, clean house, or build a fence, in a very short while, their threshold of need for the skills would come down. They'd all be back above the line, and life would be good.

However, our homes are chock-full of temptations, such as television, computers, video games, visually exciting foods, and sugary, fatty foods that can be instantly prepared.

Jack loved his flat-screen television and his huge, overstuffed lounge chair. The children's video games kept them overstimulated and zoned out. Cameron had her designer ice cream with caramel swirls or fudge brownie chunks.

Something for everyone!

The answer is to pump up our skills so we can manage whatever life tosses our way.

Each person was doing his or her best to cope with a high threshold of need for the skills and insufficient internal skills to pop above the line. But in that situation, you don't need a miracle. You just need one person who has the skill to get one molecule of his or her being above the line. That one speck can reach for these skills and pop the person's whole being above the line. Once that person is there, his or her clarity, vibrancy, and peace return, and personal balance becomes contagious. All that one person has to do is focus on staying above the line, and the results are often miraculous. That's the power of just one person's feeling brain being above the line.

You can see that it's never just one thing that sends us below the line. Stress, isolation, and temptation feed into one another. And if you add to that any genetic factors that favor weight gain—a difficult temperament, a tendency to gain weight—the extra fat simply starts growing on our bodies. It becomes *so very easy* to pack on the pounds!

Regardless of whether the threshold of need for the skills pops up, creeps up, or is continuously high, the answer is to pump up our skills. The amount of skill we need is relative, not fixed. We must have as much skill as we require to manage whatever life tosses our way.

It's Not Just Us

If you think it's harder these days to resist sitting more and eating more, you're not alone. The whole world seems to be gaining weight, and obesity in America continues to increase.[2] Around the globe, we see a nearly push-button phenomenon: when countries modernize—Egypt, Morocco, South Africa, Thailand, and Samoa, to name a few—they fatten up.[3] And the increases are so rapid in Mexico, Argentina, and Brazil that people there are poised to overtake us as the fattest in the world.[4]

Modern life is toxic. Along with modernization come lives that are more convenient but also more stressful and more lonely, and therefore more needy. At the same time, temptations abound. With urbanization and globalization only intensifying, that dynamic is unlikely to disappear.

Living in a utopian society in which we could have all the conveniences of modern life without the perils is impossible because high levels of conflict, ongoing disorder, and rapid change are integral to modernity.[5] The information overload alone is enough to make our need for the skills creep up. When television and the Internet enter homes, stimulation increases, and new values and possibilities come into view. We turn on the television and flip through the channels, encountering everything from dating contests to world violence to the shopping network's offer of a ruby pinkie ring for three easy payments of $39.99 each.

External solutions are rampant because of
modern life. It's toxic.

We work longer hours and enjoy fewer of life's natural gratifiers, such as taking a stroll, playing with children, or sitting in nature. We use food more for relaxing and rewarding ourselves. We look for gratifiers elsewhere as well. Things seem more enticing to us, and we want them more, so we spend more, which means we have to earn more, work more, and even worry about our debt more. Per capita consumer debt is five times greater today than it was in 1980.[6] There's no time left for regular exercise, a surefire stress reducer; in fact, 65 percent of us engage in *no* regular physical activity at all.[7] Ours is the most sedentary generation in the history of the world.

We also spend more time alone than our parents and grandparents did. Married couples spend less time together now than they did twenty years ago,[8] and more of us simply live alone.[9] Urbanization brings the stress of increased population density without the emotional payoffs. Since we're more below the line, we slip easily into merging, distancing, and control struggles, so that even when we live with others, we may feel lonely.

Stress and isolation make us more vulnerable to comforting ourselves with food, but the food itself makes us hungrier. We are hardwired not only for less chronic stress and more personal connection but also for an environment of scarcity. With all the sensory input of food on television, food in magazines, food in grocery stores and in restaurants, our brains respond by increasing hunger! When there *is* more, we *want* more! And there is a lot of luscious food at our fingertips. Instead of the boiled string beans and hamburger patties of the 1950s, we have gooey, captivating food served up in seemingly infinite varieties.

It's Not About the Food

Figuring out the cause of the obesity epidemic seems like a slam dunk to the casual observer. Compared to twenty years ago, we're consuming 12 percent more calories and 6 percent more fat.[10] We've switched from drinking milk to guzzling sodas—with a 60 percent increase in soda intake.[11]

Plain and simple, we're eating more.

Yet what if we didn't have an abundance of instantly available, sugary, fatty foods? What if we taxed butter, sugar, bacon, and snack foods? What if we took all sodas off the market?

Chances are, we'd just move to another excess, because the drives to do so would still be in full force. All that would have changed would be the nature of the temptations. We would have narrowed the field so that people would have fewer choices from which to select.

That happened in Russia. There was overwhelming stress with the collapse of communism in the 1980s,[12] and divorce rates soared. Although the first McDonald's in the country opened its doors in Moscow in 1991, in general, food was not abundant; in fact, it was often scarce. Russians couldn't overeat, so they chose another excess. The government subsidized alcohol and tobacco, and as a result, Russian mortality rates associated with substance abuse rose to among the highest in the world.[13] On the other hand, obesity rates dropped.[14]

During the same period, China opened itself to the world economy and modernized. As was the case with Russia, there were dramatic increases in stress, and the divorce rate rapidly increased.[15] However, the temptations were different. Cigarettes and alcohol were available, but imported high-fructose corn syrup was inexpensive compared to cigarettes and alcohol. Smoking and drinking increased somewhat, but obesity rates soared. During the same period that obesity rates in the United States increased by 40 percent, obesity rates in China doubled.[16] This suggests that food is not the problem. Being below the line is the problem that exacerbates any genetic tendency to go to excess. The symptoms vary, but the roots of the problem remain the same.

> *Dieting is stressful. Stress is part*
> *of the problem, not part of the solution.*

Not only does the prevalence of external solutions vary among cultures, but external solutions also vary within the same culture over time. For example, during the last 20 years in the United States, there has been a 25 percent decrease in total alcohol consumption[17] and about a 50 percent decline in smoking[18] and illicit drug use.[19]

During the same time, obesity has increased by about 40 percent.[20] Overspending based on per capita consumer debt increased about 50 percent,[21] and the use of prescription antidepressants increased by 400 percent.[22] Some excesses become less popular, and others become more popular.

So we can relax. The problem does not involve only food. We don't have to count every calorie or calculate every gram. Doing so is stressful, and stress is part of the problem, not part of the solution.

Instead, we can take a big, deep breath . . . and exhale, then go about rewiring our feeling brain so that we turn off the whole range of excessive appetites. We can set our sights on living life above the line.

9

The Toxic Spiral
of Weight Gain

PERHAPS WE HAVE a huge feast of a meal, a week of evenings on the couch, or a few blue days when ice cream becomes our best friend. At those times, we put a toe in the toxic spiral, but then we pull that toe out. We eat sensibly, go to the gym, and get back to a healthier lifestyle.

Except that sometimes we don't.

Instead, we take a giant step into the spiral because that one feast or blue day triggers us to go below the line. Once we are in that state, we spin out of control. A myriad of changes naturally occurs, most of which cause overeating, inactivity, metabolic slowdowns, and a pileup of problems that directly and indirectly foster weight gain.

In this chapter, you'll see exactly how we go below the line.[1] You'll see how reaching for the Solution Skills can save you from journeying further below the line and instead pop you back above the line where emotional appetite fades.

In the next chapter, you'll see the myriad of small but important changes that occur when we are below the line and that trigger weight gain or keep us fat. The remainder of the book will give you a plan to step out of the toxic spiral and jump-start lasting weight loss.

Let's begin with a snapshot of how we go below the line and how, at each moment along the way, reaching for our tool kit of these skills and using them can pop us above the line. On each and every occasion that we choose to reach for the skills and stop that slide down to life below the line, we trigger what feels like a personal awakening. That's because life above the line is conscious, grounded in the current moment, and pulsing with power. Each time we use the skills to pop ourselves back above the line, we feel a surge of "feel good" neurotransmitters that reward and nourish us without one carb, one gram of fat, or one calorie.

That power not just to know that one should be balanced and present, but to actually create that feeling in the moment—not by sheer chance but by choice—can change your life.

What Is a Feeling, Anyway?

It all begins with feelings, for the basis of every action more complex than a reflex is emotional. Knowing what to do is important, but the impulse to take action is influenced more by emotions than by thoughts. Even our most rational acts, such as checking our watches or calculating a tip, have an emotional core.

A feeling is an excitation of a nerve cell in the feeling brain. An electrical charge runs through a neuron and resonates briefly. It's like when a key is struck on a piano and the note lingers after the key has been played. The note sounds and then fades.

Feelings reflect not just our emotional state but the state of our entire being. They are deeper than thoughts and far more valuable for guiding the moment-to-moment decisions involved in giving our lives direction.

Even our most rational acts
pulse with an emotional core.

The feeling brain is our central clearinghouse, collecting information from the external world and the internal milieu and coordinating our response. Information pours into the feeling brain through our senses. Into the hopper of our feeling brain go thoughts from our thinking brain, messages about the state of our body, such as blood pressure and heart rate from our brain stem, and the emotional tendencies of our temperament. Intermingled with that input are our emotional memories and our intuition, the distillation of the truth from our entire life experiences—all of which are stored in the feeling brain.

Our feeling brain integrates and prioritizes that information, then arrives at a feeling. Although most of our feelings are unconscious, when the intensity or frequency of feelings increases, they cross the threshold of our awareness.

We feel the feeling.

A message is sent to our thinking brain. That feeling alerts us to our needs and, depending on its intensity, may provide the passion and willpower to follow through and meet that need. If we're hungry, we eat. If we're tired, we rest. If we're lonely, we call a friend.

We make tiny adjustments thousands of times a day, so that more of our needs are met. By doing so, we are more apt to stay above the line and out of the toxic spiral. If we don't bring that feeling to awareness, though, not only is the corresponding need not met, but the feeling is apt to intensify.

The Feelings Mount Up

After a feeling subsides—a note sounds and then fades—a shadow of that feeling lingers, enhancing our readiness to feel it again, but more intensely.

For example, we awake to a neighbor's dog barking and feel a flash of anger, but by the time we get out of bed and brush our teeth, the anger is gone. However, we feel irritable. Next, we spill coffee all over the morning newspaper just as our partner enters the kitchen, complaining that there are no clean towels. Now we're not just irritated, we're angry.

With each provocation, the intensity of the feeling mounts. Soon we're fuming, but we calm down and leave for work. The trouble is, we can't let go of thinking about the barking dog—and the audacity of that complaint about the towels! All the way to work, our mind will not shut off.

Thoughts trigger feelings. Repeated unconscious thoughts magnify those feelings.

Since the feeling brain can't differentiate between thinking-brain imaginings or ruminations and our sensory experience, we relive the experience emotionally again and again. By that time, the dog is sleeping peacefully and our partner has found a towel and we're sitting in the quiet of our car, yet the stress of that barking and that complaining continues to pummel our feeling brain. That reiteration of the feeling magnifies our anger.

To stop the slide to life below the line at this point, all we need to do is ask ourselves, "How do I feel?" and "What do I need?" That one choice to use the skill of checking in triggers a slight relaxation, a sense of "plugging in" to the moment, a lifting of the spirits. We're back above the line. Or one small act of Mastery Living, such as rubbing our neck or turning on pleasing music, can have a similar effect. Even a small healthful act or a simple use of the skills would disrupt the mounting overload in our feeling brain.

A Toe into the Spiral

However, let's say that we don't do anything. We allow our mind to travel in any direction it chooses, and the result is that our feelings intensify. Now we have a chip on our shoulder or a rumbling resentment within.

Then, new stresses pour into our feeling brain. The printer is out of paper, our coworker has an impossibly loud voice, and our allergies are acting up.

Anyone can have a stressful morning, with a cluster of upsets being followed by a series of annoyances. Any of us can numb out afterward and intentionally skip monitoring our internal milieu, choosing not to disrupt the mounting overload in our feeling brain.

But what determines whether that momentary lapse or longer-term separation from consciousness triggers us to eat a doughnut or order up a platter of pancakes, sausages, and eggs? What determines whether the toe that's in the toxic spiral is pulled out or drawn further in? What makes the difference?

The difference—other than genetics and circumstance—is our threshold of need for the skills and our skill level.

Our Threshold of Need

If our threshold of need for the skills is high, we're more likely to overload our feeling brain and go below the line.

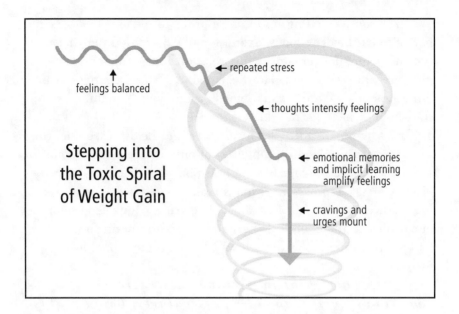

In the last chapter, we talked about the threshold of need for the skills and how it changes moment to moment based on stress, isolation, and temptations. If someone hadn't brought those doughnuts to the office, we would have been just fine!

However, we can have a threshold of need for the skills that is chronically or periodically high because of poor health, a stalled lifestyle, or a difficult temperament. If it is chronically high—as it is for most of us in modern life—we're apt to be right on the edge of going below the line nearly all the time. We teeter there, and the least thing can set us off!

> *Poor health, a stalled lifestyle,*
> *or a difficult temperament can keep us*
> *on the edge of going below the line.*

That's why it's so important to cultivate a lifestyle that keeps our threshold of need for the skills low; that is, Mastery Living. It's comparable to doing maintenance on our car: if the parts aren't working well and the engine is overloaded, it's more likely to stall or break down.

In our personal "owner's manual," many of us were not taught or shown during childhood how to take really good care of our lives.

We have some catching up to do in order to make it our personal policy to eat healthy foods, exercise daily, do something that matters with our day, create loving relationships, and take time for pleasure and relaxation. However, making those changes is now quite practical. We must take good care of our "machine" so our threshold of need for the skills is lowered.

It's why our health—both self-care and health care—matters so much: because health problems not only increase the amount of stress that pours into our feeling brain but also decrease our body's effectiveness in processing that stress. They affect our allostatic load. For example, skipping meals and eating junk food deprives our bodies of the chemicals needed for healthy brain functioning, and the resulting blood-sugar lows add to our emotional load.

Of particular importance are extremes of emotional temperament—particularly, being highly feeling-oriented or highly thinking-oriented.

Our temperament can contribute substantially to boosting our threshold of need for the skills, and even though temperament is persistent and any changes happen slowly, the long-term use of the method can have some effect in lowering our threshold of need due to temperament. As a person who has a difficult temperament myself, I can attest to the fact that just acknowledging that reality is reassuring. It helps me make sense of why it's so easy to go below the line. I'm wired differently and always have been.

Having a difficult temperament can increase the need for the skills substantially, because most stress is internally self-inflicted. Temperament describes various dimensions of personal tendencies, but of particular importance in Solution training is when emotional temperament is extreme, when we are highly feeling-oriented or highly thinking-oriented. (To determine whether you are more feeling-oriented or thinking-oriented, consider your first response to an upset—whether you feel or think.) If those tendencies are extreme and you are overloaded with either thoughts or feelings, it's harder to manage them!

Staying above the line is more challenging because we unintentionally wander into building castles of thoughts or (my specialty) grappling with such intense surges of emotion that we get exhausted! Often the two tendencies go hand in hand, as the person who is highly sensitive emotionally may unconsciously learn to put the brakes on those feelings through obsessive thinking.

In fact, most of us have a mosaic of tendencies that varies from feeling to feeling. For example, we may have a short fuse and slip quickly into hostility but struggle to access sadness or rarely experience guilt. Perhaps we're highly sensitive to fear or sadness—they echo through our brains easily and often—but when it comes to anger, we draw a blank.

> *Some people have a short fuse,*
> *others easily sink into depression.*

Yet, with the longer-term use of the method, even though the basic genetic tendencies linger, the "thinker" feels with more sensitivity and the "feeler" thinks more effectively. Even small changes in temperament can decrease our threshold of need for the skills so that we feel secure and we're not always on the brink of going below the line.

The *Skills* We Have Inside

The lower our levels of Solution Skills—all based on patterns of self-nurturing and effective limits—the easier it will be for us to have one upset lead to our going below the line and staying there for longer than we'd like.

These skills have two effects: an immediate one and a longer-term one.

You'll see the immediate effect when you use the 3-Day Solution Plan. You will reach for the skills, and in a matter of moments, you'll pop above the line. In time, you can become increasingly effective in the *intentional* use of the skills.

However, when these skills are used in the longer term, they become hardwired in the brain so that we use them *unintentionally*. They become automatic, so that we don't pop ourselves above the line only to find that the neural networks in the feeling brain aren't pleased. In fact, at the least provocation, they resume their domi-nance. When they do, there we go, back below the line. Plunk!

It's only when these skills become hardwired
in our brain that the changes last.

The neural networks that process our daily experience uncon-sciously are easily downloaded early in life, as our feeling brains then are like little sponges. They soak in the repeated contact with our environment and easily cross over the thinking-brain barrier. After all, at age two or even ten, we haven't learned to analyze our every move, nor do we have the cognitive skills—being able to think about our thoughts—that come with adolescence. After ado-lescence, it takes more contact and more repeated experiences to change those neural networks, although they can and do change.

If we had a responsive environment with lots of warm nurtur-ing stopping short of indulgence, and flexible but clear limits that were neither too harsh nor too easy, those patterns would have been downloaded into our feeling brain. We would have internalized those skills, and they would be hardwired in our brain. We would automatically bring more of our feelings to a conscious level in the thinking brain and would have downloaded a nurturing inner voice—not an indulging or a depriving one. That executive func-tioning in our thinking brain would take good care of us.

If our early environment was not responsive, these skills wouldn't be hardwired in our feeling brain, and instead, the opposite pat-terns would be—that is, depriving or indulging ourselves. Those neural networks that fire automatically would automatically numb our feelings or intensify and distort them, sending us below the line. Instead of a nurturing inner voice, we'd have an indulgent or a depriving one—and flip back and forth between the two.

When we alter our neural networks,
hostility cools and depression lifts.

These opposing neural networks shower our feeling brain with neural firings, such as repetitive negative thinking, emotional memories, and implicit learning, all of which can send us below the line. All those processes promote neurotransmitters that career out of balance, and our resulting chemical and electrical milieu turns a pleasing single note of emotion into discordant tones that reverberate and persist. Sadness slips into depression, a flash of anger becomes hostility, fear gives way to panic, and guilt turns into shame. They intensify, distort, and prolong feelings, sending us below the line and fueling our emotional appetites. The following subsections show you how.

Thoughts Intensify Feelings

Whereas some of us are swept away by feelings, others tend to ruminate, some of us more than others. We create castles of thoughts— whole worlds of "what ifs" and "whys"—and become wrapped up and tied down by obsessive, repetitive thinking. Thinking too much can be comforting, because it's familiar and we are hardwired to prefer the familiar. It's also engaging, as it gives us the illusion of control. We are doing something that can be construed as productive. However, thinking too much can also be a way to avoid feeling.

> *Obsessive thinking gives us*
> *the illusion of control.*

Not only does thinking too much remove us from an ongoing awareness of our feelings, but it can also trigger feelings to intensify and go below the line. The thoughts that shower our feeling brain don't seem at all like thoughts to it. They are reenactments of what occurred, for the feeling brain cannot differentiate between current sensory information and thinking-brain imaginings.

Most of us don't dwell on what went right during the party, the encounter, or the work incident but rather what went wrong with it. So these reenactments, analyses, and revisions of the past stir to life negative feelings, adding to the overload in our feeling brain.

All the Solution Skills disrupt that onslaught of the feeling brain by our thoughts. They give us the structure to disrupt that flow of excessive, negative, and distorted thinking by shifting our focus to feeling. Each time we take a deep breath, shift from our unconscious processing of daily life by the hardwiring in our feeling brain, and reach for and use the skills, we stem the tide of the over-load of our brain. We gently lift ourselves above the line.

Emotional Memories Are Aroused

As feelings flash in our emotional core, they arouse past memories of the same feeling. One feeling triggers other compatible feelings that send lightning across the landscape of our minds. In that way, our current feelings and our past feelings meld, and our emotional history keeps intruding on our current circumstance.

This is part of our allostatic load, the legacy of unhealed hurts that are stored as neural networks, the couplings of nerve cells. With each firing, those couplings become stronger. The more emotionally charged our experiences and the more frequently we replay them in our minds, the stronger the neural networks become. The stronger they become, the easier it is to trigger them again.

We can arouse positive memories that bring us pleasure and lift us from below the line, but if our early life was indulging or depriving instead of responsive, it's likely that within our feeling brain lies an abundance of hurtful memories. The more traumatic our childhood and the earlier the events occured, the greater the allostatic load and the more likely we are to overreact physiologically and behaviorally to stress. Furthermore, that same environment did not download the "software" that facilitates the healing of those hurts; that is, we may lack the capacity to feel our feelings and process them through effective limits, which would enable us to heal. As a result, the arousal of emotional memories is more likely to exacerbate our tendency to go below the line.

Emotional memories send us crashing below the line.

For example, consider the casual criticism about the towels. If we have a symphony of emotional memories of security and self-acceptance, that comment elicits mild irritation. A clear note of anger, a balanced feeling, sounds and it fades. We stay above the line.

On the other hand, if we have discordant tones of abandonment and self-rejection in our emotional memory, that same remark elicits a strong reaction. We feel hostility, an unbalanced feeling that tends to persist.

We go below the line.

Being below the line makes everything more stressful, and one upset leads to another. Our coworker's voice is *so* irritating. The pain from these new shoes is driving us nuts. We think, "Why am I the only person who bothers to refill the paper tray in the printer?"

> *As you take out emotional trash,*
> *there is bankable residue: compassion,*
> *emotional intelligence, resilience.*

As with thoughts, the feeling brain knows no difference between the emotions triggered by current sensory input and the emotional memories it triggers. And we carry around with us these neural networks that are our emotional history until we heal them. These neural networks travel with us from job to job, from home to home, and from relationship to relationship.

When emotional memories send us crashing below the line, we call these neural networks "emotional trash." They are the unconscious memories that reverberate in our minds and fuel our emotional appetites.

Although some of us who use The Solution Method have far more pain than others, I've never met anyone who, sooner or later, doesn't have some deep disappointment or scarring loss. Therapists' offices are filled with people whose emotional trash reverberates and overwhelms their current experience. Although healing these hurts is not easy, using Solution Skills effectively over time can heal them and free us from their excessive intrusion on our current experience.

> *It takes skill and persistence to change*
> *those neural networks, one by one.*
> *However, they can and do change.*

For there is some order among neural networks. Certain neural networks are stronger than others, and when a feeling note is struck, they compete! One feeling triggers emotional memories that have the strongest couplings and are dominant. The others submit. The triggering of that dominant neural network further strengthens it, increasing the likelihood that it will dominate the next time.

This is one reason why there are people who live primarily above the line and others who live primarily below. There are two worlds, because once the dominant neural networks in our feeling brain favor life below the line, they can be self-perpetuating, adding to our allostatic load and increasing the chances that our bodies will create a new homeostasis of imbalance.

Without our intervention, those neural networks that toss us below the line remain and strengthen. They elicit negative moods, which, in turn, generate more emotional trash, and the tone of our inner life may begin to darken. For when emotional memories are strong enough, they can shut down opposing networks so we can see only the bad times and not the good. Depression, anxiety, hostility, or shame can seduce us below the line even further.

At that point, it takes both skill and persistence to change those neural networks, one by one. However, they can and do change. You will be jump-starting that process with your 3-Day Solution Plan.

Using the second skill you will employ during these three days, emotional housecleaning, can begin to weaken those neural networks over time. It also bolsters our position above the line or keeps us from going below when we're right on the edge and heading south. I use this skill regularly when I am in emotional trouble or start to feel confused or stressed. However, the skill also has a healing effect on small pieces of emotional trash. It's best used when emotional memories create a tinge of overreaction rather than an all-out attack of it.

> *We feel the whole range of basic feelings,*
> *both positive and negative. It's cleansing!*

When we use this skill, we feel the whole range of basic feelings, both positive and negative. It's cleansing! For when a clear single note of feeling sounds, it naturally fades. We sound eight clear notes to create a natural flow of feelings: anger, sadness, fear, guilt, gratitude, happiness, security, and pride. We are more conscious in the present moment—so there's an instant reward—and those entrenched neural networks lose just a trace of their power. Every trace matters. In time and with practice, they weaken more.

Using the skill of emotional housecleaning seems to lift us up above the line because regardless of which unbalanced feeling we've gravitated to—hostility, depression, self-pity, panic, or shame—it blocks out the opposing neural networks. We can't feel any of the good feelings. In addition, that unbalanced feeling tends to obscure at least one of the basic balanced feelings, accounting for more distortion.

When we impose on our feeling brain the structure of bringing to the conscious awareness of our thinking brain all the positive and negative balanced feelings—moving through that natural flow of feelings—it inevitably has a certain balancing effect. For example, if we're depressed, the positive neural networks are quieted as well as other negative feelings, particularly anger. Emotional housecleaning triggers our feeling brain to fire up those networks.

Analyzing and figuring it out can be reassuring— but it can also be an external solution.

It's not necessary or even productive to figure out what feeling we're stuck in. The pathway to healing begins with feeling. Analyzing past hurts and gaining insight into them can be reassuring— but it can also be an external solution, because thinking can block feeling. If we bring up thoughts about past hurts and don't have a substantial supply of the internal software of these skills, the feelings it does trigger drop us below the line. We'll become depressed, hostile, panicked, or ashamed. Neither of these states—excessive thinking or below-the-line feelings—facilitates healing.

What does block both excessive thinking and below-the-line feelings is going about the business of moving those feelings above the line. This seems like such a simple tool compared to insight-oriented psychotherapy and the home variety of personal self-analysis in which most of us engage. But we can't *think* our way to emotional healing, for the doorway to healing is through *feeling*.

Emotional housecleaning enables us to step over the thinking-brain barrier, access our feelings, and go right to the core of our emotional brain. As the tool triggers us to fire up those emotional circuits, the neural networks of emotional trash that drag us below the line weaken. For small hurts, that's all we need in order to heal. We use this tool and can be gently drawn above the line.

However, some neural networks that store hurtful emotional memories are very strong. Rather than being like fine threads in our brain, they feel like ropes! They take a simple current stress and quickly and easily distort it to the point that we feel as if we were right back at the time when a loss, betrayal, change, or pain occurred. For these more substantial hurts, emotional housecleaning is not enough. When a hurt is deep enough to weave its way into our implicit memory, we need something more. We need to use the third skill: doing cycles.

Implicit Memory Fans the Flames

Our brain unconsciously extracts the rules of life from our experiences and encodes them in our implicit memory. These rules form our limits: our expectations about ourselves, others, and the world; our patterns of effective or ineffective thinking; our acceptance of life's unavoidable pain and our receptivity to its rewards.

These limits, even though we may not be able to recognize or explain them, are the bedrock of the moment-to-moment decisions in our daily lives. They are hardwired within us and are more likely to be ineffective if our life has been rocky, presenting us with considerable deprivation, indulgence, or trauma.

We may be conscious of our expectations that seem sensible. We expect ourselves to go to work, feed the dog, or scream at the neighbors if we're highly provoked! However, it's the unconscious expectations that are not sensible that hurt us the most, such as: I must please everyone; My feelings don't matter; and Whatever I do fails. They are an accurate reflection of how we unconsciously interpret our personal history because of the depriving, indulging, or traumatic turns it took. These unconscious expectations largely shape the responses to life that trigger us to go below the line. Then negative, powerless thoughts and insufficient practice at moving through life's pain rather than getting stuck in it keep us there.

Our limits are encoded in our feeling brain, based on the rules of life stored in our implicit memory.

These ineffective limits are unconscious, and even if they were conscious, without a substantial download of these skills, we may be powerless to alter them. For example, if we become aware that our basic expectation is that we can eat whatever we want to eat, knowing that that is our expectation doesn't necessarily change it. It's difficult to change that implicit learning because it is in our feeling brain. Conscious thought is in the thinking brain, and even though we tell ourselves repeatedly that we should limit our food, if our feeling brain says otherwise, we will obey it. We will "try" to limit our food, but we won't really do that—at least, not in the long term. When it comes to primitive drives, our unconscious allegiance is not completely rational.

We take action based on the limits that are at the roots of our feelings.

So we will continue to repeat the same patterns—for example, swearing off sweets in the morning, then devouring them in the evening—as long as there is a particular limit, a cluster of errant neural networks, residing within us. We change that implicit learning, those errant limits, by doing cycles. The cycle begins by plunging into our anger, sadness, fear, and guilt. That enables us to step over the thinking brain barrier and we gain far more accurate insight into our drives and motivations. Then we call on the frontal lobes of our thinking brain to craft new, more reasonable expectations. As we complete the cycle, both our thinking and feeling brain are active, effectively burning in the new learning by weakening the old neural networks and laying down new ones that favor a life of balance. It's with the repeated, effective use of the tools of method that we rewire the feeling brain and not only mature but, within the limits of circumstances and genetics, become free from the whole range of external solutions. When we retrain those neural networks, the behavior changes. Barring unusual circumstances, we wouldn't consider eating mindlessly, choosing whatever we happened to want. It's not that we're showing excessive restraint but that our hardwired neural networks have changed. We just don't do that anymore.

Let's go back to that criticism about not having clean towels. The response was anger fueled by emotional trash of abandonment and self-rejection, so the feelings were red-hot. However, wrapped around those feelings are neural networks from the implicit learning that either contain the feelings, calming them down and moving them above the line, or the opposite. Opposing networks can fuel fury, depression, panic, or shame that drop us right below the line.

> *Imagine the power to bring to consciousness your unspoken limits and tinker with them until they are just right for you.*

For example, if the wordless expectation learned from our repeated experience favors life above the line, our expectation may be something like "I expect myself to tell my partner how I feel when I feel criticized." On the other hand, if our internal limits favor life below the line, our unconscious expectation may be more like "I expect myself to fume and smolder but say nothing."

If our unconscious thinking is ineffective, it might be something like "There's no point in talking about it" rather than "It's important to talk about it."

If our implicit learning is based on responsive experiences, we will feel the essential pain, the downside of following through, reap the earned reward, and land above the line.

For example: "The essential pain is that she may be mad at me. Speaking up takes effort, but the earned reward is that my relationship will be more honest and I won't have to stress out about it all morning. I'll have gotten it off my chest."

If our implicit learning is based on repeated depriving or indulging experiences, we will unconsciously find essential pain and earned rewards that take us further below the line.

For example: "The essential pain is that I will be tense all morning, perhaps overeat, and will allow resentment to mount in my relationship. The earned reward is that I won't have to deal with it. I won't have to feel my feelings. I won't have to risk her fury or her rejection."

All this happens unconsciously thousands of times a day, based on our implicit learning, the limits that are hardwired in the neural networks in our feeling brain.

Stepping into the Spiral

When our feelings intensify, and emotional memory and implicit learning fan the flame, we go right below the line. We feel way high, way low, or numb, and for those of us prone to weight problems, appetites ramp up, metabolic rate slows, and a myriad of other changes that trigger weight gain follow. We're in the toxic spiral, and our bodies flip the switch from maintaining weight to gaining it.

With Solution Skills, you will use checking in to disrupt the internal process that's preparing to send you below the line and emotional housecleaning to gently move yourself back above the line when you're going below. You'll do cycles to take out emotional trash and rewire the neural networks in your feeling brain to create new limits, which open up vast possibilities in your life.

Imagine the power to bring to consciousness your unspoken limits and tinker with them until they are just right for you. With these skills and considerable diligence in using them, you can begin to create for yourself just the limits that will give you the power and safety you want. They will reflect how you choose to live your life. These limits are not superficial "shoulds" or "obligations" that fall flat when emotions mount. Instead, they will shimmer with passion and reside not in your thoughts but in the rewiring of your feeling brain.

You don't do cycles all the time. You do them when you need to do them, when you know you are way below the line. Cycles begin with some of the feelings you'll address in emotional housecleaning: anger, sadness, fear, and guilt. When you've expressed those most basic feelings, you've moved away from your mental functioning that has all the "shoulds" and "rules" attached, and you've explored the depths of your subconscious mind.

You've brought the unconscious to consciousness.

Those conscious thoughts are in the frontal cortex of the brain, the executive function, where you can think about your thoughts, tinker with those limits, and change them so that you create precisely the expectation that is not too harsh or too easy but responsive to you.

You feel the essential pain, move through it,
and on the other side, there is light,
energy, creativity, and hope.

Once the expectation seems right to you, you can fortify it with positive, powerful thoughts, then look the unavoidable pain of following through right in the eye. For example, you say, "He may reject me" or "I have to do something I don't want to do." Just looking at it straight on, then pausing, allowing your feeling brain to respond to it emotionally—neural networks flash, then fade—pops us above the line. The fireworks go off, the bells ring, and all of a sudden, not only are you above the line, but the reward of following through drops right into your lap!

Into your mind comes a thought, followed by the rush of a satisfying, relaxing, and fulfilling feeling.

For example, you might say, "The essential pain is that he may reject me," then pause, allowing feelings to rise up, then fade. When they do, a thought appears in your thinking brain: "Yes, he might reject me, but the earned reward is . . . even if he does, I won't reject myself! Wahoo!!! That's great!" The emotional payoff of that earned reward follows, and you are very above the line!

Or you might say, "I have to do something I don't want to do," then pause, allowing the feelings to rise up, then fade. When they do, the thought appears: "Yes, but by doing that, I will be happy. I will be healthy. My life will get even better." Your spirits are lifted, and you are above the line, full of energy and ready to take action.

That "pop" above the line burns in the new limit
that is the bedrock of personal security.

You feel the essential pain, move through it, and on the other side, there is light, energy, creativity, and hope. It's the earned reward. You have popped above the line, and now the sunshine comes out— and you have the energy and passion you need to follow through. Each cycle you do, each pop above the line that you experience counts. Each one contributes to burning in a new limit that is the bedrock of personal security.

That preoccupation with the cookie stops.

The tension is relieved, and you are flooded with a sense of peace.

Feeling the essential pain pops us above the line. We both think and *feel* at once. It is a whole-brain activity, and when both the feeling brain and the thinking brain are flashing with activity, important changes follow.

When you state and then *feel* the essential pain, your feeling brain shifts above the line, and relaxed energy flows through your body. You can see it on your face, as the facial muscles are controlled by the feeling brain.

The earned reward follows, with a wave of pleasure and promise . . . and motivation. Now you are above the line, and not only do you feel better in the present moment, but synapse by synapse, you have begun to retrain the feeling brain so that life above the line can be spontaneous and automatic more of the time.

> *In that instant, we become aware of that missed*
> *kernel of wisdom that was at the core of that hurt.*

As you begin using the method, if you are thinking-oriented, it might take you a while to access feelings, and if you're feeling-oriented, you might feel some of the feelings strongly and others not at all. Either way, mastering the skill to access feelings usually doesn't take long.

Limits, though, are a different story. The old ineffective limits are etched in the neural networks of our feeling brain, and just as they became dominant through repeated experience, it's through the repeated use of the skills that they weaken.

Each time you do a complete cycle—not just feel your feelings— you strengthen the neural networks that favor life above the line and weaken those competing neural networks that favor life below.

Finally, when the switch flips and the new neural networks become dominant, they fire up automatically. Life becomes so much easier! We are on firm ground, for those reasonable, responsive neural networks are hardwired within us, plus we have the pride of knowing that we took our life in our own hands: we created a new inner life that favors clarity, vibrancy, and peace—as well as lasting weight loss.

Some of us have lots of emotional trash and implicit learnings that seem to be embedded in our bones. They just won't go away! Healing these hurts and rewiring these limits takes time and persistence. However, the elegance of the design of human healing is breathtaking. Emotional trash can be so painful that we are motivated to keep doing cycles on it, feeling our anger, sadness, fear, and guilt over and over. Each time we do, we feel emotionally lighter and sense that we have loosened up some of those neural networks and are on our way to healing.

We watch our appetites fade,
our metabolism increase, and our weight go down.
We look and feel vibrant!

Our unhealed hurts keep bothering us, though. They keep showing up in our eating, in our loving, in our spiritual life, or at work, and that pain fortifies us with just the motivation we need to continue doing cycles about them.

Then, often when we least expect it—for me, it's frequently in the shower or in the car—we are doing a cycle and the past hurt is healed. In that instant, we become aware of that missed kernel of wisdom that was at the core of that hurt.

The wisdom and understanding that healed that hurt are not the same as book learning. They are soul-based. That healing feels spiritual, and even for those of us who do not have a spiritual base, it feels as if the earth has moved—and we are aware of the grace and mystery of life.

Now that you have a basic understanding of how we can easily slip below the line and into the toxic spiral of weight gain, we'll take a more detailed look at what happens once we're there. We spin out of control! It's all due to a myriad of changes in mind, body, and spirit that quite naturally occurs when we're below the line.

10

Spinning Out of Control

IT DOESN'T MATTER what triggers us to go below the line. Nearly anything can, but once there, we are vulnerable to a host of factors that make us gain weight.

All of a sudden, food seems to be everywhere. It all looks so luscious. The better it looks, the more we think about it. The more we think about it, the hungrier we become. The more we eat, the more we want, and the more our body seems to store whatever we eat!

It's a spiral!

And it's perfectly normal once we start gaining weight to feel as if we are spinning out of control. We may look calm and our lives may be moving along well otherwise, but slowly and surely—a few pounds here and a few there—we're gaining weight. Those small but important parts of the toxic spiral are spinning us out of control. Our metabolic rate declines, our appetite increases, and our waistline expands.

We step into the spiral because our threshold of need for the skills is too high! Our lifestyle is stalled and our skills are low, given our genetics, temperaments, allostatic load, and current stress, isolation, and temptations. We step out of it through Mastery Living and pumping up our skills. In this chapter, we'll examine what happens when we're in the toxic spiral and the science behind each part of it. Not all of the factors listed below apply to each person. You may prefer to focus only on the parts of the spiral that most apply to you.

- A change or loss triggers the stress response.
- Our appetite for sugar and fat increases.

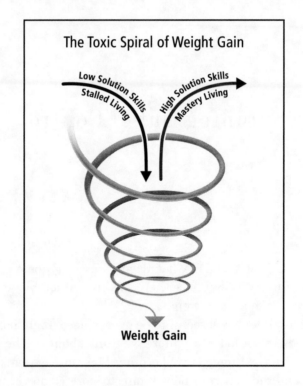

- Sugar and fat make us hungrier and fatter.
- Food variety fuels our appetite.
- Low-fiber diets make us fatter.
- Stress causes belly fat.
- Fat begets fat.
- Our neurotransmitters are drained.
- Food becomes addictive.
- We stay busy-busy-busy.
- Our physical activity decreases.
- Health declines.
- Intimacy dwindles.
- Our spiritual connection weakens.
- Body image suffers.
- Dieting makes it worse.
- Problems pile up.
- We cross over from one excess to another.

A time of gaining weight is often launched by a stress, change, or loss that sends us below the line. Although it is commonly a major life event, such as a death, divorce, or serious illness, it can frequently be a smaller change but one that hits home, that shakes us at our emotional core. For example, our cat that soothed and comforted us dies, work stops being a safe place because of the threat of layoffs, or a close friend moves away. It's usually something that shakes our world soundly or severs a major emotional artery. Then, once we're below the line, one stress leads to another . . .

A Change or Loss Triggers the Stress Response

. . . and before we know it, we're in a state of chronic stress. Rather than the kind of episodic physical stress our bodies were designed to tolerate, we're stressed emotionally with no physical release, and it's chronic—there is no relief!

The hypothalamus in the brain secretes CRH (corticotrophin-releasing hormone), which travels to the pituitary gland and causes the secretion of ACTH (adrenocorticotropic hormone). ACTH travels via the blood to the adrenal glands, above the kidneys, and triggers the secretion of stress hormones, particularly cortisol.

Glucose is released into the bloodstream from the muscles and the liver, and fat is released from the area near the portal vein of the liver. We're ready to take action, and the neurotransmitters respond. Dopamine and endorphin levels increase immediately. Dopamine, the "I gotta get it!" chemical, energizes us to act, while the endorphins protect us from pain. When the stress is resolved, serotonin, the "I got it!" chemical, floods us with feelings of well-being and satisfaction. At this point, both serotonin and dopamine levels are high, and we are in a state of clarity, vibrancy, and peace.

> *Chronic stress triggers hormone and neurotransmitter changes that pack on pounds.*

With chronic stress, however, we're subjected to ongoing elevations in cortisol that not only favor weight gain but also wreak havoc on the body. Chronic secretion of cortisol and other stress hormones increases the risk of impaired immunity, osteoporosis, memory loss, heart attack, and menstrual and fertility problems. It also draws us further into the spiral because of the effects on insulin and neurotransmitters.

Our Appetite for Sugar
and Fat Increases

Stress makes us crave oral gratifiers, only one of which is food. The food we reach for when we're drained, anxious, or impulsive is not usually bean sprouts or broccoli but sugar and fat.

Foods high in sugar and fat have a high hedonic value, something researchers use to measure the level of satisfaction a food brings. Interestingly, fat alone is not all that palatable. We don't think of eating a stick of butter but of having butter as part of chocolate chip cookie batter or disguised in pumpkin pie topped with whipped cream. Adding a little sugar to fat can cause cravings in even the staunchest dieter.

We desire just the foods that make us gain weight.

Similarly, the hedonic ratings of sugar alone are lower than those for the pleasure duo of sugar and fat. Sweet-fat cravings increase endorphins and give us that wonderful "pleasure response."

Stress ramps up our desire for fat as cortisol increases the production of galanin, the hormone that raises our appetite for fat.[1] Often the desire for fat comes after the sweet tooth has been satisfied. Eating sweets seems to prime our need for fatty foods.

Part of this pattern may reflect normal preferences that are genetically favored. We crave things that allowed our ancestors to survive. Neuropeptide Y (NPY) is distributed widely in the brain, with particularly high concentration in the feeling brain. High levels of NPY increase appetite and decrease stress. NPY levels are highest in the morning, triggering quick fueling to start the day. Unfortunately, cortisol levels are also highest in the morning, so eating refined carbs in the morning can trigger blood-sugar lows, as insulin is more readily secreted in response to cortisol. This is why having a breakfast that contains some carbs for quick energy but emphasizes protein and healthy fats is so important. Galanin levels increase by late afternoon and evening, increasing our desire for foods high in fat, such as salad dressing, chocolate, meat, and potato chips, because fat has more staying power.

Sugar and Fat Make Us Hungrier and Fatter

We respond to stress by craving fat and sugar, and eating them draws us further into the spiral.

A diet high in refined carbohydrates—particularly when sweets are eaten alone rather than in a meal mixed with protein and healthy fats—increases appetite.[2] Having a candy bar prompts the pancreas to secrete an extra shot of insulin, which lowers blood levels of all amino acids except tryptophan, a building block of serotonin. When tryptophan no longer has to compete with other amino acids to enter the brain, levels of it rise in the blood. It's easily converted to serotonin.[3] Our mood improves, and we learn that when we're below the line—way high, way low, or numb—eating sweets decreases stress and improves energy.

We feel better in the short term and hungrier soon thereafter. The insulin surge that follows the consumption of high-sugar foods shunts glucose into our cells, creating a blood-sugar low, which in turn stimulates hunger. We rush to respond, usually by eating more sugary or fatty foods.

The cycle continues with another surge of insulin and more hunger. Two hours after a meal, we reach for sugar again and perpetuate a cycle of sugar cravings, increased insulin levels, and blood-sugar highs and lows.

That blood-sugar roller coaster gives rise to mood problems—tension, tiredness, anxiety, or depression—and sugary foods are turned into belly fat, which increases cortisol levels, drains the brain of serotonin, and causes more mood problems. Those mood problems increase stress, appetite, carbohydrate intake, and weight gain.

Short-term gratification prompts
more hunger and more cravings.

Sugar is not the only culprit. Often, we think we're having carbohydrate cravings, but we may actually be yearning for fat as well. At least 25 percent of the calories in cookies, candy, and cakes traditionally viewed as "sweets" are derived from fat. Foods high in fat are so calorically dense that a relaxed wrist when pouring salad dressing, an oversize chocolate bar, or that penchant for nuts—

small handful after small handful—amounts to the calories our body needs for an entire meal. Plus, fats are far more efficiently metabolized than other foods. All food requires energy to be digested, but whereas the digestion of carbohydrates and protein uses up about 25 percent of their energy, the digestion of fat uses up only 3 percent of its energy. Calories that would otherwise be lost due to digestion are conserved.

Food Variety Fuels Our Appetite

We're surrounded by an abundance of mouthwatering foods. A sensory center in our thinking brain—the orbitofrontal cortex—responds to the taste, texture, smell, and sight of these foods.[4] The more visually exciting, highly palatable, and full of sugar and fat the food is, the more active this sensory center—and the more it triggers hunger.

In other words, watching television advertisements about junk food, looking at the dessert tray in a restaurant, or having cupboards full of chips, sodas, cakes, cookies, and pies triggers the hunger response.

Sensory-specific satiety makes
variety in food fattening.

What increases appetite is not just how appealing and delicious food is but how much variety is in the diet. The food industry is constantly inventing new products, and the more products, the more tantalized we are and the more we want to eat. When I was growing up, there was one kind of Oreo cookie. Now there are twenty-four different ways to get an Oreo fix, from Mini Oreo to Fudge Covered Oreo to Double Delight Oreo Peanut Butter & Chocolate.

We have "sensory-specific satiety,"[5] which means that food tastes great at first, but we become progressively less interested as we continue to eat it:

- Finish the salad and we're ready for the pasta.
- Can't eat another bite of pasta.
- When dessert comes, however, we have a renewed appetite.

Having simple meals and whole foods is a natural appetite suppressant, but restaurants and food companies that profit from our overeating know that variety, abundance, and tantalizing presentations make us eat more.

Low-Fiber Diets Make Us Fatter

Diets high in fat and sugar are dismal when it comes to fiber. Not only have low-fiber diets been linked to obesity in population studies,[6] but high-fiber diets have been shown to dilute calories, slow down eating and digestion, prevent insulin surges, and stave off blood-sugar roller coasters.[7]

Each time you choose 100 percent whole-grain bread (it's even better if it's chock-full of sprouted organic wheat berries) instead of the white stuff or "brown bread," you're getting an appetite suppressant in food form.

Here's how it works: that fiber in the whole-grain bread travels to the small and large intestines. The gut responds by increasing the production of many hormones. Two of those hormones, PYY (peptide YY)[8] and GLP1 (glucagon-like peptide 1),[9] suppress appetite. By consuming refined grains, we miss out on the natural organic appetite suppressants in fiber-rich foods.

Our intestines shrivel and our energy needs shrink.

A high-fiber diet is also likely to help prevent those weight plateaus that are the dieter's nemesis. We're eating well and losing weight, but then weight loss gradually comes to a halt. There are many factors that contribute to this, but one appears to be the result of a low-fiber diet. It prompts our metabolic rate to decrease because the intestines account for a quarter of our metabolic rate.

Diets that are low in fiber cause us to produce "puny stools," because with less fiber to process, the intestines shrink.[10] The hairs on the inside of the gut—microvilli—that absorb nutrients from the intestine are highly metabolically active. With a low-fiber diet, they become shorter and fewer, since the surface area of the entire intestine shrinks. In time, metabolic rate declines, and each extra bite we eat will be more likely to go to fat.

Stress Causes Belly Fat

Stress increases both insulin levels and cortisol. Insulin increases appetite and overeating, but it's cortisol that tells the body where to deposit the extra fat. The more stress in our lives and the greater our genetic propensity to secrete cortisol (the more we are "cortisol hyper-responders"), the more likely those extra calories are to be sent to the belly. That fat is not under the skin (subcutaneous fat) but under the ribs, where it cushions the visceral organs, such as the liver. Stress sends the fat directly to the place where it is released most easily into the blood. This increases the risk of metabolic syndrome, including hypertension, low HDL cholesterol, high triglycerides, and diabetes.

Here is why: when there is stress, the body needs energy to prepare for "fight or flight," and cortisol draws fat from the most accessible site, which is in the abdomen. When the stress subsides, the cortisol deposits the fat back in the abdomen; with chronic stress, the ongoing oversecretion of cortisol diverts fat storage to our bellies.

Once that fat has been deposited, cortisol inhibits its release, so more fat accumulates around our organs and we develop central obesity. That fat converts the inactive form of cortisol to the active form. In other words, the stress that got us to eat sends that extra food to a place in the body where it manufactures more cortisol. That cortisol goes to the brain and drains it of serotonin, so we have mood problems[11]—particularly depression and mood swings—creating more stress, a bigger appetite, and more overeating!

Insulin increases fat deposits but cortisol sends that fat to our bellies.

But that's not all. That belly fat releases proinflammatory cytokines, which, in turn, promote fat cells to trigger the oversecretion of insulin, leading to metabolic syndrome and diabetes.[12]

When we have periodic stress, cortisol increases insulin levels, making glucose more readily available in the blood for fight or flight. During chronic stress, however, cortisol signals the cells to ignore insulin. The cells become insulin-resistant, which, in turn, causes higher insulin levels and more overeating of high-fat, high-sugar foods. The ensuing weight gain creates more insulin resistance, more overeating, and further weight gain.

As if that weren't enough, cortisol also depletes muscle tissue,[13] and therefore our metabolic rate further decreases—so we're not only hungrier, we're also more likely to gain weight.

Fat Begets Fat

Anyone who struggles with weight gain knows it's easy to put on weight but hard to lose it. Multiple bodily mechanisms defend us against weight loss, but none protect us from regaining weight.[14]

Being fat makes us prone to becoming fatter—not just from the psychological or social fallout of the extra pounds but also due to the biological changes created by the fat tissue, including the hormone and neurotransmitter shifts it produces.

Obesity not only triggers higher spikes in insulin levels that prompt overeating but also affects the levels of two hormones, ghrelin and leptin. These hormones rise and fall in opposition to each other, so appetite is increased and weight is gained. When calories are excessive and weight is gained, the body establishes a new, higher "set point." Only when we can ratchet our weight down and keep it there for a long while, such as two years, are we more resistant to the body's propensity to regain the weight.

Body fat is not inert.
It's an organ that alters our hormones.

The fat in the body functions like an organ, with its own propensities to alter hormones. The body adapts to weight gain with a multitude of changes in an effort to rebalance itself with that extra weight. Unfortunately, many of these adaptations actually prompt more weight gain:

- The gut protein that decreases overeating, PYY (peptide YY), is lower in the obese.[15]
- Lipoprotein lipase, the enzyme that sits on fat cells and

shunts fat from the blood into the cells, increases with weight gain,[16] particularly in the presence of cortisol and insulin. The extra food we eat is more easily diverted into fat cells and stored.

- The brain adapts to obesity by becoming resistant to leptin, the hormone that tells us to stop overeating. This leptin resistance makes people more vulnerable to weight gain.[17]

Our Neurotransmitters Are Drained

Chronic stress saps the neurotransmitters that create a sense of well-being and resilience:[18] serotonin, dopamine, and endorphins.

Cortisol secretion depletes serotonin levels, and low serotonin levels increase appetite. That serotonin drain also increases depression, anxiety, irritability, and a hopeless neediness. When dopamine levels decline, we have less energy, and our moods turn toward dissatisfaction, boredom, and sluggishiness. We're also more impulsive. Low endorphin levels prompt negative moods, tension, and fatigue.

The draining of neutotransmitters disrupts mood and fuels overeating.

The overall effect of this drain in neurotransmitters varies considerably. Some people have a mild sense of disappointment or find themselves feeling grouchy. Others are so depressed that they can't get out of bed in the morning. Often this neurotransmitter drain appears as emotional fragility. Any minor disappointment could bring tears. A minor slight triggers a huge rage.

This draining of neurotransmitters is not just an inconvenience but central to weight gain. Any disruption in mood can fuel overeating. For example, the bored, sluggish mood associated with low dopamine levels may trigger the need to eat for the reward or the pleasure of it. The mentality is "I want that food, and I deserve to have it!" High-endorphin eating is often celebratory: "Food is wonderful. Life is wonderful. Let's feast!" Serotonin lows trigger eating for comfort, anxious nibbling, and eating binges. If we're helpless, hopeless, and depressed, our energy expenditure drops to near-basal levels, affecting metabolic rate, spontaneous movement, and daily activity levels. Weight accumulates on our bodies even when we're eating sensibly.

Food Becomes Addictive

When neurotransmitters are drained, we're more vulnerable to developing food cravings[19] in which the urge to eat shuts out all other urges and the urge to satisfy that need feels like inescapable pain— a survival need. Food becomes addictive, and the compulsion to eat is so strong that we can't set limits. If we can't get at our food, we're depressed, irritable, or anxious.

Current research suggests that key players in triggering cravings are dopamine, serotonin, and endorphins. The feeling brain gathers information from the external and internal environment and settles on a feeling that suggests a need. The feeling brain sends that information to a bundle of nerve cells in the brain called the nucleus accumbens.

The nucleus accumbens secretes dopamine to give us the impulse to take action, it can become sensitized due to stress, hormones, or genetic tendencies. Once the nucleus accumbus becomes sensitized, it it easily triggered to oversecrete. We're easily set off, so we don't secrete just a modicum of dopamine as well as endorphins— we overshoot our need. Or our dopamine levels are so low from genetic defects or addiction that the drive to eat is triggered by the need to return dopamine levels in the nucleus accumbens back to normal pre-addiction levels.

We get the urge to have a cookie, but we're stuck in a meeting— a very contentious, distracting, irritating meeting! Our mind turns to the package of chocolate cookies in our desk drawer. We want those cookies more and more because dopamine levels rise based on the urgency of the need. The more the dopamine levels rise, the more the serotonin levels drop. The lower the serotonin levels— and they are low in the obese and in dieters—the more painful the cravings and the more focused we become on getting that food. The stress of the craving triggers the stress response with its cascade of hormone changes and the antistress effects of NPY diminish, motivating us even more.

We eat to avoid the pain of a drop in neurotransmitters, that is, withdrawal.

We can't stand it anymore and leave the meeting to go get those cookies. We rush to our desk, rip off the wrapper, and sink our teeth into the first one. Immediately, endorphin levels rise and euphoria kicks in. Any thought about the consequences of leaving the meeting never crosses our mind. We munch on the cookies until serotonin levels rise. When both dopamine and serotonin are high, we feel satisfied. We can relax. All is well.

Except that it isn't.

Eating above the line from hunger is a survival need. But in this case, we weren't hungry. The drive didn't come from needing to respond to body hunger. It was a desire from below the line. The normal slight rise in dopamine when we're hungry followed by a rise in serotonin and endorphins and that feeling of fulfillment that signals us to stop eating didn't occur. We were driven by a "craving brain" that disregarded hunger in favor of huge rushes of dopamine and endorphins that, when combined with low serotonin, created pain, discomfort, and stress. We ate to avoid the pain of a drop in neurochemicals—that is, the pain of withdrawal.

The craving brain manifests itself when serotonin is low and dopamine is out of balance—either high or low. Serotonin is low in dieters, the obese, and binge eaters. Inescapable stress drains serotonin. Inescapable stress means experiencing a lack of control. Loss of love, chronic illness, an abusive childhood, an empty nest, a bad marriage, even weight problems can trigger feelings of inescapable stress. That stress drains serotonin, but it also sensitizes the nucleus accumbens to secrete dopamine; in fact, the secretion overshoots our needs. It also affects dopamine levels, and if our tendency is to feel depressed, our dopamine will plummet and we'll feel sluggish. If our tendency is to be anxious, dopamine will be elevated and we'll be overly energized, even manic.

Either dopamine-level pattern, combined with low serotonin, prompts food cravings. Although the origins of this chemical pattern may be genetic, chronic overeating is associated with imbalances in dopamine, elevations in endorphins, and low serotonin levels. One explanation for cravings is that once dopamine and the endorphins are abnormally elevated, the pain of withdrawal is so great that we eat more to prevent it. We ignore hunger cues because our focus is on one thing: alleviating the pain of the craving.

> *With dopamine out of balance,*
> *we may feel either sluggish or manic.*

However, about 50 percent of obese people have decreased numbers of dopamine receptors, which could have genetic origins.[20] It could also be the result of overeating, because the body is adapting to the chronically elevated dopamine but shutting off some of its receptors. This is the body's response to high insulin levels and high leptin levels associated with obesity. It decreases receptors in the fat cells and in the brain, respectively. A decreased number of dopamine receptors is also seen in alcoholism, substance abuse, smoking, attention-deficit disorder, compulsive sex, and gambling.[21]

If you believe that you have a craving brain—low serotonin, unbalanced dopamine and endorphins, a sensitized nucleus accumbens, a withdrawal-triggered stress response, and a drop in anxiety-relieving NPY—then it pays to approach this chemical mélange effectively. This means making a list of what's contributing to the problem and then, one by one, either solving each problem or doing enough cycles to neutralize the cause. That sounds so rational—and functional! Yet often if we're stuck in an addictive pattern, we don't even make out that list, let alone follow through and cure each cause. We're too below the line emotionally for that.

So the *first step* is to be sure that you are above the line about this external solution, that you don't drown in self-pity, powerlessness, shame or despair, take secret delight in the the drama involved or feel attached to having problems. It's to be above the line enough that you know you aren't minimizing the problem, avoiding or denying it, or blaming others for your situation in life. This can be a formidable but doable task, if you use these skills, and get support, if needed.

The *second step* is to commit to getting on the pathway to a Solution, not just playing with the introductory skills used in this plan, but getting the full tool kit of the skills from the complete Solution course and being sure you have lots of support and a community in doing it. Although people who don't have the extra challenge of chemical dependency take 18 months to complete the course, it will take you 2 to 3 years. The essential pain is that it takes time and work. The earned reward is a new life. This extra time is needed because biological forces will keep you addicted; that is, you will look like you are progressing but won't be, indulging the compulsion to repeat the past, substituting one addiction for another, or being perfectly "clean" then finding that one errant meal triggered a complete relapse. The good news is that you are rewiring your brain one synapse at a time, and on the horizon there is not only hope but a true Solution offering the freedoms and rewards that, without this neurological rewiring, would forever elude you.

We Stay Busy-Busy-Busy

Once we're below the line, we are magnets for external solutions. Several of the most common ones involve numbing ourselves with excessive stimulation. This overload pumps up dopamine and endorphins and gives us a stress high. When those neurotransmitters are drained, we're exhausted and turn to food for energy and as a reward.

Our society values busy lifestyles. Staying busy keeps us above the line, except when doing so becomes an external solution to internal distress. Keeping busy-busy-busy is often an effective way to escape our feelings, distract ourselves from any depth of emotional reflection, or avoid relationship problems.

Some of us are overtly active, scheduling activities every night of the week—meetings, boards, groups, and classes. Others are more quietly active, overstimulating and numbing out by playing video games, surfing the Internet, watching television, or even reading books!

Several common excesses involve numbing ourselves with excessive stimulation.

Not only does that busy-busy-busy pattern interfere with our keeping our fingers on the pulse of our inner lives, it can also affect our thinking. There are limits to our working memory and attention. We can multitask only so much!

When the mind is taxed with a high cognitive load, it compromises the functioning of the frontal lobe of the thinking brain, whose role is to guide and override the impulses and the errant drives of the feeling brain. When our thinking brain is overloaded, we're apt to lose control and overeat.

Physical Activity Decreases

When we're below the line, exercise seems like either an impossible chore or just the opposite; excessive exercise may become a solution to weight problems, distracting us from addressing the issues in our lives. Mood swings can cause us to be agitated and restless. Our metabolic rate is high, and instead of gaining weight, we lose it. However, the more common pattern, is inactivity. Being sedentary deprives us of the appetite-suppressing and mood-elevating effects of exercise[22] and the opportunity to rebalance neurotransmitters and hormones, including decreasing insulin and cortisol and increasing serotonin. The higher our weight and the more belly fat we have, the more likely we are to need that serotonin to stave off mood swings and depression.

We may miss out on the increased endorphins that cause "runner's high," but that effect only occurs when physical activity is prolonged for more than an hour. Extended exercise can also trigger a rise in metabolic rate so that energy expenditure increases for several hours after exercise, giving weight loss an added boost.

Regular exercise is as effective in treating depression as psychotherapy or antidepressants.

Heavy people generally exercise less than lean people, and their energy expenditure is lower, too, despite the fact that increased body weight results in more energy expenditure for the same activity. The heavier we are, the more prone we are to bone and joint problems. For those whose Body Mass Index (BMI) is 35 or higher or those who are over fifty years of age, it's extremely common for one bone or joint problem after another to interrupt physical activity. Just when an exercise program is working and we're losing weight, there's a turn of the ankle or a twist of the back and exercise becomes off-limits. Surgeries, recuperation, and physical therapy all enter into the mix, which makes weight loss so much more challenging.

Mood problems contribute to inactivity, too. Depression not only leads to engaging in less physical activity, but it decreases spontaneous movements. Moreover, it results in our sleeping longer and generally being inactive. We prefer sitting on the couch to going outside. We just don't have the energy!

Although regular exercise is as effective in treating moderate depression as psychotherapy or antidepressants,[23] exercise may feel emotionally risky when our mood is rocky. Moving the body arouses feelings. We can choose to be numb, but once the doors to feelings open, we are not in complete control of which ones we feel. The negative feelings come tumbling out along with the positive ones. With low levels of the Solution Skills, feelings aroused by exercise can make us feel worse. In essence, exercise avoidance associated with mood problems is a protective impulse: we don't want to feel more pain.

Regardless of the cause of inactivity, sitting all day and all evening causes our metabolic rate to lag and our muscle tissue to waste away, both of which foster further weight gain. Our mood suffers and the cookies in the kitchen drawer become more appealing. Instead of getting a boost in energy and pleasure from exercise, we get it from food.

Health Declines

Many people with extreme obesity (a BMI of 40 or more) say they are in perfect health. They go to their physicians and find that their blood pressure, lipids, and every other health marker are perfect. However, obesity increases the risk of a whole spate of diseases.

You never know whether you're going to be a robust and round 90-year-old who is completely free of every obesity-related condition. Trouble may be brewing secretly until problems arise and start draining our vitality, hampering our exercise, shattering our good spirits, and creating so much stress. One health problem seems to spawn another.

One health problem seems to spawn another.

The combination of the emotional stress of the health problem, the medications required, and all the limitations imposed—spending time going to the doctor instead of going to the gym—sends us further below the line.

What's more, the drive to overeat is very primitive and deep, so changes in the body have a disproportionate effect on weight. For example:

- Poorly controlled diabetes triggers overeating to prevent blood-sugar lows.
- Hypertension medication may affect sexual functioning, which creates stress.
- Bone and joint problems, including repeated surgeries and recuperation times, limit physical activities.
- Antidepressants or mood drugs, if not properly monitored, can blunt feelings excessively.
- Pregnancy, menopause, or premenstrual syndrome affect mood and appetite and trigger binge eating, cravings, and weight gain.

Moreover, health problems and stress can often affect sleep, which decreases metabolic rate. During the first half of sleep, growth hormone, which increases metabolic rate, is secreted.[24] When sleep is truncated or disturbed, growth hormone secretion decreases and, with it, metabolic rate. Also, sleep deprivation decreases leptin, which suppresses appetite and raises levels of grehlin, a peptide hormone that stimulates appetite and can trigger sensations of intense hunger.

What we most need when we're solving our weight problem is optimal physical vitality so we can engage in enjoyable activities that make great substitutes for overeating. When we don't feel well, we can't do that!

Intimacy Dwindles

Any basic need that is unmet can go underground only to reemerge as an excessive appetite. Intimacy problems—whether they are the cause or the consequences of weight difficulties—make matters worse. They draw us further into the toxic spiral because of the loss of intimate connection and because of all the stress that accompanies a life of isolation or loneliness. Enhancing social intimacy, emotional intimacy, and sexual intimacy is as central to stepping out of the spiral as eating veggies or going to the gym.

The aspect of health that appears most inextricably tied to appetite is intimacy.

The aspect of health that appears most inextricably tied to appetite is intimacy. Life above the line means relationships in which there is empathy, compassion, and emotional connection, without being swallowed up by the other person. Our boundaries are preserved while still allowing love to flow between us. We can tolerate the essential pain of rejection and surrender. We can stand our ground, open and loving, knowing that if we are rejected, we will still survive. It takes a lot of skill to stay close but separate.

When we're below the line, our tendency is to merge, which shows up as people rescuing others, distancing, being emotionally walled off, or even persecuting one another. Control struggles also figure into relationships that exist below the line. And external solutions weave their way into them, such as bonding by using an excess together—drowning our troubles in food—or covertly agreeing "I'll ignore your external solutions if you'll ignore mine."

Once we're in the toxic spiral,
sexual satisfaction is often hit the hardest.

Life below the line may affect sexual relationships as well. Stress, depression, obesity, and other external solutions, especially alcohol, can trigger changes in sex hormones in both men and women.[25] Stress can cause decreases in estrogen and testosterone; obesity, however, can increase estrogen due to the conversion in fat tissue of the inactive form of estrogen to the active form. In response to stress and obesity, men have decreased testosterone and increased estrogen—which, in the extreme, contributes to a more feminized appearance—and more difficulty with nervous system problems that affect sexual functioning.

Once we're in the toxic spiral, sexual satisfaction is often hit the hardest. Some couples find their sex lives enormously gratifying, but for so many, their love life drifts into sexual avoidance, low sexual desire, settling for mediocre sex, excessive use of pornography, or extramarital affairs. One of the questions participants in Solution training ask themselves is, "Are you meeting your needs for sexuality, sensuality, eroticism, and passion?" The rise in serotonin levels from orgasm, tenderness, and emotional intimacy takes the appetite away. Who wants food when you can have something so much better?

Our Spiritual Connection Weakens

All these changes in neurotransmitters, hormones, peptides, behavior, and stress send us further below the line. And the more below the line we are, the more we're apt to feel a spiritual void or to drift into using religion as an external solution—that is, adopting beliefs or practices as a substitute for feeling a spiritual awareness.

The feeling brain is the seat of the soul, and when it is out of homeostasis, any experience of rapture, connection, or appreciation for the grace and mystery of life goes on the blink. What is, for some, the richest reward of life . . . disappears. That loss impacts nearly everything, even our use of the skills. Our feelings aren't as deep and limits often shift toward overcontrol, rigidity, and negativity. The loss of that abiding connection to something makes forgiving others difficult, and revenge and persecution easily justified. When we try to conjure up a nurturing inner voice, it lacks authenticity, sounding hollow or manipulative rather than warm and secure. There is no sense of the sanctuary within, the safe place we can go to no matter what.

The feeling brain is the seat of the soul.

When that spiritual connection weakens, we may go through our days acting normal, but a part of us that may not be within our complete awareness feels abandoned, confused, and bone-chillingly alone. That void is a magnet for external solutions. One can think of life above the line as connection to spirit, and life below the line as entrapment in the ego. In that self-absorbed state, we have a bottomless appetite and rampant urges, drives, and cravings.

Our bodies are particularly vulnerable to the weakening of a spiritual connection. Certainly, our attitudes toward our body can change. Instead of it being a vessel for our soul, something to revere and take care of, it becomes an object. We treat it as such, and expose our bodies to situations, people, and substances that we otherwise would not. We're so hard on ourselves, losing any sense of compassion for our bodies. We may place too much importance on appearance, or we may do the opposite, showing little honor or pride of the body. . . .

Body Image Suffers

When we're out of balance, it's so easy to internalize society's mandate of bodily perfection that when we gain a few pounds, our self-esteem and body image can take a nosedive. Then we do to ourselves what we wouldn't do to our best friend—look in the mirror, rip to shreds every feature on our face, and magnify every bulge or dimple on our body. It's hard to feel worthy, let alone desirable. If everything is so black, why not just drown our troubles in food?

Body image and self-image are intertwined.

The more we move below the line, the more our emotional state is projected onto our body. Body image and self-image are intertwined. We aren't happy with ourselves, so we aren't happy with our body. The more isolated and the more stressed we become, the more our appearance matters too much. Each unkind thought or disparaging remark drags us further into the spiral. Any slam to the body is a bruise to the ego.

Body image can not only turn negative but also be distorted. Typically, body image is fixed in adolescence,[26] so that if we go through adolescence being overweight, we're apt to feel fat our whole lives, even long after that weight has been lost. On the other hand, we can dissociate from our current body size and see ourselves as far thinner than we are.

Many people who suffer from extreme obesity say that they can't see their weight. Their body image is distorted and their mind shuts off to their current body size. Stepping out of the spiral takes time, and as the skills gently deepen, often an awareness of the extent of obesity unfolds slowly as we have the skills to handle it.

When we're above the line, we strive to lose weight out of self-love. We care about our happiness and ourselves. We love our bodies and want to enjoy them! However, when we're in the toxic spiral, we lose weight out of body disgust, self-hate, or because the health consequences are so dire. So we go on a diet . . .

Dieting Makes It Worse

. . . and severe dieting lowers serotonin, dopamine, and endorphin levels,[27] which can set up a rebound effect. After severe food restriction, binge eating or another substitute behavior wipes away the benefits of all our hard work. Trying to restrict what we eat in an environment in which the sights, sounds, and smell of foods are abundant is extremely difficult because of our biology. Through conditioning, the presence of delicious food triggers increases in dopamine,[28] giving us the urge to eat. At the same time, the stimulation of the occipital lobe that triggers a dopamine release increases cravings. The sensory center in our thinking brain—the orbitofrontal cortex—responds to that sensory input by stimulating more hunger!

Rapid weight loss triggers multiple mechanisms in the body to restore its weight to former levels. Being in a starvation state prompts dieter's rebound. For example, when body-fat stores are depleted too rapidly, leptin levels lower and turn on fat cravings. Once we're consuming fewer than 1,200 to 1,500 calories per day, metabolic rate decreases. Although we're eating less, we're also burning fewer calories.

When the diet is out of balance, neurotransmitters,
mood, and appetite are affected.

Other nutrients that affect emotional balance, metabolism, and weight are often deficient. In particular, neurotransmitters are nutritionally sensitive, as they are composed of either amino acids or fatlike substances called choline that are obtained from food. When the diet is out of balance, the body limits production or activation of neurotransmitters, and mood, appetite, and thinking are affected. Similarly, vitamins and minerals—such as vitamins C, E, and B; selenium; and iron—are required for the synthesis, activity, or storage of neurotransmitters.

What's more, weight-loss diets are often low in omega-3 fatty acids[29] and calcium,[30] both of which facilitate weight loss. Our ancestors ate diets of lean meats (not today's marbled steaks), nuts, seeds, leaves, honey, and fish—a diet high in omega-3 fatty acids. The brain is 50 percent fat, and omega-3 fatty acids aid brain functioning, including compounds that release chemicals such as serotonin.

Many dieters stop drinking milk, which not only contains high levels of trypotophan, a precursor of serotonin, but is also high in protein and calcium, which are converted to calcitriol, which facilitates fat burning. By switching from milk to diet sodas or water, dieters miss out on a 200-calorie-per-day advantage in losing weight that they get from milk.

Any diet that is rigid, that doesn't allow for fluctuations in intake based on hunger and for variations in the kinds of food based on personal needs, sets us up for dieter's rebound. The solution to weight problems is to be more sensitive to our feelings and needs and any diet should reflect that priority. This is particularly true because energy needs can vary dramatically day to day, so if we stay with a rigid diet, we're apt to overindulge on some days and undereat on others. For example:

- In the second half of the menstrual cycle, women need as many as 500 calories more per day.[31]
- The weekend athlete who plays three sets of tennis on Saturday and Sunday needs as many as 600 calories more per day than during the week.

Many of us are on the brink of information overload most of the time, and having another thing to think about—restricting food, calculating grams, and avoiding tasty foods—can overload the frontal lobe and result in abandoning restraint and binge eating!

Worst of all, diets are unlikely to produce lasting weight loss. We work really hard to lose weight, only to regain the weight, then blame ourselves and feel less happy, less powerful, and more apt to reach for food for comfort.

Problems Pile Up

When we're in the toxic spiral and feeling as if we're spinning out of control, there's not just one problem—our weight—but a lot of them. Even if we have no particular problems, we'll have disappointments or important areas of life in which our needs go unmet.

We have a whole crop of difficulties and problems, with one symptom substituting for another because they all arise from the same source. They're all part of life below the line. For example:

- The same limits that make us too easy on ourselves about food also cause us to be too easy on ourselves about overspending.
- Our lack of a nurturing inner voice triggers a negative body image as well as a reluctance to make new friends.
- The harsh limits that make us expect our appearance to be perfect also cause us to demand perfection from others, thus interfering with intimacy.

So instead of tackling one problem we have a whole cluster of difficulties to deal with. Treating the myriad of symptoms caused by a feeling brain that is out of homeostasis can be a full-time job. We're exhausted! Worse, doing so shifts our focus from inherent strength, goodness, and wisdom, that is, what is right about us, to reinforcing what is wrong with us. It's easy to become so beleaguered by our situation that we don't use the power we do have to make our lives better.

We Cross Over from One Excess to Another

Mixed in with this pileup of problems may be some external solutions that stay stubbornly stuck because we have a craving brain. The role of the nucleus accumbens is to ensure the survival of the species through strong cravings for safety, food, and sex. We're not left to languish around watching ourselves waste away. We are neurologically motivated and on target to meet our survival needs.

Mixed in with this pileup of problems
may be strong cravings for survival needs.

The problem is that this survival response is transferable to almost any other behavior by association. The survival drive is so strong that when we can't get that need met, we're desperate! We reach for something else to satisfy that craving. Or perhaps, by chance, we engage in another behavior and discover that it works to stop the craving.

For example, we are hungry and we go to the freezer for that pint-size carton of chocolate ice cream. We have our spoon in hand, poised in anticipation of that sweet, chocolaty treat, then we realize, there's no ice cream there! We're on a diet!

With dopamine out of balance and serotonin low, we yearn for relief. Since its a survival need, we do something—anything—to feel better. We have a beer, turn on the shopping network, or reach for a cigarette.

The more often we use this new behavior to soothe the pain of our cravings for a survival need, the more we associate that behavior with the relief of our pain. The more we use it, the more things we associate with it—the sight of the credit cards, the pack of cigarettes, the bottle of beer—and in time, the sight, smell, or touch of something associated with that external solution lowers serotonin and alters dopamine levels.

Some external solutions are more chemically motivated than others.

We create the chemical changes of a survival need; however, serotonin levels may not rise. Even if they do, we might not pay attention to those feelings of satisfaction. They won't signal us to stop the behavior, because the drive and the preoccupation are caused by the craving, not a true survival need.

That's why if we're addicted to food, once we start eating, it's so hard to stop. Likewise, when we're in the groove with overly restrictive dieting, eating a cheeseburger and fries sounds abhorrent. The survival need to eat has crossed over and become the need to restrict.

Some behaviors are more addictive than others. Yet this crossover effect, given the right mix of genetics and conditioning, can make "addicts" out of the best of us. That's one reason why there are no judgments in Solution training. Those excesses are just external solutions, some of which are more chemically motivated than others.

So that's the toxic spiral. There are so many layers to it!

It's important to appreciate how easy it is to step into the spiral in which one thing leads to another and another, but it's more important to go about the business of stepping out of that spiral.

Let's move on and use the 3-Day Solution Plan to do exactly that!

11

Stepping Out of the Toxic Spiral

DURING THESE THREE days, you will learn how to live above the line and begin to step out of the toxic spiral. The Solution Skills will lift your mind above the line, and Mastery Living will move your body above the line. Using these powerful skills and this lifestyle plan together will turn off the drive to overeat and give you a jump-start on the pathway to lasting weight loss.

Getting a new start takes three days because you are orchestrating powerful effects on both your mind and your body. The mind skills affect not only the feeling brain but the thinking brain as well. Over the course of these three days, you will have many thinking-brain "aha!" moments—insights and discoveries—but the most riveting moments will come from accessing your feeling brain with the skills you are about to learn.

There are three basic Solution Skills, and it takes at least one day to familiarize yourself with using each of them. The feeling brain does not respond well to quick fixes. Lasting changes require practice and persistence. Your body will also need three days to begin to detox from sugary, fatty foods and any other external solution on which you decide to work on during this time.

By the third day, life will be different and the drive to overeat will have faded. You will see that there is tremendous power in making small changes in many important areas of life all at once. The changes will not be linear, such as a number on the scale or a new fitness routine, but will be systemic. Your entire body, mind, and spirit will feel different. The world will look different to you in ways that are subtle but at the same time absolutely monumental. You will savor the taste of a new life—life above the line.

What follows is a brief description of each day's focus and purpose. The remainder of this chapter touches on the three Solution Skills as well as all five elements of Mastery Living. This will help you to prepare for and plan your three-day experience. Next, Chapter 12, "Checklist: Preparing for a Solution," will help you set up and individualize your three-day plan by giving you ideas about how to make this plan easier so that you will achieve the best results.

When you've finished reading this chapter and have completed the checklist in Chapter 12, you can begin the three-day program. I'll guide you through it each step of the way, coaching you on what to expect and how to focus your energies to make the changes easier and more powerful.

Included in the appendix are three pocket reminders for the plan, one for each day. One side of each pocket reminder shows the Solution Skills for the day, and the other is a checklist for Mastery Living.

After you complete your 3-Day Solution Plan, you will decide whether you want to continue using the method, and you can continue with Phase 2 of the plan, days 4 to 14, which is less intensive. If you decide to rewire your feeling brain and create a solution in your life, you can continue with Phase 3 of the plan, becoming involved in Solution training, with Internet support, professional training, or self-help circles.

Later in the book, you can read the stories of some people who have continued with Phase 3 of the plan. You'll also find information about 1-2-3 Eating, including food lists (Chapter 22), menus (Chapters 16 and 18), and wonderful recipes from Solution participants (Chapter 19).

For now, let's focus on the next three days.

Solution Skills: Day by Day

Your Solution Skills will build, day by day.

• *Day 1—detox:* On the first day, you will develop the skill of checking in; that is, checking how you feel and what you need. You will also work on identifying whether you are above or below the line. The act of checking your feelings alone will give you an idea of whether you're above the line or below, but you will look for other signposts as well. You will check in with yourself 10 times on the first day. Doing this lays the foundation for the skills you will use on days two and three of the plan.

• *Day 2—connection:* On the second day, you will strengthen your checking in skill, again checking in 10 times. This second day of checking in helps you develop a pattern of keeping your fingers on the pulse of your inner life, checking in with yourself regularly, and at a deep level. You will also add a second Solution Skill, emotional housecleaning. Each time that you check in with yourself and determine that you're above the line, you won't need to go any further. You'll be aware of your feelings and your needs and will be able to respond to them.

However, if you are below the line, you will use emotional housecleaning. This skill is not difficult to learn, and it disrupts those repetitive thoughts and balances out emotions. This skill is not nearly as powerful as what you will do on the third day—cycles—but using emotional housecleaning on your second day is the perfect preparation for being able to do a cycle on the third day.

• *Day 3—vibrancy:* On the third day of the plan, you will use the skills from days one and two and add the third skill, cycles. You will now have two skills to use when you check in with yourself and find that you are below the line. If you're just a little bit below the line—slightly upset or somewhat stressed—you can lift yourself above the line by using emotional housecleaning. If you are clearly below the line—very upset or quite stressed—you'll do a cycle. You'll pop yourself above the line! Your inner life will be ready to do a cycle successfully because of the learning you will have done on the first two days.

After these three days, you will have been introduced to the three basic skills of The Solution Method. You will know how it feels to make staying above the line your first priority, and you'll have a starter kit of three skills that will enable you to stay there more of the time.

Knowing how to keep yourself above the line is a huge accomplishment, something that many people never manage to do. Yet you will do this in just three days.

Mastery Living: Day by Day

The lifestyle surgery part of the method will make it far easier to use the Solution Skills effectively. If your lifestyle is stalled, it's almost impossible to access your balanced feelings, because they're buried under a pile of problems, numbed by food, and distorted by unhealthy living.

Each of the three days will include all five elements of a masterful life: body work, 1-2-3 Eating, meaningful pursuits, time to restore, and intimacy time. However, each day's plan includes various ways to apply each element. By experimenting with a range of options, you can discover which ones are most effective in turning off your drive to overeat. In essence, your charge for these three days is to create a lifestyle of such delight, satisfaction, and vitality that you don't want the extra food.

You'll also begin to detoxify your body. Right now, your insulin levels may be elevated, resulting in faulty hunger signals. You may feel hungry when your body really doesn't need the extra food. As you begin to live life above the line, you'll discover how much food you really need, and you'll stop wanting excess food. As you know, many of us are very afraid of not getting enough to eat.

At the same time that your insulin levels are elevated, your serotonin levels may be low, giving you the feeling of not being fully satisfied, particularly as the day turns into evening. Your dopamine levels may also be out of balance—with a tendency to be either too low or too high. If they are low, you may feel drained, tired, and depressed as the day goes on, and if they are high, your tendency will be to have excessive energy and more anxiety. Either way, you will begin to balance your serotonin and dopamine levels during these three days.

• *Day 1—detox:* The focus of your first day of Mastery Living is to experience all five elements of the plan. It is also to begin detoxifying, for you will not be relying on regulating your energy and mood with sugar, fat, alcohol, or caffeine. You will be using your lifestyle and the Solution Skills instead.

On this first day, you're likely to be more sensitive to the effects of detoxing. You are changing! It may be an adjustment to take an hour of exercise and an hour of restorative "me time" in your day as well as setting aside time for intimacy. If you usually work too much or don't have enough work, working in a focused way for no fewer than six hours and no more than eight hours also takes getting used to. The 1-2-3 Eating is easy and delicious, though it is not the typical American diet. You can always have more food, if you *really need* it, but chances are you won't need much more than is suggested.

You are adjusting to this entire plan today. It's a lot to manage, so be gentle with yourself. Doing a reasonable—but not necessarily perfect—job of each part of the plan will be enough to get you off to a good start.

• *Day 2—connection:* On the second day of the plan, you will continue to use all five elements of Mastery Living. However, although the most challenging part of detoxing has passed, today you will probably feel as if you are missing something. Staying with it will not be easy.

During this day, you will pump up your serotonin levels and continue to rebalance your dopamine and insulin levels by eating from above the line and by having an absolutely wonderful time doing so. This is a day of pleasure, fulfillment, and fun, and even though you're spending six to eight hours in meaningful pursuits, the various activities of the day will be apt to leave you feeling very, very satisfied.

• *Day 3—vibrancy:* You made it to the third day! By now, the cumulative effects of the skills and a masterful life are becoming apparent to you.

The focus of day 3 is to continue with the plan so that the benefits escalate and you achieve a systemic change. You feel different all over—mind, body, and spirit. Today you will experiment with ways to satisfy and please yourself that are different from the first two days, with an emphasis on emotional intimacy. By the end of the day, you will have had a sampling of the whole array of life's joys that turn off the drive to overeat and rebalance your hormones and neurotransmitters.

By the evening of the third day, you will know how it feels to live life above the line and to turn off the drive to overeat from within.

These three days will be an adventure that can prove to be the start of a new life. The rest of the chapter shows you how to use each aspect of the plan.

Solution Skill 1: Checking In

Checking in is the most fundamental of the three skills. (For additional information on this skill, turn to pages 158 to 163.) When this skill becomes automatic, and you have a Solution, you will use the skill almost unconsciously. You will constantly know how you feel and what you need, keeping your fingers on the pulse of your inner life all the time.

To use this skill, ask yourself three questions:

1. How do I feel?
2. Am I above the line or below the line?
3. What do I need?

When you ask yourself "How do I feel?" you step over the thinking-brain barrier and access your feeling brain. You are right at your emotional core and are able to identify the feeling that is strongest.

The basic feelings are the messages from our feeling brain that indicate a need. Because the feeling brain is the clearinghouse for all our senses, thoughts, drives, implicit learning, and emotional memories, these messages are diverse. Since all stress is pain, and since the feeling brain feels that pain regardless of its origins, and since we go below the line if there is too much pain, we need to monitor and respond to diverse emotional messages.

The Basic Feelings

Angry	Grateful
Sad	Happy
Afraid	Secure
Guilty	Proud
Tired	Rested
Tense	Relaxed
Hungry or full	Satisfied
Lonely	Loved
Sick	Healthy

On the list above, you can see the major feelings to which we need to have access to in order to survive and thrive. In this method, we try to find the *basic* feeling, not the subtle feeling. Most of us have learned to be very articulate about our feelings, choosing words that express emotional nuance. That is not helpful when you are using this method.

It's best to use words that express the basic feelings, such as *anger*, rather than shades of that emotion, such as *frustration* or *irritation*. Even saying "a little angry" is more effective than using other words to express a feeling that has an emotional core of anger. By training yourself to identify the most basic feelings, you will more rapidly reveal important patterns in your inner life. Instead of getting lost in articulating your disappointment, discouragement, melancholy, and dejection, you will notice that you're sad (a little sad, sad, or very sad). This supports your clarity as you master the skills.

As you begin using the skill of checking in, identify only one feeling—the strongest one. If you're feeling-oriented, that won't be difficult. If you're a "thinker," it may be more challenging, as you'll list many feelings. However, our feeling brain sends us feelings that are emotional motivators to take action. The strongest feeling signals the most important need, so find the feeling that is strongest.

In the left column of the "Basic Feelings" list are all the basic negative feelings, and in the right column are the basic positive feelings. Both these types of feelings are "good" feelings, in that they will help you to identify your most important need.

After you have identified the strongest feeling, ask yourself, "Am I above the line or below the line?" and "What do I need?"

If you are above the line, the logical need often comes to mind, such as "I feel tense; I need to relax," or "I feel sad; I need to feel my sadness and let it fade." If you're above the line, it is much easier to identify what you really need.

If you are below the line, finding your need is far more difficult. It's easy to find your want, but not your need. When you are asking yourself "How do I feel?" and "What do I need?" also ask yourself "Am I above the line or below the line?"

You can tell when you're below the line because your feelings will be either very high, very low, or numb and are usually associated with other symptoms of being below the line. Common signs are having cravings or strong urges for external solutions. Or you might notice that you are passive or aggressive, feeling lost or abandoned, or obsessing about the future or the past.

Balanced feelings, such as the basic ones shown on the list, are not necessarily mild feelings. In fact, they can be quite intense. You can feel very sad about something or very, very angry. However, if the feeling is above the line, you are aware of that feeling in the present moment. Instead of feeling as if your mind has traveled to the past or the future, you're aware of your mind and body in the current moment.

When you're above the line and are in the presence of other people, you feel an appropriate amount of closeness. You don't merge with them—that is, lose yourself in them so you know how they feel and what they need but lose track of your own feelings and need. You don't feel drawn to rescue them or to "people-please." Nor do you have a strong drive to distance from them and have difficulty empathizing with them—that is, being aware of how they might feel in this situation and what they might need from you. In both merged and disengaged relationships, fear is prominent, and due to that fear, we vie for power. Our struggles for control just send us further below the line.

If you are below the line, you feel confused, upset, and stressed, and at first, you may not even know you're below the line! So if you have any question about whether you're above or below the line, consider yourself below! It can't hurt, because the skills you use when you are there help even if you're above the line. They strengthen the neural networks that favor a life of balance.

When you're below the line, your need is to get above the line. There is no use trying to figure out what you need when you're below the line. You'll identify a want, not a need. For example, if you check your feelings when you are below the line, you might find that you aren't sad; you're depressed. Then you'll ask, "What do I need? Pasta." Or "How do I feel? Exhausted. What do I need? Television and chocolate."

On the first day, when you are learning how to use the checking-in skill, if you find yourself below the line—a little below or way below—just contain the feeling with an effective limit. Tell yourself something like this: "It's reasonable to expect that I'll go below the line at times. This is progress. At least I know that I'm below the line!"

On all three days of the plan, you will check in with yourself 10 times each day. Every time you check in, you are disrupting the neural networks of confusion, lethargy, and conflict that favor life below the line and opening up the possibility of strengthening the networks of clarity, vibrancy, and peace that are above the line. You are disrupting the party below the line in favor of throwing a new party above the line. Checking in is a quiet act of courage. That personal decision—time after time—to disrupt business as usual in your feeling brain and tinker with your inner life with these skills will, over time, create a revolution from within.

The feeling brain prefers business as usual. It didn't ask to be rewired. On the contrary, it's in a groove and wants to stay there! Hardwired in our feeling brain is a huge compulsion for us to repeat the past. The frontal cortex of our brain (behind our forehead) is what separates us from the apes. It's what enables us to *choose what to think about.* It's what we are using when we are in the middle of the stresses of our day and stop everything; take a big, deep breath; and then we go inside with our tool kit of these skills to rewire our inner lives.

But our frontal cortex is not accustomed to doing this! And not only does it have to do this, but it needs to do this often throughout the day for many days to rewire the brain. It would be so much easier if we already had a Solution! But we don't, so we have to force the issue on our inner lives. Our brain prefers business as usual. It won't remind us to check in and won't necessarily welcome our using the skills. The thinking brain easily checks out of doing this, and the feeling brain, being at times either a hotbed of chaos or a chilling void, isn't always helpful either!

So in order to check in daily 10 times during these three days, we will need a way to remind ourselves. Some people check in hourly between 9:00 a.m. and 6:00 p.m., triggered by automated reminders, such as setting their watch, their computer, or their cell phone. Other people use natural pause points during the day. Find some method that works for you.

Once you've checked in with yourself, you will refer to your pocket reminder, both for information about how to use the skill for the day and to record your findings. Again, on the first day, you will use only the skill of checking in. On the second day, you will add to that the skill of emotional housecleaning, which you'll use when you are below the line. On the last day, you'll add to those two skills a third skill: doing cycles. When you're below the line just a little, you'll use emotional housecleaning; otherwise, when you're below the line, you'll do a cycle.

As you start using the skills, keep in mind that you don't need to have perfect answers to the questions. You don't even need to have an answer! Just trust that if you ask the question, the answer, in time, will come. Appreciate that these skills will get stronger and stronger with practice.

The whole process of learning the skills is messy and confusing at times—which is particularly hard if we're smart, accomplished, well educated, analytical, or perfectionists. We don't like not knowing! We don't like being "wrong"! The essential pain of starting to use the method is that we have to tolerate irresolution, not knowing everything, and feeling imperfect. The earned reward, in addition to self-acceptance, is lasting weight loss, turning off the drive to overeat, and reaping more of life's richest rewards.

Besides, using the skills only becomes easier! Most people start off using the method and find it difficult, then they go through a "honeymoon" in which they think they have a Solution. After that, they usually have a dip back into reality and start the long-term layering of the skills that leads them to a lasting Solution.

Examples of Checking In

- I feel angry. I'm above the line. I need to cool off.
- I feel hungry. That's above the line. I need to eat. No, I need to wait 30 minutes, then check again. I'm not that hungry.
- I feel depressed. I must be below the line. What do I need? To get above the line.
- I feel lonely. I need ice cream. Am I above the line? Well, ice cream fixes hunger, not loneliness. I must be below the line. What do I need? To get above the line.
- I feel happy. Am I above the line? Yes. What do I need? To enjoy the feeling.
- I feel angry. I need to get back at her. That's aggressive. I must be below the line. I need to not talk to her until I get above the line. My need is to get above the line.
- I feel afraid and grateful. I'm above the line. I need to feel my fear and let it fade. I need to thank her for what she did to help me.
- I feel guilty. No, I feel ashamed. Being ashamed is below the line. I need to get above the line.

When you have a Solution, you will automatically and spontaneously check in with yourself nearly constantly. You will walk through your day knowing how you feel and what you need most of the time. Going inside will feel like neither a hotbed of chaos nor a chilling void. In fact, it will feel warm, comfortable, and secure because you have a sanctuary, a safe place within that you created for yourself by using these skills.

Solution Skill 2:
Emotional Housecleaning

Emotional housecleaning is the skill to use when you are a little bit below the line or feel yourself in danger of slipping below the line and want to prevent it. You feel and express eight of the most basic feelings. There are four positive feelings and four negative ones. These eight feelings facilitate a "natural flow of emotion" that has a balancing and healing effect. (For additional information on this skill, turn to pages 189 to 191.)

> I feel angry that . . .
> I feel sad that . . .
> I feel afraid that . . .
> I feel guilty that . . .
>
> I feel grateful that . . .
> I feel happy that . . .
> I feel secure that . . .
> I feel proud that . . .

All this skill requires is for you to go with the flow, completing each sentence that expresses each feeling, one after another. It's amazing what will come to your mind. Remember that feelings don't have to make sense. Just say the first few words of each sentence and then pay attention to what comes into your mind.

For each feeling, you may have only one statement. Or you may have five statements for some or all of the feelings. If you have more than five statements, it's possible that the feeling is getting stuck and going out of balance, so it's best to go on to the next feeling. Also, keep your sentences short and choppy—no need for long, intellectualized statements. Don't be smart, just be basic. It's the four-year-old in us who has those feelings, and we need to speak in that basic four-year-old language to express the feelings deeply and pop ourselves back into balance.

To use emotional housecleaning, start each of the sentences listed above, and your feeling brain will complete it! For example, say to yourself or to another person, or write down, "I feel sad that . . ." Then wait for the words that complete the sentence to appear.

What you're likely to find is that you have no control over what comes out. You may encounter some surprising feelings that were previously below the conscious level: the excitation of the nerve cells hadn't reached a conscious level, or in other words, the bell had not yet sounded. Some very practical feelings will come up, such as, "I feel angry that I forgot to take out the trash." That's valuable information! However, other sentences you complete may reflect the deepest musings at your emotional core, such as, "I feel grateful that I am alive."

If no thoughts come to mind, you can either say the first half of the sentence one more time and wait again, or you can immediately go on to the next feeling.

There are eight feelings in emotional housecleaning. Four of them are negative feelings, or "essential pains":

1. Angry
2. Sad
3. Afraid
4. Guilty

There are also four positive feelings, or "earned rewards":

1. Grateful
2. Happy
3. Secure
4. Proud

You won't have to memorize these feelings because you can consult the pocket reminder on page 336 for the second day of the plan. I'll show you a few examples of how to use emotional housecleaning, and then I hope you'll consider using it yourself. In the first example below, notice that the feelings are completely unrelated to one another. That's good! In fact, this is one of the most fascinating ways to use this skill. You might say, "I can't believe I have that feeling! I wasn't even aware . . ."

Here's some emotional housecleaning I did when I was feeling balanced and was just being curious about what was inside:

I feel angry that . . .	my kitchen is such a mess.
I feel sad that . . .	there is war.
I feel afraid that . . .	my children will get hurt.
I feel guilty that . . .	I haven't taken the cat to the vet.

I feel grateful that . . .	the house is peaceful.
I feel happy that . . .	my parents live nearby.
I feel secure that . . .	the universe will provide.
I feel proud that . . .	I paid my bills last night.

Here's another example. This time, I was a little more below the line, and although I was attempting simply to go inside and emotionally clean house, many of the feelings found their way to the same topic. I wasn't far enough below the line to need to do a cycle, but almost. Notice the short, choppy sentences. Keeping the sentences short and simple—nonintellectualized—is most effective.

I had just taken my daughter to the airport. She was going halfway across the country to do some work that is important to her, and she wouldn't be coming home again for three months. She was 24 years old, but that seemed like a long time for her to be away. . . .

I feel angry that . . .	she is gone.
I feel sad that . . .	she is gone. I miss her already.
I feel afraid that . . .	she will get hurt.
I feel afraid that . . .	her airplane will go down.
I felt guilty that . . .	I'm being so negative.
I feel grateful that . . .	she is my daughter.
I feel grateful that . . .	I have a daughter.
I feel happy that . . .	we had so much laughter yesterday.
I feel happy that . . .	we took the dog for a walk together.
I feel happy that . . .	she loves me.
I feel secure that . . .	she is following her spiritual path.
I feel proud that . . .	I encourage her to live her life to the fullest.

After that, I felt much better. I still felt sad, but I was back above the line. The Solution does not take away the unavoidable pain of life, but it enables us to avoid the unnecessary pain we cause ourselves when we are below the line. Feeling negative feelings is still difficult, but feeling *balanced* negative feelings makes those times as good as they can get.

Now, if you like, consider giving it a try. You may need to use this tool a few times before you become comfortable with it. The idea is simply to be curious: "I wonder what feelings are going to come up?" And when one does, just say to yourself, "Wow, that's interesting!" No judgments. Complete authenticity. No censoring. Just start the sentence and see what words come to mind. If nothing comes to mind, that's fine, too. Just go on to the next sentence. If you're way below the line and don't feel comfortable using this tool, don't use it. To make using this skill safer, consider limiting the number of statements you make for any one feeling to five, such as:

I feel angry that . . .	I have to deal with my weight.
I feel angry that . . .	eating what I like makes me fat.
I feel angry that . . .	I wasn't born skinny.
I feel angry that . . .	I have to diet.
I feel angry that . . .	I can't simply eat whatever I want.

That's five feelings. Just move on!

I feel sad that . . .	I am alone.
I feel afraid that . . .	I will fail again.
I feel afraid that . . .	I won't do it perfectly.
I feel afraid that . . .	I'll get started but then quit.
I feel guilty that . . .	I didn't solve this problem a long time ago.

I feel grateful that . . .	I have a 3-Day Solution.
I feel happy that . . .	there is a way to turn off the drive to overeat.
I feel secure that . . .	I will do the best I can.
I feel proud that . . .	I'm trying this plan.

Before you try emotional housecleaning, please find a way to have uninterrupted time for five minutes. Then go inside yourself, connect with your feelings, use a supportive inner voice, and bring to mind the first words of each sentence. You can say these words to yourself, or if you prefer, say them aloud. You can also write the words on paper or on your computer screen. Do whatever works best for you. Just begin. . . .

I feel angry that . . .
I feel sad that . . .
I feel afraid that . . .
I feel guilty that . . .

I feel grateful that . . .
I feel happy that . . .
I feel secure that . . .
I feel proud that . . .

Solution Skill 3: Doing Cycles

You can use the skill of doing cycles in many different ways to take out emotional trash, cultivate a nurturing inner voice, cope with current stress, and stay above the line in order to live in a masterful way. (For additional information on this skill, turn to pages 212 to 214.)

Doing cycles is actually a blend of two skills: the nurturing skill that enables us to know and honor ourselves and the limit-setting skill that gives us power and safety in the world. In the best of all worlds, these skills would have been hardwired in us naturally by growing up in a responsive—not indulging or depriving—environment. But no matter how much our parents may have loved us, we may not have learned this skill growing up. Love is an emotion, and this is not about emotion but about skill. If our parents didn't have these skills, they could not pass them along to us. And even if they did have these skills, and we did acquire them at a young age, with the stresses, isolation, and temptations of modern culture, having more of these skills comes in very handy.

Doing a cycle begins with thoughts. First, state what you are upset about, whatever that might be. It's just a statement. Don't include your feelings yet. State the simple facts, and those thoughts from your thinking brain will begin stimulating feelings in your feeling brain. When the feelings are all churned up, then you begin doing the cycle, starting with the natural flow of feelings: anger, sadness, fear, and guilt. Once you've gone to your emotional core and brought up those feelings—many of which may have been completely subconscious before—you can be more rational.

If you are thinking-oriented, this is the fun part, because you will create a new limit for yourself, even though the process involves both thoughts and feelings. However, you may tend to be too harsh on yourself. Instead of setting reasonable limits that will keep you above the line in a state of balance, you may tend to set harsh ones that you will rebel against, procrastinate about, or push through at too great an expense—including the unwanted effects on your appetite.

If you are feeling-oriented, the natural flow of feelings may come easily to you, although some feelings may be more challenging than others. But for you, setting new limits will not be easy. Your tendency may be to set expectations that are too easy or too difficult or not to have any clear expectations. It's hard to have any security in life when you lack clear, flexible expectations and the power to follow through, so when you do start to set effective limits, it's likely you'll feel much better!

When you begin to create a limit for yourself, it helps to pause for a moment and reflect on the feelings you just expressed. However, it's at the end of this cycle that you will find you have popped yourself above the line—with a sense of body relaxation, lifted spirits, and calm energy—a feeling that will become familiar in time. After you create a reasonable expectation, fortify it with encouraging words (we call that positive, powerful thinking). Then pause again and ask yourself, "What is the essential pain? What is the downside, the hard part, the reality of the human condition I would have to face in order to follow through with that reasonable expectation?" It's usually something developmental, such as an acceptance of one of life's realities that was not learned in childhood; for example, "Life is difficult," "Not everyone will like me," or "I have to do things I don't want to do."

Once you look that truth straight in the eye, it loses its power to block your energy. In fact, once you face it, you pop above the line, where you can feel, receive, and enjoy the earned reward, the pay-off, the benefit—your reason for following through.

You are above the line, and it feels wonderful! That "popping" above the line is not only a means of rewiring the feeling brain but a natural, predictable way of triggering an increase in "feel good" neurotransmitters. There is no research that elucidates which neuro-chemicals are affected, but you can explore some possibilities for yourself. Does that "pop" feel like a satisfaction of serotonin, the energy of dopamine, or the pleasurable high of endorphins?

You have done this for yourself. You can ask someone to listen to you do a cycle, because these skills grow best in a loving environ-ment, but having the skill to pop yourself above the line on your own is incredibly empowering. Though many difficult moments arise when you are bone-chillingly alone, and it's important to be able to pop yourself above the line even then, you can ask someone to listen to you do a cycle when you have the opportunity to do so. We call that doing a Community Connection. The person doesn't interrupt, give advice, or comment. He or she is simply asked to be a loving presence while *you* answer the questions. It creates a lot of intimacy (and it can also begin to retrain your listener's feeling brain in the process).

Once you're above the line, you feel better, but you're not done yet. You also need to take whatever actions are necessary and make whatever shifts you need in order to follow through with the ex-pectation.

Ask yourself, "What do I need?" If you had asked that ques-tion before, when you were below the line, you would have come up with a want, not a need. For example, "I feel miserable. I need ice cream." But when you are above the line, you can identify your true need and, if appropriate, ask for support. So the last two questions of a cycle are: "What do I need?" and "Do I need sup-port?"

Here is a cycle that was done by Kara. Notice that Kara first states the facts—no feelings—about what is upsetting her. When she is done with this "thinking journal," in which she states all the facts that she needs to express in order to awaken strong feelings in her feeling brain, and her feelings are red-hot, she launches into her cycle.

Kara's Cycle

I know I should be exercising, and I keep telling myself I'll start a walking program, but I don't do it. I come home from work at night, and I really mean to put on my running shoes and go for a run, but I'm too tired. I hate to push myself more after I've already been through commuter traffic. Plus I've worked all day long!

Kara's Natural Flow of Feelings

I feel angry that I have to do one more thing.

I hate it that there is never time to relax.

I hate it that I feel guilty in my own home because I want to watch television and sit on the couch instead of going to the gym.

I hate going to the gym.

I feel sad that there are so many demands on me.

I feel sad that I have no energy at the end of the day.

I feel sad that I have to work so hard.

I feel afraid that I'll just keep putting it off and never be in shape.

I feel afraid that my weight will keep going up.

I feel guilty. . . . I don't feel guilty. I work a 9-hour day and have a 3-hour commute, and I do not feel guilty for not exercising.

I feel guilty that . . . in the best of all worlds, I wish that I had the energy and time to exercise.

I feel guilty that I work as much as I do.

Kara's Limits Cycle

What's my unreasonable expectation under all those feelings?

My unreasonable expectation is that I can be gone for 13 hours a day and expect myself to go to the gym when I hate to go to the gym anyway. Hah!

What's reasonable?

As long as I have a 13-hour workday, it's not a reasonable expectation that I'm going to exercise.

I expect myself to find some kind of exercise that I really enjoy and to do it daily.

Positive, powerful, and encouraging words I need to hear?
Your health is more important than the extra hour at work.
The essential pain I must face in order to follow through?
I must leave work at 6:00 p.m.
The earned reward?
I get to leave work at 6:00 p.m. I will have time for exercise.
I will be more fit and will feel better about my body.

Kara's Needs and Support

So what do I need?

I need to leave work at 6:00 p.m. and figure out some kind of exercise that I really like. That's easy. I want to line dance. I want to join a hiking group.

Do I need support?

Yes, I need to talk with my friends about signing up for a dance class.
I need to call about the hiking group.
I feel great. Thanks for listening to my cycle!

Now for Chuck's cycle:

Chuck's Cycle

My life is such a rat race. I am in the car driving the kids to school in the morning, rushing to work, then rushing home and getting the kids and feeling pulled in all directions. Nothing is going well, and I can't quit my job, but I'm sick of feeling tired and sick of rushing around.

Chuck's Natural Flow of Feelings

I feel angry that I don't have a life.

I feel furious that I take care of everyone and everything and I'm left with the crumbs.

I feel furious that my life is so rushed.

I feel angry that there is never time to breathe.

I hate it that my life is going by in a blur, which also makes me sad.

I feel sad that I never have any time for myself.

I feel sad that I am always so tired.

I feel sad that my kids are being raised with all these pressures.

I feel sad that I have no control over my family.

I feel sad that I am tired.

I feel afraid that I'll just keep rolling along, living a life that is exhausting.

I feel afraid that my kids will grow up and I will have missed it.

I feel afraid that they will not have happy memories of their childhood.

I feel afraid that I won't have happy memories of their childhood.

I feel guilty that I talk about it and complain about it but that I don't do anything about it.

I feel guilty for being so passive.

Chuck's Limits Cycle

What's my unreasonable expectation under all those feelings? I'm not sure. Let's see.

My unreasonable expectation is that I have no power.

My unreasonable expectation is that no matter what I do, life will be rushed and unsatisfying.

My unreasonable expectation is that my feelings don't matter.

Well, no wonder I'm out of balance, with all those expectations.

Let's see, what is reasonable to expect?

I expect that my feelings matter.

I expect that I do have some power in this situation.

What do I expect of myself?

I expect myself to use the power I do have to create a less rushed, more fulfilling life for my family and myself.

What are the positive, powerful thoughts and the encouragement I need to hear?

You have more power than you know.

The essential pain, the hard part of following through?

My children may be mad. My children may reject me.

The earned reward, the benefit, the payoff of following through?

I won't reject myself.
I will know that I am being a good father.
I will have more balance in my life.

Chuck's Needs and Support

What do I need?

I need to develop a plan that makes our life more livable.

I need to talk with my wife and come up with plans that we can both live with.

Do I need support?

Yes, from my wife. I need to talk with her.

Summary of How to Do a Cycle

Again, the process of doing a cycle is:

1. *The facts:* State the facts of what you're upset about. No feelings, just the simple facts of the matter. Here are some more examples:
   - My mother is coming to live with us for a week, and when she comes, she always demands that we give all our time to her.
   - I just had some medical tests done, and I won't know the results until next week.
   - I don't know what to do with my life, but I know that I am unhappy.
2. *Natural flow of feelings:* Keep stating the facts until the feelings are strong, then go on to the natural flow of feelings. Make your sentences short and choppy, not intellectual.
   - I feel angry that . . .
   - I feel sad that . . .
   - I feel afraid that . . .
   - I feel guilty that . . .
3. *The limits cycle:* Ask yourself:
   - What is my unreasonable expectation?

- What is a reasonable one—not too easy but not too harsh?
- What positive, powerful, encouraging words do I most need to hear so I will follow through?
- What is the essential pain, the hard part, the reality of the human condition I must face to follow through?
- What is the earned reward—the payoff, the benefit of following through with this new reasonable expectation, the reward that comes from it that matters to me?

4. *Check feelings and needs:* Now that you're above the line, you can accurately identify what you really need. Your response to "What do I need?" is what you need to do in order to follow through with that new reasonable expectation. Do you need support? Do you need help from others (not from yourself) to make following through with that expectation easier? By asking for support, we step off that lonely pedestal of self-sufficiency and have more intimacy in our lives and get our needs met. Ask yourself:

- What do I need?
- What support do I need from others?

Now you know how to do a cycle! If you are anxious to try it now, by all means, begin! You need not do one, though, if it seems as if it's too much for you. On the third day, if you prefer not to do a cycle, just use emotional housecleaning instead. You don't have to be perfect to be wonderful. Just do what you can do. It will work out fine. The method is not going away, and you can always do a cycle later on.

Which of the three skills do you reach for when you are wandering around the kitchen wondering if you should snack on ice cream, cookies, or leftover spaghetti?

All of them!

- *Skill 1:* Use checking in and ask yourself, "How do I feel? What do I really need?"

- *Skill 2:* If you still have a desire for the food, use skill 2, emotional housecleaning. Standing right there in the kitchen, write down or say aloud all eight sentences.
- *Skill 3:* If you still want the food, use skill 3, doing cycles. Better yet, ask someone to listen to you do a cycle—a friend by telephone or an adult with whom you live.

Still want to eat? Then do. You probably really need it! Eat without a shred of guilt and enjoy every bite.

Body Work

The last thing that a person who is below the line wants to do is exercise. It brings up too many feelings. If he or she does exercise, it's usually compulsive or numbing. It's running on the treadmill mindlessly or getting high in a spinning class where you race to an instructor's drill-sergeant commands. It's *not* balanced!

During these three days, you will spend one hour of the day in physical activity that is above the line. On day 1, you will combine exercise with either being out in nature or listening to music. Both music and nature increase serotonin levels, so you get a boost from exercise and from music or nature. On day 2, you will choose an activity that brings you more closeness with yourself. Day 2 is a day of intimacy and pleasure, and the preparation for intimacy with others begins with intimacy with ourselves. On day 3, you will *play*—you will do some form of exercise that is playful, fun, and brings out the kid in you.

This is a time to try new things, so if you're used to walking on the treadmill at the gym for 45 minutes, try something new on the first day that combines music and/or nature with exercise. Likewise, do something different on each of the three days. Walking on the treadmill could be justified as an "intimacy with myself" activity for day 2 and play on day 3. But since this is the start of a new life above the line, try different things each day. Open up to new possibilities during these three days!

As you can see, the goal is not simply to exercise. It's to enjoy your body and move your body from above the line. It's to feel integrated. It's not about going to work all day as if you were just a "head," then going to the gym and sweating bullets as if you were just a body.

The point of exercise, beyond physical fitness, is to feel integrated and whole, to move your body, mind, and spirit all at once. Your spirit might be competitive, wanting to shoot hoops or lift another ten pounds of weights. It might want to express its playfulness by dancing, playing games, or taking up sports. Perhaps you want to run in nature, hike, kayak, row, climb mountains, or dig in the garden. Or maybe what gratifies you is learning ballet, jazz dancing, line dancing, or pairing exercise with intimacy, having a heart-to-heart talk while walking with a backpacking partner or experiencing the camaraderie of a whole team.

In other words, body work is not just exercise. Exercise alone is the most powerful way of naturally balancing your neurotransmitters. In addition, body work boosts your levels of serotonin, dopamine, and endorphins. That boost is the result of doing something that is intensely pleasurable, something that soothes your soul, delights the child in you, or gratifies your dark side.

That's right, dark side. One of the reasons we eat so much is that we are so terminally *good*. We are such people-pleasers. We are good guys who meet the deadline, make everybody happy, raise perfect children, and meet everyone's needs but our own. We're left with a part of us that is needy, aggressive, indulgent, rebellious, or gloriously villainous! That side of us comes out in our eating. We *reward* ourselves with food. We believe we *deserve* to overload our bodies with fat, sugar, and calories. Fortunately, exercise gives us an easy way to act out that dark side without hurting ourselves or others, so we don't have to express it through our eating. For example, kickboxing, running, climbing hills, paddling boats, stomping our feet, dancing wildly, pumping iron, playing soccer, digging in the garden, and clipping hedges.

In your 3-Day Solution Plan, you'll be devoting one hour a day to physical activity. So it's important to plan something that doesn't meet just your body's needs but the needs of your mind and spirit, too. It's not effective merely to plug in to the treadmill or go on a mindless walk in a visually bankrupt environment. Your task is to find various options for spending an hour to not only move your body but to express yourself. Instead of repressing your aggression or expressing it by hitting your boss, strike a punching bag or scream and stomp. Honor your vile tendencies, delight your senses, or soothe and gratify yourself. Music, nature, self-expression, emotional intimacy, or belonging to a team are all serotonin enhancers.

Sample Body-Work Plans

On day 1, I will take a hike at sunset, my favorite time of day. On day 2, I will take a horseback-riding lesson, because being close to horses always makes me know myself better. If I'm anxious, the horse picks up on that right away. On day 3, I will play basketball with my son. We can meet at the school, and I'll bring the ball.

The first day, I will go to the gym for some free weights and the StairMaster with my headphones blasting reggae music. On the second day, I will go to a yoga class. The last day, I'm going to go to the beach in my shorts, run for a while, and walk in the breakers, finding shells and playing with the waves.

On the first day of the plan, I'm going to play basketball at the court down the street from work. There is a noontime group there, and I'm going to join it. The second day, I'll go on an early-morning hike before anyone is up. I'll see the sunrise and have that peace. On the third day, I'm going to turn up the music after dinner and get our family dancing. I'm not going to stop. They can do the dishes while I wail!

Body time takes one hour, unless your physician does not recommend you exert yourself for that length of time. If you've
been inactive recently, consider starting with 45 minutes and go
slowly. Very slowly! To decrease the risk of injury, choose physical
activities that are low-impact and that don't require strenuous
movements that go beyond the normal range of motion of your
joints. However, in these three days, you are jump-starting a
pattern of committing to moving your body for one hour daily,
such that when you are done each day, you say to yourself, "Life
is good."

Solution 1-2-3 Eating

The easiest part of the plan is the eating. I've included menus in the
plan that are popular, easy to fix, and will give you the nutrition you
need. If you prefer another menu, though, you can substitute any
one of 14 options for each meal. Included in each daily plan is a
menu for three meals and two snacks—one in midmorning and another in midafternoon. Your evening snack will not be food. The
sustenance you give yourself in the evening will be far more satisfying: time to restore and intimacy time.

Although the Solution 1-2-3 Eating is flexible, it reflects the
truth about nutrition. What you eat is extraordinarily important to
your vibrancy and mood. A few extra forkfuls can lead to lethargy
and emotional numbness, just as too much hunger can also be
numbing or emotionally distorting.

The basic concept is to eat only when you are hungry and to
stop eating when you are just satisfied, not full. It's to eat only those
foods that are pleasurable and make the foundation of your diet
healthy foods that you enjoy. Eat the less healthful foods only if you
really need them. If you do, abandon guilt and enjoy every bite of
them. In fact, one of the optional menus in 1-2-3 Eating is the Self-
Acceptance Meal, to use every once in a while when you really need
it. You don't eat your meat, your broccoli, your lima beans, and the
candy bar. You just eat the candy bar. You go for dessert and skip
the dinner rather than overloading your body with both.

To use this plan with success takes facing the essential pain, the reality of the human condition, that eating lots of fatty, sugary, greasy foods doesn't make for a happy, healthy life. It takes facing the essential pain that we can't have whatever we want when we want it unless we're willing to deal with the consequences.

It means redefining what is edible. Food is not sugary, fatty fabrications produced by the food industry. It's the genuine article—whole foods—except just the ones that give us the most pleasure. Whatever whole foods delight and satisfy you become the mainstay of your meals and snacks. Perhaps it is strawberries, gnarly whole-grain breads, ripe peaches, thinly sliced steak, huge green salads, or luscious ears of corn.

At each meal, you create balance by having a food that you enjoy from each of the three groups: You have something from *The Fiber Group,* such as fruits, veggies, and whole grains. You have a small amount of *Healthy Fat,* such as olive oil, canola oil, avocado, seeds, or nuts. And you have some lean *Protein Group* foods, such as fish, lean poultry, lean meats, low-fat and nonfat milk products, beans, and soy foods.

You combine the foods you find appealing from each of these three groups. Have large amounts of vegetables and fruits, some whole grains, and solid portions of protein foods. Accent those foods with small amounts of Healthy Fats. A tablespoon of olive oil and a few nuts balance out a meal. You will learn more about what is a reasonable portion size of various foods from the menus and recipes in Chapters 16, 18, and 19.

If you really need *White Stuff*—a collective term for sugary, fatty, refined carbs, alcohol, trans fats, saturated fats, caffeine, and salty foods—then you can have them, but only if you really need them.

Eat snacks when you're hungry. The trouble is that it's so easy to feel hungry when we see food. The question becomes not "Am I hungry?" but "Am I hungry for that delicious piece of cake?" It's fine to snack if you're hungry, and by snacking on healthy foods, it's easier to avoid eating for entertainment or self-soothing. So it's best to snack on healthy foods, 1-2-3 Foods, particularly veggies and fruits that cause less of a rise in serotonin. That way, we'll get less of an emotional payoff when we eat and won't snack when we're really not hungry.

Because calcium intake is important to weight loss, some snacks on the plan contain milk. You can use soy if you're vegan or if you prefer it. Fruits and vegetables are high in fiber and low in calories, which makes them good choices, but some people find themselves hungrier when they eat fruit. They are better off emphasizing vegetables, milk, and nuts for snacks. Having a few nuts as part of a vegetable or fruit snack adds staying power. However, nuts have a high caloric density (calories per bite). They are also salty, crunchy foods that are often craved as comfort food. Include them only if having a few nuts doesn't lead to eating too many.

When you have White Stuff, particularly refined-carbohydrate White Stuff, it will have less of an impact on your insulin levels if you consume it with a meal rather than as a snack. Having a small candy for dessert with lunch is smarter than snacking on it in midafternoon.

It's easy to use 1-2-3 Eating because it's very clear-cut. For a food to be on our 1-2-3 Food Lists, it has to have considerable nutritional merit. It has to promote wellness and prevent disease. During your 3-Day Solution Plan, there's no need to learn more about 1-2-3 Eating because the menus have already been prepared for you. However, there is more information about 1-2-3 Eating in Part 5 of this book, including the 1-2-3 Food Lists (Chapter 22) and more ideas about eating for lasting weight loss (Chapter 21).

Many of those who tested this plan spontaneously chose to clean out their cupboards before they started and set up a 1-2-3 kitchen. They took out most of the foods that aren't on the 1-2-3 Food Lists and brought into the house the foods they like that are on the lists. Consider the possibility of using the 3-Day Solution Plan to create a house or family food policy, either now or after you complete the 3-Day Solution Plan.

Some families that wouldn't think of having marijuana, cigarettes, or alcohol in the house have cupboards stuffed with sugary, fatty foods! They tell their children not to smoke or take drugs, then serve up fried foods, cookies, and candy. These foods are *not* drugs when eaten now and then as part of a whole-food diet, but when eaten excessively, they can have profound effects on mood and health. As you saw in Chapter 10, "Spinning Out of Control," for those with weight in the middle of their bodies, the combination of stress, obesity, and a high-fat, high-sugar diet can contribute to mood swings and depression as well as the potential for addiction to overeating.

Consider the merits of turning your home into an environment not of shared indulgence but of an abundance of delicious healthy foods that have low addictive potential and that nourish your body and please your palate. Consider doing this in a healthy way—not a compulsive way. After all, it is just food! You are always free to eat the other foods, but most of the time, you simply won't want to.

Many families settle on a trial policy that they will keep the house clean of excessive White Stuff for two weeks. After that trial period, they can redecide what is right for the family. This cleaning up the food environment can be great fun. Choosing luscious fruits at the local farmers' markets or finding stores that have wonderful produce departments can be an adventure. Your home can become lavish with healthy foods, and most family members will be surprised at how great the food tastes and how much better they feel.

If you set up a 1-2-3 kitchen or a trial food policy for your home, be sure to stop short of making this change feel depriving. Ask each family member what White Stuff is important to him or her to have in the house. Limit each person to two or three things that are really important to him or her, then be sure to have those foods available.

With 1-2-3 Eating, shopping becomes so much easier. When you go to the store, you put in the basket 1-2-3 Foods and only the White Stuff that is really important to you or another family member. There's no more random or mindless tossing of junk food into the shopping cart and no more impulse purchases of processed foods.

For now, just think about the 3-Day Solution Plan. Think about how it would be to eat only when you are hungry and to stop when the hunger has disappeared but before you are full. Think about how it would be to commit to giving your body whole foods that nourish and satisfy, and to replace the gratification of excessive sugar and fat with the excitement and joy of life above the line.

Consider doing this but still knowing that when you really need that sweet or creamy treat, you can have it, guilt-free. You are more important than your food.

Meaningful Pursuits

During your 3-Day Solution, you must do something that is not easy, something on which you must focus that has rewards for you, for six to eight hours per day. It doesn't matter what your occupation or whether you are a student, caring for children, or running a corporation, the biological need is the same.

We have a hardwired need to work. We need to make an effort that increases dopamine levels, followed by receiving a reward that increases serotonin. Effort that is followed by rewards balances our neurotransmitters and keeps us above the line. It's a survival need.

On the other hand, expending effort without a reward is depriving and making no effort but still getting a reward is indulging. Both send us below the line, and neither has a balancing effect on our neurotransmitters.

So what you do during the day and whether it takes you above the line shows up in your appetite. A depriving day is often followed by an indulging evening. An indulging day can just roll along and turn into an indulging night.

This does not mean that you need to have a nice boss or do altruistic work. It's not about what is objective but what is subjective. It's about how we process that experience and whether we stay above the line. If we are above the line about our work, it is meaningful. If it weren't meaningful, we wouldn't be doing it. If the earned rewards of being there on that day did not outweigh the downside, we wouldn't engage in that activity. When we're above the line, we don't distort the downside of our work—feeling sorry for ourselves, mentally denigrating our coworkers, disparaging our pay—we accept the downside. We move through it and feel the earned reward of being there. Once we feel the earned reward, we can focus, do our very best, and get so much more work done with less stress. There are fewer side trips into unnecessary busywork, control struggles, and slowdowns. It makes for a great day.

For your 3-Day Solution, you will need to work in a focused way for no fewer than six hours per day and no more than eight hours per day. The work should be intense and should require your full attention, but allow you to check in with yourself periodically throughout the day. That will probably mean adjusting your work schedule and perhaps also your level of focus. You'll want to be very productive but not to work so intensely that you lose yourself in the process.

To get above the line about meaningful pursuits, consider doing some cycles. Here are a few examples. The first subsection presents Tom's cycle.

Tom's Cycle

I am working on projects for my boss's boss, and it's infuriating my boss because she's not getting enough credit. My boss's boss is very demanding. I'm dealing not only with that, but I'm also putting up with emotional turmoil because my boss is picking on me, stressing me out, and not including me in department meetings. Everyone in our department is on her side: when I walk in, they ignore me, and when I talk, they act uninterested.

Tom's Natural Flow of Feelings

I feel angry that my boss has the authority to treat me like this and get away with it.

I feel angry that I have so much work but don't get recognition or more money.

I feel angry that my coworkers can treat me badly and my boss promotes it.

I feel angry that I have to play this ridiculous game with my boss in order to keep my job.

I feel angry that my work is excellent but my boss is trying to ruin my reputation.

I'm sad because I've put in a lot of work and no value is placed on what I've done.

I feel sad because I want to find another job.

I feel sad that there is no future here for me.

I'm sad because other people will criticize me.

I feel afraid that I won't be able to support myself and my family.

I'm scared that no matter where I go, the same thing will happen.

I'm scared that I'm getting older, so it's harder to get a job.

I'm scared at how much money I need to make to support my family.

I feel guilty that I didn't play the "game" better from the beginning.

I feel guilty that I didn't make more friendships outside of my department.

I feel guilty that I don't want to be part of the corporate ladder anymore.

Tom's Limits Cycle

My unreasonable expectation: I expect to be in a work environment where politics is not an issue.

Another unreasonable expectation: I expect that my boss will be moral, intelligent, and fair.

A reasonable expectation: I may never get a good boss. If I ever do, there is such a revolving door that they'd soon be promoted, moved somewhere else, and then I'd get another buffoon as a boss.

An unreasonable expectation: I can alienate my boss and coworkers and get their acceptance.

A reasonable expectation: I can make an effort to get along with them.

What do I expect of myself?

I expect myself to be healthy and to let go of the impossible situation.

I expect myself to relax and learn how to deal with this.

Positive, powerful thinking? The encouraging words I need to hear are: Get over it! You're not the only one who hates their job.

The essential pain?

Life is difficult.

My situation is not perfect.

I have to do things I don't want to do.

I can't get love from my coworkers.

The earned reward?

I can get love from myself. I get acceptance from my family.

I can stop stressing out and feel better.

I will have a paycheck that supports my family.

Tom's Needs and Support

What do I need?

I need to do my work and try to get along.

I need to accept that this work situation can eat me alive.

I need to take time for my health and not ruin my life over my job.

Do I need support?

Yes. I need to talk with my wife.

Tom did a great cycle, and he will need to continue doing them. Any situation that triggers a feeling of inescapable stress sets off the survival mechanisms of the oversecretion of dopamine in the presence of low serotonin and boosts the drive to go to excess. With the 3-Day Solution Plan, how Tom spends his hours outside of work will begin to change, which will help, too.

The next subsection presents a cycle that was done by a young mother, Meredith, who is staying home with a two-year-old and a four-year-old and expecting her third child.

Meredith's Cycle

I have two young children and my husband goes to a challenging job all day, but it's a long day for me. I have my children in playgroups and I get together with the other mothers, but there is a lot of time when the three of us are home together. I get really tired and bored at times, and sometimes I'm short with the children. Before I had the children, I was an interior designer, and I liked being attached to the energy of what was happening and the customers. I put on makeup and bought clothes. Now it doesn't matter what I look like.

Meredith's Natural Flow of Feelings

I don't feel angry.

I feel sad.

I feel sad that all I have to talk about is what's on sale at Target.

I feel sad that I have lost touch with the world.

I feel afraid I am losing myself in my kids.

I feel angry that there are no good options.

I feel angry that I have the kids all the time.

I feel guilty if I leave them.

I feel angry that Steve doesn't help out more.

I feel angry that when he comes home from work, he wants to relax. *I* want to relax!!!

I feel furious that I do everything for everyone but myself.

I feel angry that nobody thinks about me—they only think about themselves.

I feel sad that I am so bored.

I feel afraid that I am going to turn into a witch or a very boring person.

I feel guilty that I let my husband get away with doing nothing.

I feel guilty that I don't set better limits with the kids.

I feel guilty that I eat cookies in the afternoon.

I feel guilty that I haven't created a day that meets some of my adult needs.

Meredith's Limits Cycle

My unreasonable expectation is that taking care of myself isn't important.

My unreasonable expectation is that Steve should read my mind and meet my needs.

What do I expect of myself?

I expect myself to do something that gives me energy and drive, and not to be bored as much as I am.

I expect myself to ask Steve to take care of the kids more in the evening.

Positive and powerful thinking? Having urgency and excitement in my life matters.

The essential pain?

Steve may be angry about having to do more at home.

I won't have a reason to complain. I won't have an excuse to overeat.

I'll have to put effort into planning what I want to do.

The earned reward?

A happier, more vibrant life.

A more honest relationship with Steve.

Turning off the drive to overeat.

Meredith's Needs and Support

What do I need?

Help with the children.

To brainstorm about what I can do to get more stimulation in my life.

Do I need support?

Yes! I'll talk with Steve and call my friend.

Unlike Tom, Meredith didn't have enough stimulation in her day. Some jobs are like that, but most people adjust by using their time off to do things that meet their needs for urgency. Some jobs have no redeeming social value at all, but doing volunteer, community, or other altruistic work during off-hours can meet that need to balance neurotransmitters and turn off the drive to overeat.

For these three days, schedule yourself to do something for six to eight hours that requires you to focus with intensity, knowing that after that rush of intensity, your serotonin level will increase and give you an intrinsic reward.

Time to Restore

During these three days, you will take an hour each day to restore yourself, when you are completely off-limits to everyone and everything and you can do whatever you want. You will focus on restoring yourself physically, emotionally, intellectually, and spiritually. You will do whatever nourishes you. If it restores you, then do it.

In addition to taking an hour per day for time to restore, you will go to bed early. You will stay in bed for a total of nine hours. That will give you eight hours to sleep and an hour to transition, contemplate the day, check your feelings, honor the awakening of the day, and the closing of it at night.

According to researchers, a majority of Americans are currently getting 60 to 90 minutes less sleep a night than they should. Sleep deprivation is highly correlated with weight gain in both children and adults. Tape your favorite late-night shows if you like, but carve out nine hours for sleep and transition for these three days.

The high-risk time for overeating is between 4:00 p.m. and 8:00 p.m., when dopamine and serotonin are low and endorphins are shot, too. We're restless, bored, ungratified, depressed, or empty and . . . hungry!

Some people relax by switching to a different activity—from the sales job during the day to painting class in the evening. Other people need "chewing-gum" activities, doing absolutely nothing, such as taking a nap, watching television, flipping through the newspaper—anything that requires no effort whatsoever.

For some of us, overeating serves as a "reward-deficiency syndrome"; that is, we're just not getting the gratification we need from life, so we get it from food. Since there are so many demands on our time, this one golden hour needs to deliver! We must devote that time to something with high "reward density"—the greatest payoff per minute possible!

If you were dieting, that wouldn't be necessary because the strategy would be to *force* yourself to eat less. That's not what you are doing with this plan. You're creating a life that is so fulfilling—in both your internal life and your external lifestyle—that you naturally and unconsciously stop wanting the extra food.

That puts a lot of pressure on you to be sure that you spend the moments getting the most satisfaction. That still may involve resting or daydreaming, but the difference lies in being aware that you need to spend that time doing exactly what will restore you the most.

Try asking yourself, "What can I do for one hour a day that will satisfy me as much as the extra helping of mashed potatoes?"

It probably isn't watching television. Perhaps it's taking a hot bath, playing the guitar, gardening, hiking in nature, making a point of seeing the sunset. The fallout of a low-dopamine/low-serotonin configuration in life is that at the end of the day, we are remarkably uncreative. So it takes planning and some insight. It takes saying,

"What *really* gratifies me?" then planning for it, doing it, and reaping the rewards: pushing away from the table.

Intimacy Time

Survival needs—safety, sex, and food—spawn intensity: we've "gotta get it." Safety is the most important survival need, and the way we are genetically programmed to create that safety is by being together—literally, being in the presence of others.

We may think we are connecting to others by e-mail or telephone, but when we look at our genetically determined equipment to create connection, it suggests that something essential is lost. The facial muscles are the only ones in the body that are attached to the skin, facilitating a flurry of subtle emotions that enables us to be seen and to see. The eyes channel directly to the feeling brain, and we become attuned to other people's inner state. When we look into each other's eyes, it is a multilayered experience, the resonance between two feeling brains. With more endorphin (opiate) receptors in the feeling brain than any other part, we see firsthand the magic of connection and the pain of loss.

When we're below the line, we're alone, even if we are surrounded by those we love. When we can't connect with ourselves, we don't have the foundation in place for connection with others. At least if we are alone, we are at peace with ourselves, but our genetic destiny dictates that we need to be involved with people, neighborhoods, communities, interest groups, or pets: we *need* them.

During these three days, you will take time for three kinds of intimacy: social intimacy on day 1, sexual intimacy on day 2, and emotional intimacy on day 3.

Social intimacy is the easiest to achieve because it can be cognitive. You can have shared interests, but the emotional pipeline between you may be closed. Still, there are benefits, principally drawing from our herding mentality and need to belong to a tribe. On the first day, you will take time for social intimacy with any group or individual outside your family with whom you have a shared interest or need.

Sexual intimacy is more challenging because, as much as with food regulation, when we wander below the line, sexual intimacy goes with us. Common sexual external solutions are: sexual avoidance, sexual preoccupation, problems with sexual functioning, excessive pornography, having sex when you don't want it or in ways you don't want, settling for mediocre sex, and betrayal in a committed, sexually exclusive relationship. Since emotional intimacy, sexual intimacy, and food problems are all wound up together, there can be an endless variety of problems.

Instead of focusing on the problems, for these three days, consider being practical and positive. Your relationship might not be great, your sexual satisfaction may not be high, and your body may not be perfect, but we have bigger fish to fry. We have to turn off the drive to overeat, and the most primitive expression of sexuality is oral. If we do not take responsibility for honoring our needs for sexuality, sensuality, eroticism, and passion, we're going to be eating pasta, cinnamon rolls, or ice cream. So for these three days, within your ethical and spiritual limits, go for it!

Emotional intimacy refers to emotional closeness. It's when the boundary between you and another person is tissue-paper-thin. You feel safe and close, but you don't lose yourself. You know that you will not surrender to the other person, and if he or she rejects you, you would feel hurt, but you would not reject yourself. In other words, you would experience closeness without unhealthy dependency.

If you are above the line and your partner, spouse, or friend is not, then emotional intimacy will suffer. In Solution training, we suggest waiting one year before making decisions about any non-abusive relationship. Once you start moving above the line, that state is often catching, but that contagion takes time. If you have others close to you who have an interest in giving the method a try, then they can learn the basics of the skills, too. It puts you on more of an even playing field, in which all of you have the basic tools to enhance intimacy in your lives.

There are two intimacy time options on the third day, Two Chairs, involves you and another person's sitting in two chairs, knee to knee, eye to eye, and leaning forward. We call this using "connecting body language." You take turns listening to each other do emotional housecleaning. When each person is done, the other makes a nurturing comment, what we call a tender morsel. Opening the emotional pipeline between the two of you is satisfying, more satisfying than a sugary dessert.

The following subsections present examples of brief cycles that Anne and Clay did to get above the line and increase the intimacy in their lives.

Anne's Cycle

I'm divorced and live in New York City, where getting a date when you're over 40 isn't easy. I have lots of male friends but nobody that I'm involved with sexually. I know that my sexual frustrations get taken out on food because I can't stop eating in the evenings. It's a catch-22. I don't feel like dating because I'm too fat, and because I don't date, I eat more and stay overweight. I have emotional intimacy with my women friends and a couple of my male friends. I have too much social intimacy; I belong to too many groups, but I don't have sexual intimacy at all.

Anne's Natural Flow of Feelings

I feel angry that I'm 45 and can't get a date.

I hate it that I'm an attractive woman but men aren't attracted to me.

I am furious that I'm alone.

I can't stand it that my prime years are going by without a man.

I feel sad that I'm missing out.

I feel afraid that I'll be alone forever.

I feel afraid that I'll compromise again and let someone use me.

I feel guilty that I am not more creative about my sex life.

I feel guilty that I don't enjoy my body more.

Anne's Limits Cycle

My unreasonable expectation is that because I'm alone, I can't honor my needs.

A reasonable expectation?

I expect myself to honor my needs for sensuality, sexuality, and passion!

Positive and powering thinking?
My needs matter.
Essential pain?
All of my needs will not be met.
I don't have a partner.
I am alone.
Earned reward?
I have myself.
I can be creative.
More of my needs will be met!

Anne's Needs and Support

What do I need?

I need to ask Thomas to go to dinner. At least, I can give and get a back rub from him. We have a great friendship, and who knows?

I need to dig out my old erotica books and find some candles for the bathroom when I take my late-evening sensual bath.

Do I need support?

Yes, I need to ask Thomas to come to dinner!

Anne was successful in putting together a plan for meeting her needs and being creative in doing so. When we're below the line, relationships frequently suffer. Some couples use the 3-Day Solution at the same time, so they're each invested in making the needed adjustments and compromises to create sexual intimacy. Reaching that point, however, often takes doing cycles, as Clay's cycle illustrates.

Clay's Cycle

My wife and I have made our children the center of our marriage. They're now teenagers, but over the last 15 years, with each of us working full-time, we've accepted that there is not much left over for our marriage. My wife is too tired to make love except a couple of times a month, and I don't think she enjoys it then. I think she is making love with me out of guilt and trying to get it over with. I take out my frustration by overeating. She cooks diet food, or when I'm off a diet, we're back to having pasta and pizza. Sometimes I think she likes me to be fat and happy so I won't pester her for sex. All of this makes me plenty mad. . . .

Clay's Natural Flow of Feelings

I feel angry that she has no interest in sex.

I hate it that I've let her get away with it.

I can't stand it that I've become nothing more than a paycheck and someone to take care of the kids.

I feel angry that just because she has no interest in me, she thinks that I have no needs.

I feel angry that I am so horny.

I feel tired of using pornography and taking a shower.

I feel sad that 15 years have gone by.

I feel afraid that things won't change.

I feel guilty for making it okay for our marriage to become sexless.

Clay's Limits Cycle

My unreasonable expectation?

That I can teach her it's okay to have a sexless marriage and still have great sex.

A reasonable expectation? What do I expect of myself?

I expect myself to create a sex life for myself that gratifies me.

I expect myself to talk with my wife and get whatever help is needed to make our love life better.

I expect myself to gratify myself with lovemaking, not with pizza and beer.

Positive, powerful thoughts, the encouraging words I most need to hear right now?

Even if she doesn't think sex is important, I do. Sex is important to a marriage.

The essential pain?

I may lose my marriage.

I may be alone.

My wife may be hurt. She may cry. She may lash out at me. This may be uncomfortable.

The earned reward?

More satisfaction.
A better marriage.
Less need for pizza and beer.

Clay's Needs and Support

What do I need?
To talk with my wife.
Do I need support?
Not now. Maybe later. If we have to go to counseling, I'm up for it. I'll do whatever it takes. If she won't go to counseling, I will.

Your intimacy plan doesn't have to be perfect to be wonderful. Imagine each moment of intimacy being a designer appetite suppressant without the side effects. You will take one a day—or more, if you like!—during these three days.

After this introduction to the basic elements of the plan, just complete the necessary planning (discussed in the following chapter) and start your 3-Day Solution!

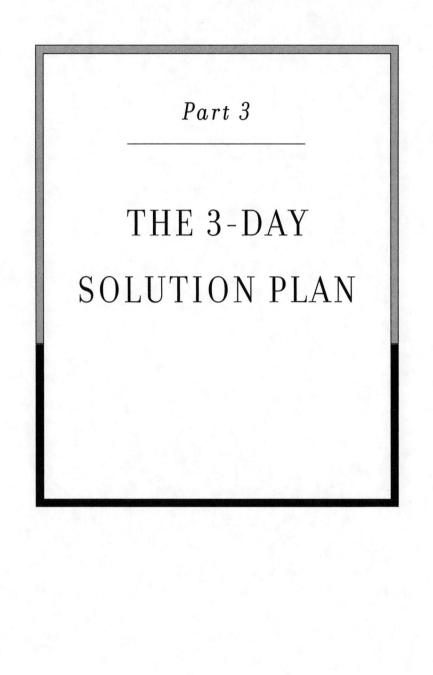

Part 3

THE 3-DAY
SOLUTION PLAN

12

Checklist: Preparing for a Solution

ALTHOUGH NOT A lot of work is required to get ready to start your three-day plan, please take a few moments to prepare for it so you can get the most benefit from these three days! They will be the start of a new life for you and will give you a jump-start on mastering this method so you can lose weight and keep it off.

Schedule Your 3-Day Solution

Identify a date to begin! Schedule it at a time when you can devote your energies to the plan for three days in a row. Breaking it up just does not work. The benefits of the plan build day by day. Many people schedule their 3-Day Solution Plan for Wednesday, Thursday, and Friday, when work may be less demanding than earlier in the week.

This is not a retreat where you go away somewhere and have a fantasy life. It's not even about a time to restore yourself and get away from reality. It's a time to be in your real-life situations but alter them slightly based on Mastery Living and respond to them differently with your Solution Skills.

If your tendency is to do everything perfectly—perfectionism is an external solution—and that keeps you from scheduling a day to begin, consider facing the essential pain: I am not perfect. This experience will not be perfect. Then reap the earned reward: I am human. This experience, though not perfect, will be wonderful!

Find Someone Else to Do This Plan with You

See whether at least one person you know—a friend, relative, neighbor, or coworker—has an interest in doing this, too.

If you live with an adult, consider inviting him or her to join you in this 3-Day Solution Plan. Having two or more people in the home using the plan makes it easier—and more fun. Plus, you'll have a chance to create a systemic change so that your whole family begins to live life above the line.

This plan also works well to use with a close friend or a small support group of friends, neighbors, or coworkers, who can get together either in person or by telephone. For example, you and several others can form a 3-Day Solution group or throw a Solution party to celebrate life above the line. You can get together once by telephone or in person before you do your plan, then check in daily during the plan by telephone. Afterward, you can get together again to celebrate your accomplishments.

If you do that, some people in your Solution party may decide to continue with the method and find a Solution in their lives. You may want to, too. If you do, you and the others can complete the Solution course to acquire the remainder of the skills and layer them step by step until you have a Solution. You would have the advantage of an already-established "buddy system."

Part of using this method in the long term and reaching a Solution is having a list of Solution buddies with whom to do cycles. A Solution buddy is someone who is on the pathway to a Solution and has learned how to use the Solution Skills effectively and knows the safety guidelines of the method. When you want to do a cycle, you call and ask your Solution buddy whether it's a good time to listen to you do a cycle. If it is, your buddy will listen; if not, he or she won't. Your buddy can do the same, calling you to do a cycle. Doing a cycle with a listener who knows how to stay within the safety guidelines—such as no interrupting, no giving unasked-for advice—can deepen the effectiveness of the cycle. Plus the experience offers intimacy, caring, support, and community—all of which motivate us to stay on the pathway until we have rewired our feeling brain and have a Solution in our life.

If you prefer to do this alone, then do it alone! However, you may have questions or want confidential support. If you do, there is a free part of our website (www.thepathway.org) for anyone who has a copy of this book that includes a discussion board for those using this plan. Professional support is also available, including daily coaching by telephone from a Solution provider to support you through the 3-Day Solution Plan. Visit our website for more information.

Ask for Support from Those Close to You

During these three days, you will be changing your lifestyle, and that will affect those around you. To the extent that you feel safe doing so, speak with each family member and, if you like, one or more close friends and let them know that you are trying a three-day plan for your health. Share with them what to expect and ask for support.

One of the symptoms of being below the line is feeling as if you have to do everything yourself and not sharing the realities of your life experiences with those close to you. To get off to a good start with this plan, share this information with others and ask for their help. When you move above the line, they will be affected. You will be so much more relaxed and satisfied that they will feel grateful that you are using the method. Get their support now so that it will be easier for you to experience the full benefits of the plan. For example, you might say something like this:

> For three days, I'm going to be taking really good care of my health, making adjustments in my lifestyle, and using skills that will give me motivation. It is an intense plan, and I hope to do it well and get the full benefits of the plan. In order to do that, I need your support. I need you to [for example]:
> - Take the children to school.
> - Come home by 5:00 p.m. and make dinner.
> - Get the sugary, fatty foods out of the house.
> - Be aware that I will not be home until after I finish exercising.
> - Keep up with washing the dishes and doing the laundry.
> - Anticipate that I will be gone on the first evening, doing something social.
> - Do an activity with me on the second evening that involves sensuality.

- Do an activity with me on the third evening that involves sharing feelings.
- Be positive and supportive about my using this 3-Day Solution Plan.

Would you please tell me how you feel about giving me that support? I really appreciate your help on this and understand that this may not be exactly what you feel like doing. But your help means a lot to me. Thank you.

Make Sure This Plan Will Be Safe for You

Safety is our first consideration. Any abrupt change in the chemicals that we put into our bodies can pose a risk.

- It's fine to drink one 6-ounce cup of coffee daily during this three-day plan. If you are drinking more than one 6-ounce cup of coffee per day, during the 3-Day Solution, continue drinking coffee but cut the number of cups in half. If you cut down any further or quit, you're likely to have a caffeine-withdrawal headache for all three days.
- It's fine to drink two 6-ounce cups of tea with caffeine during this three-day plan. If you drink more than that, cut the number of cups in half to avoid a caffeine-withdrawal headache. There is no limit on the reasonable consumption of decaffeinated and caffeine-free tea, and decaffeinated coffee.
- If you drink alcoholic beverages, limit your consumption to one drink (5 ounces of wine, a 12-ounce beer, or 1.5 ounces of liquor) per day during the 3-Day Solution. If you usually drink more than two drinks a day and don't think you can stay within the one-drink limit for three days, you may have a drinking problem. If so, it's more effective to deal with the drinking problem first, then use this plan.
- If you smoke more than 10 cigarettes per day, do not quit smoking while on this plan. Instead, quit smoking with

the support of your physician and a nicotine patch, before or after using this plan. If you smoke 10 or fewer cigarettes and want to quit smoking, you may or may not want to quit during these three days. Trust your gut feeling. It reflects the wisdom of your implicit learning in your feeling brain.

- If you are taking any medications that you think are unnecessary, do not stop taking them unless you have your physician's approval. *Stopping many medications can lead to severe or even life-threatening consequences.* Do not try to be your own doctor. Call your physician before making any changes.
- If you have emotional difficulties, medical problems, or are under unusual stress right now, postpone using this plan until you are feeling better.
- If you have a serious addiction to a substance, do not use this plan. Instead, get support to withdraw from the substance before using this plan.
- Before starting this or any health program, get your physician's approval. If you have any reservations that this might not be safe for you, do not use this plan.

Also, if you have formidable roadblocks to feeling good, consider addressing them in part before you begin the plan. For example, if you have insomnia, hormonal imbalances, or bone or joint pain, consider talking with your doctor about ways to get relief. If you are taking drugs for your mood that prevent you from feeling your feelings, speak with your physician about the merits of making small adjustments. Do not stop taking your medications, but check with your doctor to see if any adjustments can be made so that you can safely and easily access your feelings.

Do not use this plan if you are pregnant, as weight loss is not advised during pregnancy. If you are breast-feeding or if you have any medical condition in which nutrition plays a central role, check with your physician before using the plan and make any modifications he or she recommends. For example, if you have type 1 diabetes, the carbohydrate intake for this plan may be too low for the level of insulin you are currently taking.

If you have any doubts about the safety of this plan, speak with your physician before starting it. If at any time during your use of the plan, you don't think it is right for you, stop using it.

Do Some Lifestyle Surgery on Your Home, Car, and Office

Make it easier to eat and live above the line by cleaning up your environment. Here are some ideas to consider:

• Take all the foods that are not on the 1-2-3 Food Lists out of the house, out of your car, and away from your workplace. Throw them out, give them to a food bank, or store them in the garage or in the freezer, but keep them out of reach.

• Bring foods that you have checked off that you like on the 1-2-3 Food Lists into the house. Have them available at work and in the car. If there is White Stuff that you really need, be sure you have just the items that please you. Get rid of the rest.

• Be sure to have plenty of water and other sugar-free, caffeine-free beverages available wherever you are. Remove fruit juices, vegetable juices, and sodas from your home and car. Limit diet sodas to one per day. Try seltzer water or try mineral water with a slice of lemon, lime, or cucumber or with a dash of fruit juice (two ounces plus six ounces of mineral water).

• Shop almost exclusively on the perimeter of the grocery store, where the lean-protein foods, nonfat and low-fat dairy products, and fresh produce are. Buy organic when possible, shop at farmers' markets, and find other food stores that emphasize healthful foods.

• Have on hand an *abundance* of fruits and vegetables that you *love*, even if they cost considerably more than the tired, mundane alternatives. Having ready access to foods like strawberries, peaches, blueberries, baby carrots, and melons will make it easier to stay above the line with food.

• In addition to body work, identify ways in which you can become more active, particularly ways that are woven into your normal daily life, such as climbing stairs, walking to work or from the bus, or taking a walking break at lunch. Find a coworker who is willing to walk around the block with you during your lunch break or bring your walking shoes and your CD player and earphones to work and take a stroll all by yourself.

• Create more peace in your home and avoid information overload. If you live alone or those with whom you live agree, turn off your phone or screen your calls. Turn off pagers and cell phones. You might even change your outgoing message on your voice mail for these three days to let people know that except in the event of an emergency, you will not be returning calls for three days.

• Review the role of television in your life. It does not provide intimacy or activity. Limit your television viewing to no more than one hour on these three days. Better yet, turn it off completely. Make that easier by disconnecting the television or, if you have more than one, storing some of them in the garage.

• Review the role of the Internet and computer games in your life. They do not provide intimacy or activity. Limit your computer time after 5:00 p.m. to no more than one hour. Better yet, skip it altogether. If the computer is in a dominant place in your home, consider moving it to another location. Total "screen time" per day—that is, the time after 5:00 p.m. spent using computers, playing video games, or watching television—is limited to two hours.

• Protect yourself from information that does not meet your needs. Review the papers and magazines you read and the news programs you watch or to which you listen. Are they helping you turn off the drive to overeat? If not, do not expose yourself to them.

• Set an alarm on your watch, your computer, or your bedside clock so you will establish a rhythm of sleeping and waking. Schedule sleeping for at least eight hours and allow one additional hour of transition time. That gives you 30 minutes to stretch and create a mental expectation of your day in the morning and 30 minutes in the evening to review your day, check whether you stayed above the line, and become aware of the ways in which you feel grateful, happy, secure, and proud.

• Find a way to remind yourself to check in 10 times daily. Use natural pause points during the day or check in hourly between 9:00 a.m. and 6:00 p.m. daily with an automated reminder. Set your watch or cell phone to go off on the hour, each hour. Set your computer to remind you hourly. There are inexpensive watches available at most drugstores that can be set for an hourly check-in. If you want one that is preset to go off hourly or other ideas for reminding yourself to check in, visit our website.

• Toss out the scale. Being obsessed about weight is part of the problem for many of us. If you are interested in knowing how much weight you lose during these three days, weigh yourself the morning of the first day before breakfast and the fourth morning before breakfast. Otherwise, do not weigh. On an ongoing basis, what is best for many people is to weigh weekly. Then, if their weight begins to increase, they can deal with it right away. Although you should do what seems right for you, weighing more often can lead to weight preoccupation, which doesn't improve health or happiness.

Have on Hand, Clothes That Support a Positive Body Image

What you wear during this time is important because body image and self-image are intertwined. What if you're accustomed to paying no attention to your appearance or to dressing the way others think you should dress? Then do something different these three days. Enjoy your body and your appearance. Have fun with it. Wear clothes that reflect your personal style and that say, "I like my body" or "I have fun with my appearance."

Wearing clothes that are clean, fit well, and express your pride in your body enhances your sense of feeling whole, joyful, and integrated. Please check to see that you have clothes that reflect your body pride for all the intimacy time and body-work activities.

After all, you're starting a new life—above the line.

Select Your Menus for These Three Days

Although the menus for each day are presented and discussed at the relevant points throughout Chapters 13, 14, and 15, the menus are also collected separately in Chapter 16, "Menus for the 3-Day Solution Plan," for your convenience. Turn to Chapter 16 and peruse the menus. These foods will give you the balance of nutrition you need to stay above the line and turn off your drive to overeat. They were chosen because they are either easy and quick to prepare or generally available at most restaurants. For those who want to see more weight loss right away, the Chapter 16 menus provide slightly fewer calories than those in Chapter 18.

If these menus don't meet your needs—perhaps you're vegetarian or don't care for these foods—choose alternate menus from the ones in Chapter 18. It's important that you eat for both health and pleasure during the three days of the plan.

The menus for the three-day plan without additional White Stuff provide about one thousand calories per day. The alternate meals and snacks provide about twelve hundred to fourteen hundred calories per day. Your needs may differ based on your activity level, size, body composition, health status, and gender, but these levels are the recommended intakes advised for most people for ongoing weight loss. If you have any particular health problems or special needs, please consult your physician and/or a registered or licensed dietitian (see www.eatright.org for dietitians in your area).

Plan Your Daily Physical Activity

Think about what you will do for exercise. Each day, you will exercise for an hour unless you have health problems or have not exercised recently. In that case, exercise for the length of time that your physician recommends and exercise only with his or her approval.

However, if you are able to exercise, on the first day, you will do something that is either in nature or involves listening to music while you move.

The second day, you will do something that either helps you connect with yourself, such as yoga, dancing, or a solitary walk or run, or else something that helps you connect with another person, such as walking with a friend or playing on a basketball team.

The last day takes the most preparation because it involves some kind of exercise that is pure play—for example, ride horseback, play soccer or squash, go for a hike, fish, climb a mountain, dance to oldies, or dig in your garden. Just have fun and move at the same time.

Although the plan shows the major physical activity of the day in the afternoon, it can be done any time of the day and can be broken up into two or three segments, if you prefer.

Consider Options for Intimacy Time and Time to Restore

Planning time to restore is easy because your job is to do whatever is really relaxing and satisfying to you. Options are given for each day. The first day's focus is pleasure, the second day's is relaxation, and the last day's is inspiration.

Intimacy time, however, often takes some planning and, except for the first day, is usually done in the evenings. Begin thinking now about what would give you a sense of belonging to a group outside of work and family. What form of social intimacy on day 1 would be deeply satisfying to you—satisfying enough that you wouldn't want extra food?

On day 2, plan for sensual/sexual intimacy. This can range from a sensual experience with yourself—say, getting a massage or taking a hot bath with candles and music—to sexual activities alone or with a spouse or partner.

For day 3, consider how you will arrange for emotional intimacy. This requires another person who is willing to listen to you express your feelings and willing to share his or her feelings with you. If you live with someone, I suggest asking that individual about his or her willingness to do this, especially if the relationship is not perfect. Or if you prefer, ask someone else who you think might be willing. Both people use emotional housecleaning so there is a set process for each person that can be mutually rewarding.

Clip the 3-Day Solution Plan Pocket Reminders from This Book

In the appendix, there are three pocket reminders to guide you through the activities for each of the first three days. There is also a fourth pocket reminder for you to use during the second phase of the plan. For now, just clip the pocket reminders for the first three days, and use one each day.

The plan detailed in the next three chapters includes specific guidance for each aspect of each of the three days, so I recommend that you keep this book with you during these days. You can use the pocket reminders when it's time to check in with yourself, for quick access to the skills, and to keep yourself focused on the most important aspects of the day.

Review the accompanying checklist to make sure your preparations are complete, and that's it! Now it's time to begin your 3-Day Solution Plan!

Checklist: Preparing for a Solution

I have:

☐ Scheduled my 3-Day Solution for the following days:

_____.

☐ Found someone else to do this plan with me.

☐ Asked for support from those close to me.

☐ Made sure that this plan will be safe for me.

☐ Done some lifestyle surgery on my home, car, and office.

☐ Made sure I have on hand clothes that support a positive body image.

☐ Selected menus for these three days.

☐ Planned daily physical activity.

☐ Considered options for time to restore and intimacy time.

☐ Clipped the 3-Day Solution pocket reminders from this book.

13

Day 1: Detox

Introduction: The First Day

THIS IS YOUR first day of the 3-Day Solution Plan. By the end of the third day, your drive to overeat will have faded. You will have two important tools, Solution Skills and Mastery Living, which will jump-start lasting weight loss. You'll be fully equipped to do a cycle—the most powerful of the three Solution Skills—and will experience "life above the line," where you will have more clarity, vibrancy, and peace than you can remember. What's more, you'll lose weight: as much as five pounds.

For each of the three days, there is a step-by-step plan. Each plan has an introduction, so you will know what to expect, how you will feel, and the rewards you will experience on that particular day. Each plan outlines exactly what to do, from the moment you awaken in the morning until you go to sleep in the evening. Each day has its own pocket reminder that guides your progress; you also use it to record how you're doing. A checklist on which to record your progress also appears at the end of each day's plan.

Although these three days will be exciting and fulfilling, they will not always be easy. There may be times when you want to quit and when your critical inner voice tries to convince you that this will never work, that you aren't doing it perfectly enough, or that doing this plan doesn't matter.

It does matter. This is an opportunity to stop dieting and to start living more abundantly—and to acquire the skills that are the missing link in our lives. If you stick with this plan for three days, by the third day, you will feel so healthy and so happy—

and so empowered—that you will probably never want to go back. You will want to make these three days the start of a new life.

The purpose of the first day, detox, is to begin cleansing your body of the extra fat, sugar, salt, and calories you have been consuming and to begin separating from the reliance on food to destress. You will have clear guidelines for what to eat and drink, and a plan for the day that enables you to experience more fully the natural rewards of life. This day will also serve to rebalance your hormones and neurotransmitters. Plus, your Solution Skills will begin to retrain your feeling brain, making the lifestyle changes far easier to accomplish.

It's only three days. You can do this for three days!

What You Will Do Today

Solution Skills

Having a clear expectation and intention for the day will give you greater strength and clarity. You will start your day by bringing to mind a basic expectation for the day that expresses your vision of how you want your day to be. You will do this each morning on the plan, and the expectation will change and develop over the three days. This expectation will give you an internal limit, a focus for the day. It has a way of burrowing into your feeling brain and prompting a greater depth of change in your life.

After breakfast and your morning body work, you will begin using the first Solution Skill, checking in. You will use it hourly, 10 times today and 10 times a day over each of the next two days. Today, you focus on checking your feelings and needs and determining whether you are above the line. Once that foundational skill is put in place today, you can build on it during each of the next two days.

Here's how you will do this:

Step 1: Have your Solution day 1 pocket reminder in hand.
Keep your pocket reminder with you all day. A sample filled-in copy of both sides of the first day's pocket reminder appears on the following page.

Use one side to record your Solution Skills, your 10 daily check-ins, and your reflections at the end of the day. They are: "Checked in 10 times today?" "Did my best to stay above the line?" Use the other side to check off the 5 elements of Mastery Living. You'll also find a list there of all the basic feelings.

As you check in with yourself, refer to the Solution day 1 pocket reminder and check for any of the basic feelings. Then record your strongest feeling on the pocket reminder. Also record your needs and whether you are above or below the line. Do this each time you check in, using one line each time.

Step 2: How do I feel?

Each time you begin to use checking in, shift your focus to inside. Bring up a nurturing inner voice, and then ask yourself, "How do I feel?" Turn over your pocket reminder to the list of the basic feelings. Find the *strongest* applicable feeling listed and write that feeling on your pocket reminder on the first line under "How do I feel?"

If you don't know how you feel, put a question mark (?).

If your strongest feeling appears on that list, you're probably above the line. If you're above the line and a word other than those that describe the basic feelings comes to mind, try to use one of the basic feelings instead. For example, write in *angry* rather than *irritated* or *sad* rather than *disappointed.*

If you're below the line—such as feeling depressed, powerless,

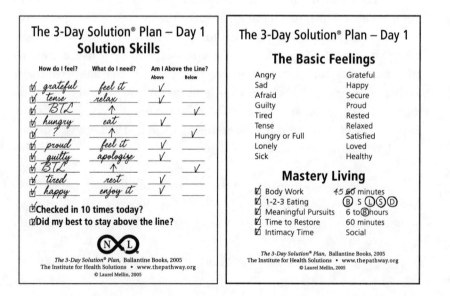

all-powerful, self-pitying, rebellious, hostile, panicked, ashamed, numb, or elated—just mark in *BTL*, to indicate below the line.

If a "smoke screen" such as feeling stressed, upset, miserable, or bored comes to mind, go under that smoke screen and see what is there. Smoke screens are clusters of feelings. If you can't figure out what feelings are under that smoke screen, write down *BTL* under "How do I feel?" If you can find several feelings that are under that smoke screen, identify the strongest one. If it's an above-the-line feeling, write it down under "How do I feel?" If it's a below-the-line feeling, write down *BTL*.

For example, you might say, "I'm stressed. That's a smoke screen. What feelings are under that smoke screen? Tense, angry, lonely. Those are all above-the-line feelings, but they are all merged together, making it difficult to determine your need. The strongest one at the moment is anger. I will write *anger* on the pocket reminder under 'How do I feel?' and check off 'Below' under 'Am I above the line?' "

Another time, you might say, "I'm miserable. What feelings are under that? I'm depressed, afraid, and tired. The strongest feeling is that I'm depressed. That's a below-the-line feeling. So I'll write down *BTL* under 'How do I feel?' and check off 'Below' under 'Am I above the line?' "

This system may sound complicated, but once you start using it over these three days, it will become far clearer. Rather than worrying that you're not doing it right, just jump in and try, referring back to this page when you need to. From the first time you check it, there is a positive effect. Even if you come up with no answers to any of the questions, simply asking them is progress, since it awakens your feeling brain.

Step 3: Am I above the line or below the line?
Next, ask yourself, "Am I above the line or below the line?" If the strongest feeling you identified was a basic feeling—it appeared on the list of basic feelings—you're probably above the line. To be more certain that you are, notice whether you have any of these symptoms of being below the line:

- *Extreme mood:* feeling very high or very low, with the mood accompanied by other signs of being below the line.

- *Staying stuck:* noticing that the feeling persists for hours or days rather than feeling the feeling and having it fade.
- *Obsessive thinking:* having obsessive, repetitive thoughts or having no feelings—that is, being emotionally numb.
- *Body awareness:* feeling aware of your mind but not your body, as if your body were only meant to carry your head around.
- *Passive or aggressive:* tending to be passive or aggressive rather than being assertive.
- *Merging, distancing, or control struggles:* being overly close or very removed or getting into control struggles.
- *Future or past:* focusing obsessively on the past or the future rather than on the current moment.
- *External solutions:* having strong urges or cravings for food or for another external solution.
- *Crossed wires:* identifying a need that has nothing to do with the feeling, such as feeling sad but perceiving that you "need" ice cream.

If this all seems very confusing, don't worry, because as you use it during the next three days, it will become clear to you. For during these three days, you'll probably keep going above and below the line all day long. That's normal!

Knowing when you're below the line is essential, because over the next three days, starting with day 2, you will use additional skills when you're below the line. You will not use those skills today, because you must first strengthen the skill of checking in, which will establish the foundation for the more advanced skills.

If you think you're below the line, put a check (✔) under "Below" on the first line on your pocket reminder under "Am I above the line?" If you think you're above the line, put a check under "Above." If you don't know, just write in a question mark (?)

Step 4: What do I need?

Next, ask yourself, "What do I need?" If you are above the line, identify the logical need, such as, "I feel hungry. I need to eat," or "I feel tense. I need to relax," or "I feel lonely. I need to call a friend." Identify that need and write it in the space under "What do I need?" for the first check-in on your pocket reminder. To the extent that you are able to meet that need, do so—for example, eat, relax, or call a friend.

If you are below the line, it's harder to know what you need. Or you may think you know what you need, but it's actually that you know what you want—after all, what you need and what you want are not always the same thing. A *want* is a below-the-line need.

What we really need when we're below the line is one thing: to get above the line, where our appetites fade and where we can identify what we *really* need! Nothing much good happens when we're below the line, so the priority is to reach for the skills, use them, and get above the line.

So if you're below the line, just mark an upward arrow (^) under "What do I need?" An upward arrow indicates that your need is to get above the line.

That's all you do. On this first day, you don't worry about getting above the line when you are below it—you just recognize that you're below the line. That is the most important thing you can do today: check your feelings and needs and determine whether you're above the line or below. Once you've practiced this skill for one day—the feeling brain changes only through practice—it will be easier to add the skills you will use on each of the next two days.

How can you feel better on the first day when you find that you're below the line? Just make a statement to yourself that begins to create a limit and gently guides you above the line. Try saying to yourself one or both of these statements when you find yourself below the line:

- "Just recognizing that I'm below the line is progress."
- "I expect myself to do my best to get above the line."

You will be checking in regularly today, for a total of 10 times. You can do it hourly with a watch alarm, a cell-phone reminder, a computer message, or another reminder that works for you. Or you can check in during natural change points in your day, such as when you're on your way to work, after you get settled at your job in the morning, when you take a restroom break, or before you eat. As long as you check in about once an hour during the day, find whatever rhythm of check-ins works best for you.

It is important to check in regularly and often, because that is where your power lies. Each time you check in, you will be disrupting the "party" that is going on below the line and throwing a new one above the line. You will begin to weaken the neural networks that support overeating and life below the line and strengthen the ones that turn off that drive and favor life above the line. Each time you do that, there is an effect. *Each time matters.*

Again, when you check in, just shift your attention from whatever you are doing. Take out your pocket reminder and ask yourself, "How do I feel?" "What do I need?" and "Am I above the line or below the line?" Mark your results on the pocket reminder for day 1. Then go on and meet your need and continue your day until the next check-in, either when your alarm sounds one hour later or during your next natural check-in time.

If you'd like more information on checking in, please turn to page 104. If you want more support, visit www.thepathway.org, where there is free access to a discussion board for those with a copy of this book.

Mastery Living

The Mastery Living part of the day is intentionally gentle. You'll be engaging in meaningful pursuits in an intense and focused way for six to eight hours and taking between 45 minutes and one hour for lunch. You will take one hour of time to restore that will involve doing whatever is pleasurable to you. Body work for one hour will involve exercising outside in nature or exercising while you listen to music. Your intimacy time will involve something social that you enjoy.

This might sound like a lot to fit into a day! However, you are engaging in only six to eight hours of meaningful pursuits, so there is much more time than you might think. Also, this is a three-day intensive training in the method, not something you expect of yourself on an ongoing basis. When you complete your third day, you can begin the plan for days 4 to 14, discussed in Chapter 17. It is much less challenging but stays true to the same principles. You'll be doing something for 1-2-3 Eating, meaningful pursuits, time to restore, and intimacy time each day. However, you will touch on each of them rather than devoting as much time to each.

Some people come to these three days wanting quick weight loss. The menu plans that are preselected (see Chapter 16) will produce that for you, particularly if you minimize your intake of White Stuff. The menus require minimal cooking and easy shopping. All of the meals have simple variations that can be ordered in most restaurants. The advantage of quick weight loss is initial encouragement. It's motivating to see results right away. Most people who use these menus report a weight loss of three to five pounds.

If you are less concerned about rapid weight loss and would be happy to lose two to three pounds in three days, choose menus from Chapter 18, "More Menus from Solution Providers." These menus offer greater variety and contain slightly more calories and carbohydrates.

If you are eating out, the menus for the three-day plan meals in Chapter 16 include restaurant options.

Some salads and vegetables are so simple that they don't require a recipe. The vegetables that are in the recipes in the plan can be eaten freely, as their caloric density is low and their nutritional benefits are high. They can be cooked any way you would like, avoiding trans and saturated fats and using no fat or modest amounts of healthy fats. Steaming is best. Add no more than one teaspoon of oil to the vegetables you consume in any particular meal. Similarly, fresh greens and the vegetables in salads can be eaten in unlimited amounts, but keep the dressing to no more than one tablespoon of oil for your portion of the salad at any meal.

If you want rapid weight loss, stay with the portion sizes shown in the menus. However, if that is less important to you, eat what is shown on the menus or a little bit more, if you are hungry. Portion sizes matter, particularly now when your hormones, neurotransmitters, and peptides are in harmony with a higher weight and intake of food. Later, when your body has adjusted to a lower body weight and a lower intake of calories, fat, and carbohydrates, you will be better able to trust that the signals your body gives you are correct. You will be better able to eat in response to hunger, and trust that portion sizes will vary slightly as a result, and that is fine.

Again, during this time of detoxing and adjusting to losing weight rather than holding on to it, be aware of portion sizes. Each day's recipes and menus have specific amounts shown. But even though the signs your body is giving you may not be accurate right now, don't abandon yourself. If you really feel that you need more food, then by all means, have it.

These menus are packed with nutrition. Having optimal nutrition is essential to your weight solution, and to boost your nutritional intake, I suggest taking these nutritional supplements daily during the plan: one therapeutic dose of a multivitamin/mineral supplement (for example, Centrum), 500 milligrams of calcium, and 1,000 milligrams of omega-3 fatty acids. The therapeutic dose of multivitamins and minerals supports your overall health, well-being, and weight loss. It takes optimal nutrition to release body fat! Also, although the plan includes about 900 milligrams of calcium per day, taking an extra 500 milligrams each day is prudent for fat burning as well as mood, since calcium decreases muscle tension. If you are post-menopausal, take 1,000 milligrams of calcium. Omega-3 fatty acids prevent heart disease and bolster emotional balance. If you have heart disease or a family history of heart disease, take 3,000 milligrams of omega-3 fatty acids. As with all vitamins or nutritional supplements, please check with your physician before taking them.

How You Will Feel Today

On this first day of the plan, you may have lots of strong feelings. You may feel high, elated that you are starting, but also fearful that the plan will not work or that you will quit. You may feel angry that you have to do it at all or grateful that there is a plan and hopeful that this will be the start of something—finally—that will offer a true Solution.

Because you are not dampening your feelings by overeating, you may feel a whole range of strong feelings today. That's great! The feelings are starting to emerge, which is progress. You are no longer pushing down the feelings or connecting with external solutions rather than connecting with yourself.

Of the three days, this is the one in which you will be most sensitive to the transition. To the extent that you are not accustomed to eating healthy foods and exercising regularly, your body will notice the change. If the changes make you worry that this plan is not right for you, then stop using it and consult your physician. But do expect that you will feel different. That's how transformation occurs. You may, in fact, feel wonderful. You may relish the chance to take really good care of yourself and jump-start a new life.

The Rewards You Will Reap Today

The most important thing you will do today is to begin. Even if not everything goes exactly the way you want it to go—you miss your time to restore, or your intimacy time social activity falls through— at least, you have begun. By the end of three days, it will be more than worth it.

The rewards from this particular day will be substantial. By the end of the day, not only will your hormones and neurotransmitters have started to shift, but you will also have put into place the basic foundation of your Solution Skills. The key aspects of a lifestyle that turns off the drive to overeat will be starting to take hold, too.

It will be an extremely productive day!

Now you are prepared to begin. Just do the best you can to follow the plan. Even if you don't do it perfectly, just jump in and start!

Morning Expectations: Creating Your Day

Creating Your Day

Create a basic expectation for your day.

Awaken

As you awaken, bring to mind that this is the first of three days that will lead to life above the line, where the drives to overeat have faded. You eat less because those cravings and drives have subsided. You've stopped wanting the extra food.

Connect Inside

Take time to transition from sleep to wakefulness, breathing deeply and shifting your awareness inside. Become conscious that there is a safe place inside you, even if that place is very small. It is a place that feels comforting to you, a sanctuary. During the next three days, you will move your attention often from what is outside you to that place inside. That's where you will find a supportive inner voice that will ask you the questions of the Solution Skills.

Create Your Day

When you are ready, begin to turn your attention to your day. Take several minutes to consciously create your day—the way you want it to happen. Make solid an intention that will guide you through this day. Use the following intention or a similar one that works for you.

I expect myself to do the best I can to stay above the line.

Visualize yourself walking through your day, staying above the line. There will be upsets, temptations, and distractions, but you will keep on target. You will not focus on pleasing others, getting everything perfect, or being in complete control. Instead, all you intend is that you will stay above the line.

By creating your day, stating an expectation or intention that is your focus, your feeling brain awakens. The neural networks that focus on staying above the line strengthen.

Morning Body Work: Wake-up Stretch

> ## Wake-up Stretch
>
> - *Shift your focus:* Shift your focus to inside yourself. Be aware of the center of your body, a safe place within, your sanctuary.
> - *Move as you please:* Notice any urge you have to stretch and honor it. Perhaps stretch your hands to the ceiling, then to the walls, do foot circles, point your toes, stretch your heels. Honor each impulse to stretch, and move slowly and notice the joy of it.
> - *Full-body stretch:* Do one last stretch of your full body. Make your body into the shape of an X with your arms and legs as far apart as possible, gently stretching your entire body.
> - *Relax!* Notice a sense of relaxation and peace flow through your body.

If you keep that basic expectation in the back of your mind throughout the day, you will notice it affecting your experience. You will notice small things change. You will notice that you stay above the line or are able to do things that amaze you.

Right now, you may not be sure what being above the line means or how to get above the line when you are below. That does not matter. Having that basic expectation in place begins to change your feeling brain, and your feeling brain is where the drive to overeat resides.

Before you go on with your day, take one additional moment and state that expectation to yourself: *I expect myself to do the best I can to stay above the line.*

Begin Your Day and Stretch

Start the day by honoring your body. Even a short morning stretch can give you a good start to the day and integrate your mind and body. Stretching your body in the morning helps you start the day feeling whole—and it feels good!

There will be a different morning body work each day, so you can experiment with different body awakenings. Today, you will do the wake-up stretch, described above.

After you stretch, have your great-start breakfast and shower and dress. As you wash and groom, pay particular attention to taking good care of your body, appreciating what you like about your appearance, and wearing clothes that support your body pride.

Eat a Great-Start Breakfast

As you eat, focus on enjoying your food. That's difficult to do when the television is on. Turn it off. Do not read the paper when you are eating. Look at your food; notice it going into your mouth; savor the textures, flavors, and smells; and enjoy swallowing each bite.

Great-Start Breakfast: Light Eggs and Fresh Strawberries

Light Eggs and Fresh Strawberries

Light Eggs (see recipe on page 265)
1 cup of fresh strawberries

Water, decaffeinated coffee or tea, or herbal tea, with 1 percent low-fat or nonfat milk and sugar substitute, if desired

White Stuff: 1 cup of coffee, 1 teaspoon butter for cooking eggs, or whatever you really need

It's above the line to start eating when you are hungry and stop eating when the hunger disappears. When you are not aware of signs of hunger, your body hunger is satisfied. If you wait 10 minutes, you will feel full. If, instead, you eat until you are full, after 10 minutes, you will feel very full and you will have overeaten. If you start eating when you do not have body hunger or eat past the time the body hunger disappears, that is overeating. That is eating for emotional hunger—that is, appetite—not for body hunger. That is below the line.

Pumping up your skill to be sensitive to signals of body hunger is extremely important. It's really hard to get a good body-hunger reading if you are eating too rapidly. The feedback mechanism in your body includes sensors in your esophagus, stomach, and intestines as well as blood sugar, and all these signals take time to register in your brain. If you tend to bolt food, slow down your pace of eating by taking a midmeal break. Eat half your breakfast, read the paper or do a chore for three minutes, then eat the second half of your meal.

During these three days, you will begin to sharpen your ability to eat in response to hunger, not appetite. You already know about the times when you eat and realize that you aren't hungry, but what about the times when you feel hungry but your body doesn't need food? For example, you can feel hungry because your insulin levels have sent you on a blood-sugar low. Although you have plenty of fat stored and don't really need extra food, your blood sugar is low, so you feel hungry. If your neurotransmitters are out of balance, you'll crave food, but that craving has little or nothing to do with your body's actual need for nutrition.

So, as you begin this three-day plan, you may not always know whether you're hungry. Despite all these complexities, the following basic limits are essential to having a weight solution:

- Eat when you feel body hunger.
- Stop when the hunger disappears so that you feel just satisfied, not full.
- Don't eat when you do not feel body hunger.

This will soon become easier because both the skills and this lifestyle rebalance neurotransmitters and hormones to make reading hunger signals more accurate. You will become increasingly sensitive to your hunger signals as you move through these three days. At some point, when you have a Solution, you wouldn't consider eating when you were not hungry—not a grape, not a stick of celery, nothing! You don't eat when you aren't hungry. That will be a very strong limit that is automatic and spontaneous and carved into the neural networks in your feeling brain.

Breakfast is the time of day when cortisol is the highest. It's cortisol that triggers increases in insulin and glucose, so it's really easy for a high-refined-carbohydrate breakfast to trigger a spike in glucose and insulin followed by a midmorning blood-sugar low. This breakfast—which includes protein, fiber, and healthy fat and is low in carbs—will have staying power throughout the morning.

If you use sweetener, choose Splenda or stevia, if you can. Some people are sensitive to aspartame, as it can cause nerve cells to overfire. Some people who use large amounts of aspartame or are particularly sensitive to it have symptoms such as headaches, dizziness, memory loss, slurred speech, numbness, mood swings, depression, insomnia, fatigue, hearing loss, low blood sugar, and decreased sense of taste that disappear when they stop using it. Sucralose (Splenda) or the herb stevia appear to be safer sweeteners.

If you drink coffee rather than tea or decaffeinated coffee, limit it to one six-ounce cup. If you drink tea that contains caffeine rather than decaffeinated tea or caffeine-free herbal tea, limit it to two six-ounce cups. Caffeine increases the tendency to have a midmorning blood-sugar low.

The rationale for light eggs, tossing out one or more of the egg yolks when you have several eggs, is to boost protein without increasing cholesterol. Egg whites are a fat-free source of protein, and egg yolks contain high concentrations of cholesterol. Cooking the eggs in nonstick spray plus a small amount of canola-oil margarine or even a teaspoon of butter, if you don't have heart disease, boosts the fat and the staying power of the breakfast without adding the cholesterol in another egg yolk.

If you prefer, use egg substitute, but the calories and fat are substantially lower, so be sure to cook them not just in cooking spray but in a small amount of canola margarine. Including a bit of Healthy Fat in the meal reduces the need for excessive protein intake and provides calories that are not from carbohydrates. This helps turn off the drive to overeat and keeps blood-sugar levels more stable. Healthy Fats are free of saturated fats and trans fats and their deleterious effects on blood vessels. Because they contain more than twice the calories of carbohydrates and protein, you will use Healthy Fats in small amounts, but it is important to use them.

This is a 1-2-3 Meal:

1. The Fiber Group: Strawberries
2. Healthy Fat: Canola margarine
3. The Protein Group: Light Eggs

White Stuff

Of all meals, breakfast is the most important meal at which to limit White Stuff. However, you are more important than your food. If you really need White Stuff, you should definitely have it. How do you know whether you really need it? Later on, you will learn how to do a cycle and get above the line, so you will be able to tell whether you really need it.

For now, it's better to skip the White Stuff because you're trying to detox. But if something is really important to you, ask yourself, "Do I really need it?" That's not "Do I *want* it?" but "Do I *really need* it?" If the answer is a resounding "Yes!" then have it. Otherwise, skip it. The essential pain? You can't always have what you want when you want it. Change is difficult. The earned reward? Detoxing. Turning off the drive to overeat. Life above the line!

After eating your breakfast and enjoying your food, continue on to morning meaningful pursuits!

Morning Meaningful Pursuits: Hourly Check-ins

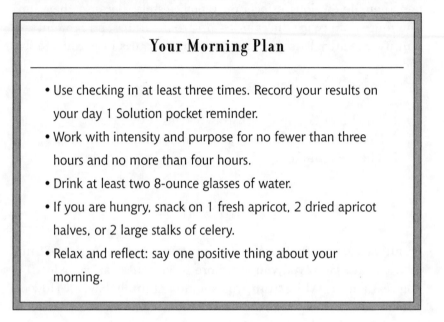

Your Morning Plan

- Use checking in at least three times. Record your results on your day 1 Solution pocket reminder.
- Work with intensity and purpose for no fewer than three hours and no more than four hours.
- Drink at least two 8-ounce glasses of water.
- If you are hungry, snack on 1 fresh apricot, 2 dried apricot halves, or 2 large stalks of celery.
- Relax and reflect: say one positive thing about your morning.

Use Solution Skills

On your way to your morning's meaningful pursuits, begin checking in. Just go inside yourself and check how you feel and what you need. Decide whether you are above or below the line. If you don't know, put a question mark. If you are above the line, identify your logical need, then meet it. If you are below the line, your need is to get above the line. Just say to yourself, *"I expect myself to do the best I can to stay above the line."* Then watch what occurs!

Do this once an hour all morning, using whatever reminder works best for you—an alarm set hourly, a reminder on the computer, or even a Solution buddy calling to remind you. You can also use normal transitions of the day, such as checking in on your way to work and then, just after you settle into your tasks, checking in again. Or you might check in each time you go to the restroom. At least three times this morning, check in with yourself and record your findings on your pocket reminder.

Work with Intensity and Purpose

You will be engaged with intensity and purpose for three to four hours this morning. In order to turn off the drive to overeat, you need to get serotonin from something other than food. You will get that flood of satisfaction from doing meaningful pursuits, regardless of whether it is taking care of children, building a house, slaying computer dragons, or waiting tables. Focus and intensity increase your dopamine levels. It's only with a rise in dopamine that when you take a break, you will relax, reflect on your accomplishments, and feel the satisfaction of a rise in serotonin. No focus, no reward.

As you engage in meaningful pursuits, keep in mind the day you are creating for yourself: *I expect myself to do my best to stay above the line.* Don't worry if you aren't sure whether you're above the line or don't know how to get above the line if you're below. Just allow the expectation to wander around in your feeling brain and begin to change it.

Have Water and a Snack

During the morning, drink at least two 8-ounce glasses of water or some other beverage that contains no caffeine or calories, such as tea, either decaffeinated or herbal caffeine-free tea. Add a slice of lemon, lime, or cucumber in a glass of mineral water, or have decaffeinated coffee with a splash of low-fat or nonfat milk in it. Just a reminder from earlier on: diet drinks are White Stuff, as they are sweetened with aspartame, which can spike insulin levels. But if having diet sodas is important to you, limit them to one per day. If you are hungry, snack on an apricot, fresh or dried, or if you'd prefer more volume, have two large stalks of celery.

Pause and Reflect

After you have worked with intensity and purpose for at least three hours and not more than four hours, stop working. Even if there is more to do, turn away from work and toward having a balancing lunch.

However, before you start lunch, pause and reflect. All morning, you have been focused and intense. If you continued that for the rest of the day, your dopamine and serotonin would be drained by late afternoon and you'd be vulnerable to overeating. It would be far more difficult for you to respond to your body's hunger, and you'd be far more likely to respond instead to an excessive appetite. You would have less energy to engage in activities that naturally re-balance your neurotransmitters—enjoying nature, art, music, and other pleasures that are calorie-free.

Take a moment to pause and reflect. This will boost serotonin, which will trigger a decrease in dopamine. Just take one minute to take a big, deep breath and reflect on your morning. Then say one positive thing to yourself about your morning. After you do, allow your body to relax and feel that surge of satisfaction that your positive thoughts created!

Balancing Lunch: California Chicken Salad

California Chicken Salad

California Chicken Salad (see recipe on page 269)

Water, decaffeinated coffee or tea, or herbal tea, with 1 percent low-fat or nonfat milk and sugar substitute, if desired

White Stuff: diet soda, 1 cup of coffee, or whatever you really need

By now, it's reasonable to expect that you are hungry.

Notice your hunger level. If you're not hungry, you may have overeaten for breakfast or had a snack when you didn't need one. That's important information from which to learn for tomorrow. Or you could be on an endorphin or dopamine high that may take away your appetite for lunch and set you up to crash during midafternoon or in the evening. If you are, count on slowing the pace and intensity of your work. If you are ravenous, that's something else to notice. Perhaps you needed that midmorning snack.

It's fine to be a little bit hungry, because you are taking off weight, but it's important not to let yourself get too hungry, because that affects your ability to check in with yourself and identify your feelings. Also, excessive hunger can trigger overeating.

Eat a Balancing Lunch

Take a moment to relax before you start eating and appreciate that, to turn off the drive to overeat, it's important to savor every bite and to eat slowly. Look at your food. Smell your food. Take small bites and chew each bite well. Notice how it feels to swallow the food. Can you feel the food in your stomach? Stay conscious and attentive to each aspect of the experience of eating, from the time you take your first bite to the time you swallow your last.

You will have started eating when you felt hungry. During the second half of your meal, check in after every bite and ask yourself, "Do I still feel hungry? Do I still sense feelings of hunger?" When the answers are no, stop eating. Wait 10 minutes. You will be full. If you are not full, you can choose to eat a few bites more.

Because you are detoxing today and may be for a while, your hormones and neurotransmitters may distort the accuracy of your hunger cues. So if you are still hungry after eating a reasonable amount, eat more but make it a big plate of leafy greens, with lots of tomatoes. That will trigger hormonal changes that send the message to your brain that you are full.

If you still feel hungry after eating the California Chicken Salad and an extra plate of greens and tomatoes, stop eating. Your body has had enough food to satisfy body hunger. Your hormones and neurotransmitters will adjust in time. Right now, they are still misfiring and sending you signals that are not accurate. Push back from the table and continue with your day.

This is a very balancing lunch. By having a healthy portion of fiber, protein, and Healthy Fat at lunch, you will stay focused with energy all afternoon. You can have access to this meal almost anywhere. It doesn't have to be on the menu at a restaurant. If you go into any restaurant that serves salads, just ask for a bed of greens with grilled chicken, with a slice of avocado and tomatoes on top. Request an olive oil–based dressing on the side and sprinkle on your salad one tablespoon of dressing. This is also an easy dish to make at home or to take with you to work. Drink plenty of liquids.

This is a 1-2-3 Meal:

1. The Fiber Group: Greens and tomatoes
2. Healthy Fats: Olive oil vinaigrette, avocado
3. The Protein Group: Chicken breast

Prepare for Your Afternoon

After you've eaten, take a walk, call a friend, or go outside and get some fresh air. Do not stay at your place of work for the entire lunchtime. Take at least a few minutes to have a change of scenery.

Be sure to continue your hourly check-ins during this time.

If you tend to push yourself too hard during the day, shift gears during lunchtime. You are at risk of getting on a "worker's high" and depleting your dopamine and serotonin by midafternoon. Use this lunch break to restore yourself. Even 10 minutes of fresh air and moving your body can break the escalating stress. Breathe deeply. Check in with yourself. Relax.

On the other hand, if your pursuits are not demanding or structured enough, the risk in the afternoon is that you won't have that energy and intensity that turn off the drive to overeat. You won't get that increase in dopamine that is essential to releasing the flood of serotonin that will satisfy you.

Afternoon Meaningful Pursuits: Hourly Check-ins

Your Afternoon Plan

- Use checking in at least three times and record your findings on your day 1 Solution pocket reminder.
- Work with intensity and purpose for no fewer than three hours and no more than four hours.
- Drink at least two 8-ounce glasses of water.
- If you are hungry, snack on 1 small apple and 5 cashews or almonds.
- Pause and reflect: say one positive thing about your afternoon.

Take a moment during this lunch break to consider the pace of your afternoon, either increasing it or decreasing it so that, three or four hours from now, your neurotransmitters will be reasonably balanced and your drive to overeat will be low.

You have eaten a balancing lunch. Continue with afternoon meaningful pursuits!

Use Solution Skills

After a satisfying lunch break, you are more above the line. The challenge is to stay there. Stress has a way of piling up during the afternoon, so it's important to be careful to check in with yourself often, if not hourly.

Start your afternoon by bringing to mind your most basic expectation: *I expect myself to do the best I can to stay above the line.* Notice how having that expectation—rather than the expectation that you have to be perfect, to please everyone, to be in complete control, and all those other below-the-line expectations—eases your tension.

About 80 percent of problems disappear if you just stay above the line, and the other 20 percent are far easier to manage from there.

Work with Intensity and Purpose

If there are *too many* demands on you this afternoon, pace yourself. Slow down and focus. Take five-minute breaks every hour, simply to cut the tension. Although the feeling brains of those around you are naturally apt to seduce you below the line, stick with your basic expectation of staying above the line. Others can be as below the line as they choose to be. Your job is to draw a border in the sand around yourself and stay above the line.

If there are *too few* demands, find things to do that excite, energize, and fulfill you. Find something you care about doing and push yourself to do it well. Find something that challenges you, so that after focusing for three to four hours, you can feel that flood of satisfaction and pride. Even if your job is not perfect or intense, create that intensity for yourself. Seek higher ground. Notice how you move your body, how you speak to people. Focus intensely on being more authentic, remembering more, being more efficient, using the skills more deeply or more often. Create an afternoon of intensity and purpose.

Have Water and a Snack

Drink plenty of water or other sugar-free, caffeine-free beverages— at least two 8-ounce glasses. Have a snack if you are hungry. If your body work is planned for late afternoon, even if you are only slightly hungry, have a small snack.

Pause and Reflect

After another three to four hours of focused activity, stop working. Check off "Meaningful Pursuits" on your pocket reminder. At that point, leave your work behind you. Take your body away from your work site, and take your mind off work, too.

It is time to create a different sort of fulfillment in life, engaging in activities that nourish your body, mind, and spirit effectively, so that you can return to your work tomorrow and rock!

At this point in the afternoon, your dopamine and serotonin may be somewhat drained. As you did this morning, take a moment to pause and reflect. Say one positive thing to yourself about your afternoon. Allow the good feelings and relaxation that follow to please you.

You may have four or more check-ins yet to do. That's fine. Just do them, approximately one per hour, until you have checked off 10 for the day.

Afternoon Body Work: Nature or Music

Nature or Music

For 45 to 60 minutes:

- Move your body in *nature:* walk outside, hike, cross-country ski, play basketball, ride a bike, or garden.
- Exercise while listening to *music:* work out wearing headphones, go to a dance class, or turn on music and dance.

Exercise for 45 to 60 Minutes

Your eating is above the line. You've been checking in with yourself and engaging in meaningful pursuits, and now it's time to reward yourself by taking one hour to move your body. If you're just beginning to get fit, you may need to limit the time to 45 minutes; otherwise, move for one hour.

The goal is to do something that has three benefits:

1. You move your body at the intensity that is right for you. If you have not been exercising, move very slowly. If you have been moving, exercise more vigorously. Safety is the first consideration.

2. When you finish the hour, you feel integrated and whole. You sense a harmony among mind, body, and spirit.
3. You give yourself a serotonin boost. Exercise that is not exhausting boosts serotonin and balances dopamine. In addition, you will give yourself a greater "reward density"—payoff per minute—by combining exercise with another known serotonin enhancer.

Today, you will choose to add being in nature or listening to music to your exercise. Or if you prefer, do something outdoors that also involves music.

Today is an especially important day to exercise because you are detoxing from eating too much food, too much fat, too much sugar, or using too much of another external solution. Your neurotransmitters may be sending you cravings, or you may even feel disoriented and sense that you are grieving a loss. You may fear that without the fat, sugar, alcohol, or whatever, you can't possibly get by. This activity will help to balance your chemicals and keep you above the line.

Healthy Dinner: Flank Steak and Green Beans

Flank Steak and Green Beans

Grilled Flank Steak Teriyaki (see recipe on page 280)

Spicy Garlic Green Beans (see recipe on page 288)

Butter Lettuce with Feta and Cucumber (see recipe on page 277)

Cantaloupe slices topped with raspberries

Water, decaffeinated coffee or tea, or herbal tea, with 1 percent low-fat or nonfat milk and sugar substitute, if desired

White Stuff: 5 ounces of fine red wine, whipped cream on dessert, or whatever you really need

By the time you have finished the hour of exercise, you should not be exhausted. It's important not to overexercise. Instead, notice a certain sense of *happiness* about you and pride in your body. You *feel* good. It can be subtle, but that's what you're shooting for: having distinct feelings of pride in your body and a sense of being at peace with yourself.

This is the most challenging day. It will get easier after this! Keep in mind the earned reward: No more diets! Lasting weight loss. Life above the line!

Eat a Healthy Dinner

Your body needs healthy foods in the evening, for the physical activity of the day is done, and the evening is often sedentary and followed by a period of sleep. However, at the end of the day, dinner often feels like your reward. Intimacy time and time to restore are our rewards, but dinner must taste good and sustain you until morning.

By not overeating in the evening, you'll have the energy for pleasurable activities all evening. Even your family or household responsibilities will be easier to accomplish. The extra food will not weigh you down and make you feel lethargic.

Evening is the time when overeating can be the least advantageous. Insulin levels are high in the evening, and loading up on sugary foods will further spike them and cause more fat deposition while you are asleep. If you decide to have White Stuff, notice that if you choose the very best quality foods or beverages and consume them slowly, savoring each bite or each sip, you won't need so much.

Enjoy bite after bite until your hunger disappears. If you are still hungry after eating today's dinner menu with a serving of meat about as large as your fist, you're probably not experiencing body hunger. You may *want* more food, have an appetite for it, but your body doesn't *need* it.

It's okay to eat in response to wanting the food even though your body doesn't need it, but it's hard to lose weight if you do that. If it's really important to you to continue eating, then by all means, do. If the essential pain of stopping eating feels *huge*—bigger than the benefit of staying above the line, feeling vibrant, and losing weight—then eat more. However, choose 1-2-3 Foods rather than

White Stuff, and preferably veggies and fruits. But, if you really need White Stuff, then definitely have it.

When your hunger disappears, push away from the table. Your survival need for food, your body hunger, has been satisfied. Take a few moments after you eat to relax and turn your attention to meeting your next survival need, which is safety: taking time to restore yourself and time for intimacy.

This is a 1-2-3 Meal:

1. The Fiber Group   Beans, mixed greens
2. Healthy Fats   Pine nuts and olive oil
3. The Protein Group   Grilled flank steak

Use Solution Skills

Before you continue with time to restore and intimacy time, please check your pocket reminder and make plans for doing any checking in you have left to do. By the time you go to bed this evening, it's important to have checked in with yourself and recorded your findings 10 times.

If you're having difficulty fitting everything in, you're not alone. It's a big adjustment! You don't have to do this perfectly. Just do the best you can. Consider asking for more help. It's below the line to be passive or aggressive. It's above the line to be assertive and to ask for help.

Now, go on to the next activity. You've almost completed your first day on the plan!

Time to Restore: Pleasure

Pleasure

Spend one hour of uninterrupted time doing whatever pleases you.

Take Time to Restore

Spend at least one hour doing whatever gives you pure pleasure. Check in with yourself to see how you feel and what you really need. It's a reasonable expectation that at this point in the first day of your 3-Day Solution, you could feel anything from sick, depressed, panicked, and hostile to healthy, happy, grateful, and proud. You may feel all of these things!

However, in the back of your mind, you are keeping that basic expectation: *I expect myself to do the best I can to stay above the line.* Staying above the line means taking care of your health and your happiness, so take this one hour to be "off-limits" to those around you and to do whatever pleases you. Do the best you can to find something that really "does it" for you, that gives you just what you most need.

Examples include reading a book that gives you a mental vacation; doing something creative, such as painting a picture or working on a craft; taking a long, hot shower or bath; or puttering in the garden, meditating or praying, or spending one entire hour simply relaxing all by yourself!

Do whatever brings you pure pleasure for a full hour.

Intimacy Time: Social Intimacy

> ### Social Intimacy
>
> Engage in a social activity that enhances your sense of belonging.

Take Time for Intimacy

Today's suggested intimacy activity focuses on social intimacy, on honoring your belonging to a group outside of your family that shares a common focus or interest. Staying connected to others is a survival need, just like eating.

Our genetic comfort zone is to be in a tribe, which means having nearly constant physical proximity and deep emotional affiliation and interdependence. That's why, when we gather with others and have a sense of safety and belonging, our serotonin levels increase and our appetites fade.

There is no need to engage in any social activity that is demanding or that brings up your need to please others or your desire to distance. You don't have to go to a cocktail party if you don't like cocktail parties! Instead, choose something that is easy, fun, and comfortable. It's best to be with others physically, but do what is possible for you.

Some examples: visiting with neighbors, having coffee or dinner with a friend, attending a community gathering, attending a lecture or book signing, going out to a club and listening to music, going to a sporting event, going to the park with your dog and visiting with other dog owners, going shopping with a friend, going to a religious study group, or calling a very special friend and catching up.

Sometimes time to restore, intimacy time, and healthy dinners overlap. How do you know whether it still "counts" when you multitask? It has to do with whether your needs are met. For example, if you had a quick dinner with a friend, you could check off both intimacy time and healthy dinner. However, did that quick meal satisfy your need for social intimacy, giving you a sense of belonging and being part of something outside yourself? If it did, then it counts for both, but if your need was not met, it does not. Go home and find another way to be sure your need to feel part of a group with a shared interest or goal is met.

Be sure to check in with yourself during this time, to complete your 10 check-ins for the day.

Reap Your Rewards

Complete your day by making the final check marks on your pocket reminder. Check whether you did your best to stay above the line today, did 10 check-ins, and did something for each element of Mastery Living.

Evening Check-in: Earned Rewards

Earned Rewards

Ask yourself:

    Did I do my best to stay above the line?

    Did I check in with myself at least 10 times?

    Was my eating above the line?

    Did I take time for exercise, work, intimacy, and relaxation?

Feel the earned rewards:

    I feel grateful that . . .

    I feel happy that . . .

    I feel secure that . . .

    I feel proud that . . .

You have completed your first day of the 3-Day Solution.

This was the most difficult of the three days. What you accomplished today will give you a foundation for the progress you will make in the next two days.

If you have a tendency to be hard on yourself, you might minimize your accomplishments. You might say, "I didn't do it perfectly. I forgot to do this. I couldn't squeeze that in."

That's *so* below the line. It's not easy to attempt this—especially the first day, when you are detoxing and transitioning to a new lifestyle! You have completed your first day of the 3-Day Solution Plan. Congratulations!

Conclude your day early. Allow for plenty of time to get to sleep and sleep a minimum of 8 hours. Spend one more hour of quiet time in bed, as you retire or before arising.

As you drift off to sleep, do your evening check-in, asking yourself:

Did I do my best to stay above the line?
Did I check in with myself 10 times?
Was my eating above the line?
Did I take time for exercise, meaningful activities,
    intimacy, and relaxation?

After you answer those questions, pause for another moment
and feel the earned rewards of your day, completing the sentences
with whatever words come into your mind:

I feel grateful that . . .
I feel happy that . . .
I feel secure that . . .
I feel proud that . . .

Then turn off the light and relax into sleep. After your first day on
the plan, you are on your way to turning off the drive to overeat and
living life above the line! Day 2 will be very rewarding and far easier.

Day 1: Detox Checklist

☐ Morning expectations:	creating your day
☐ Morning body work:	wake-up stretch
☐ Great-start breakfast:	Light Eggs and Fresh Strawberries
☐ Morning meaningful pursuits:	hourly check-ins
☐ Balancing lunch:	California Chicken Salad
☐ Afternoon meaningful pursuits:	hourly check-ins
☐ Afternoon body work:	nature or music
☐ Healthy dinner:	Flank Steak and Green Beans
☐ Time to restore:	pleasure
☐ Intimacy time	social intimacy
☐ Evening check-in:	earned rewards

14
Day 2: Connection

THIS IS YOUR second day of the 3-Day Solution Plan. This day was designed to bring you an abundance of positive feelings so that the drive to overeat continues to decrease.

You will be strengthening your Solution Skills and learning to pop yourself above the line, and you will have the most personal pleasure this evening, when the drives to overeat would otherwise be increasing.

What You Will Do Today
Solution Skills

You will begin your day by creating an expectation that reflects what you want for yourself, in life and on this particular day. This expectation reflects the rewards you most value in life. Keeping this expectation in the back of your mind affects your feeling brain and creates an internal limit and purpose for your day.

You will also build your Solution Skills today. Now that you have a sturdy base of checking in regularly throughout the day, you are ready to expand your skills to include emotional housecleaning. For a more complete description of this skill, please turn to page 113.

After breakfast and your morning body work, you will begin using the skill of checking in. As you did yesterday, you will check in 10 times, but today, when you are below the line, you will use emotional housecleaning.

Today, when you check in, if you're below the line, you will have a skill to use that will pop you up above the line. Using it can take two to five minutes. Also, you're better off having some privacy when you do emotional housecleaning. If you have a piece of paper handy, you can write out your emotional housecleaning. Otherwise, just follow the guidance on your Day 2 pocket reminder and complete all eight sentences in your mind. It works!

If you want some privacy while you use emotional housecleaning, take a restroom break, find an empty office where you can close the door, or walk around the block. Go out for "coffee" and find a quiet table where you can write. On the other hand, you can make it quick. Just run through the feelings in your mind.

Before long, you will be skilled enough in using emotional housecleaning that you can do it on the bus, on the street corner while you're waiting for a bus, or while you're doing errands. But today, if possible, give yourself the comfort of some privacy and time to use this skill.

When they first use emotional housecleaning, the two feelings that many people struggle to express are anger and guilt.

If it's hard for you to express anger about someone, you might find it easier to express anger about a situation. Anger is a balanced feeling and extremely important, for without anger, sadness turns into depression, powerlessness, self-pity, and immobilization. Anger is very different from hostility, which is associated with aggression. Anger is a balanced feeling: you feel it and it fades. If we were raised in an environment in which anger was not permitted—that is, there was so much hostility that any anger felt unsafe—or an emotionally repressive environment in which anger was not applauded as a normal human feeling, then it might be more difficult to express it. Just practice it! Pump up your "I feel angry that . . ." skill by using it. It's just a feeling, and it will fade.

Likewise, guilt is a balanced feeling that gives us power. When we know what we contributed to a situation, we have the beginnings of making different choices. It is very different from shame, which suggests not just regret at our actions but self-rejection. If it's difficult to express guilt, try saying instead, "In the best of all worlds, I wish that I had . . ." or "What I contributed to it was . . ."

Today, you will check in with yourself just the way you did yesterday, but now you'll have two options for responding:

- *Step 1:* Have your Solution Day 2 pocket reminder in hand.
- *Step 2:* Ask yourself "How do I feel?" and record your findings.
- *Step 3:* Ask yourself, "Am I above or below the line?" and record your findings.
- *Step 4:* Take appropriate action, depending on your findings:

    If you're above the line, identify your need, record it, and do your best to meet it.

    If you're below the line, your need is to get above the line. Do emotional housecleaning to move yourself above the line. The basic feelings are listed on your pocket reminder.

Mastery Living

The Mastery Living part of today is very gratifying. Your body will continue to detox, and you will enjoy activities that give you a great deal of pleasure. It's essential to have that pleasure in order to re-balance your neurotransmitters and turn off the drive to overeat.

Today, you will be engaged for no fewer than six hours and no more than eight hours at a meaningful pursuit, and you will take forty-five minutes to an hour for a lunch break. Your hour

---

The 3-Day Solution® Plan – Day 2
Solution Skills

How do I feel?	What do I need?	Am I Above the Line?		
		Above	Below	EH?
?	↑		√	√
lonely	call friend	√		
BTL	↑		√	√
angry	speak up	√		
hungry	eat	√		
tired	take a walk	√		
sad	feel it	√		
BTL	↑		√	√
secure	feel it	√		
tired	go to sleep	√		

☑ Checked in 10 times today?
☑ Did my best to stay above the line?

ⓃⓍⓁ

The 3-Day Solution® Plan, Ballantine Books, 2005
The Institute for Health Solutions • www.thepathway.org
© Laurel Mellin, 2005

The 3-Day Solution® Plan – Day 2
Emotional Housecleaning

I feel angry that . . .
I feel sad that . . .
I feel afraid that . . .
I feel guilty that . . .

I feel grateful that . . .
I feel happy that . . .
I feel secure that . . .
I feel proud that . . .

Mastery Living

☑ Body Work	60 minutes
☑ 1-2-3 Eating	Ⓑ s Ⓛ s Ⓓ
☑ Meaningful Pursuits	Ⓖ to 8 hours
☑ Time to Restore	90 ~~60~~ minutes
☑ Intimacy Time	Sensual

The 3-Day Solution® Plan, Ballantine Books, 2005
The Institute for Health Solutions • www.thepathway.org
© Laurel Mellin, 2005

of body work and time to restore will involve doing things that you enjoy alone. The purpose of that is to strengthen your connection with yourself in order to have a more intimate experience in the evening. Intimacy with self is the foundation upon which intimacy with others rests. Time to restore is scheduled before intimacy time today, to give you time to relax and prepare for an intimate evening.

The evening plans for intimacy time are very important and very gratifying. Regardless of whether you are involved in a relationship, this time can be one of the high points of the 3-Day Solution Plan. The activity that involves feeding each other may sound alarming, but it is an experience you will never forget. I still remember doing it and how shocked I was that I was full after eating half my food! Do what you can to find someone close whom you can invite to do this activity with you. And if you prefer not to do it, there are several other great options from which to choose.

If you are using the preselected menus designed for rapid weight loss, make sure that you are eating enough. If this calorie level is too low for you, then you won't feel well and it'll be more difficult for you to check in with yourself. Consider consuming a little bit more food. On the other hand, if you are using the menus from Chapter 18, "More Menus from Solution Providers," and are feeling too full, cut back on the amounts or switch to the preselected meal plans.

Take each element of the plan seriously today. Sometimes it's easy to slack off on the second day, but to get that sensation of having turned off the drive to overeat by day 3, it's important to stick with the plan as much as you possibly can. You will feel so wonderful by tomorrow!

How You Will Feel Today

On this second day of the plan, the elation of the first day is over, and you're settling in to still needing to check in with yourself 10 times a day.

In Solution training, it's common for participants to say, "You mean I have to *keep* doing it? I've done it for one day. Isn't that enough?"

Awakening your feeling brain to checking in often is not easy.

People eat, drink, spend, and smoke—they do anything to avoid their feelings. It's wonderful that you are doing this. Please appreciate that it will only get easier.

When you have retrained your feeling brain so that the neural networks that support life above the line are dominant, they fire up automatically. You just *know* how you feel and what you need and only use the skills intentionally now and then.

Right now, there is a huge, riotous party going on down there below the line—a party of all those neural networks that spontaneously and automatically trigger you to go below the line. Most of us have many of these below-the-line neural networks. That's why it's so easy, in the blink of an eye, to go below the line! It takes a lot of repeated checking in to break up that party and throw a new party above the line. But by the conclusion of these three days, you will begin to notice that some of the skills are becoming unconscious, even if it is just now and then.

You may still be grieving somewhat today, missing the old ways. Those neural networks that support life below the line care less about how happy and healthy we are and more about repeating the past. They don't like change. So expect to feel as if you are asking yourself to do something that feels a bit unnatural. However, in time, this way of experiencing life will be the natural, spontaneous norm.

The Rewards You Will Reap Today

Day 2 is an incredibly productive day. By the conclusion of this day, you will start to feel far more of the benefits of the plan. You will have strengthened the habit of checking in and will now be able to move yourself above the line by adding the skill of emotional housecleaning to your repertoire.

Your body will feel more balanced, and you will notice that you are starting to lose weight. Weight comes off in unpredictable ways, which is why we recommend only weighing yourself before breakfast on the first day of the plan and then not again until the morning of the fourth day, before breakfast.

In any case, you will probably start feeling lighter and more vibrant today.

Morning Expectations: Creating Your Day

> ### Creating Your Day
> ___
>
> Create a basic expectation for your day of what you will bring to yourself.

Awaken

As you awaken on this second day of the 3-Day Solution Plan, give yourself time to relax and prepare for the day. This is a day of pleasure and connection that will have a substantial effect on your drive to overeat.

Connect Inside

Take time to transition from sleep to wakefulness, breathing deeply and shifting your awareness inside. Become conscious that there is a safe place inside you and bring up a voice that is supportive; that knows you, respects you, and likes you; the voice that is willing to give you the benefit of the doubt.

Create Your Day

When you are ready, begin to turn your attention to your day. Think about the day that is awaiting you and consider what you would like to create for yourself during this day.

Today, please build on the intention you created yesterday, which was: *I expect myself to do the best I can to stay above the line.*

The question becomes, why? Why do you want to stay above the line? Literally, what is in it for you? Why will you make the effort?

Shape a new intention for today that expresses what you want to create *for yourself*—not for others—by living life above the line. For example:

> *I expect myself to do the best I can to stay above the line and . . .*
>   *. . . have more clarity, vibrancy, and peace in my life.*
>   *. . . have freedom from external solutions.*
>   *. . . create a life of health and happiness.*
>   *. . . enjoy my life to the fullest.*
>   *. . . turn off the drive to overeat.*
>   *. . . lose weight and keep it off.*
>   *. . . or whatever is true for you.*

After you settle on the intention that is right for you, take several minutes to visualize yourself walking through your day making that a reality. This is your purpose for yourself today.

This day's expectation focuses on what you want for yourself in life. Tomorrow's expectation will focus on what you want to give back to others or to the world. It's easy when we're below the line to focus on one of these two things—ourselves or others—but not both. If you tend to give too much, it may be difficult to craft this expectation. However, see whether you can create one that resonates for you and seems deeply true.

Keep that basic expectation in the back of your mind throughout the day. Notice that it has reverberated in your feeling brain and is beginning to appear in your words, actions, and gestures. The neural networks in your feeling brain affect your experience. Notice small ways in which you are changing that would never have occurred if the very core of you did not hold this personal intention.

Before you go on with your day, please take another moment and state that expectation to yourself.

> *I expect myself to do the best I can to stay above the line and . . .*
>   *[your purpose].*

Morning Body Work: Sensual Stretch

Sensual Stretch

- *Shift your focus:* Look at the palms of your hands. Place them on your face, massaging your face, then your neck, then moving your hands to your shoulders and massaging them. If you like, continue moving your hands down your torso, all the way to your legs. If you would like, massage your feet! Notice how much pleasure you derive from massaging yourself in just the way that pleases you.
- *Full-body stretch:* Stretch your full body into the shape of an X, arms and legs as far apart as possible, gently stretching your entire body.
- *Relax!* Watch the sense of relaxation and peace flow through your body!

Begin Your Day with a Sensual Stretch

On the first day, you awakened and stretched to feel more whole, to feel integrated in mind, body, and spirit. Today you will do the same thing, but you will also honor the power of touch. Just the simple act of rubbing the palms of your hands together or stroking your arm—taking your right hand, putting it on your shoulder, and with a gentle caress, stroking your arm—is comforting. It increases serotonin levels and brings us a sense of peacefulness.

Life below the line brings with it a sense of disconnection from our bodies. The intense scrutiny of body fat and objectification of the body further separates us from having body *joy*—just loving and accepting and even delighting in our bodies, imperfections and all. It doesn't mean we aren't striving to improve, but, truth be told,

we love ourselves and our bodies regardless of their "imperfections."

This morning's stretch honors the power of touch and our need
to appreciate our bodies. Start by looking at the palms of your
hands, then placing them gently on your face. Continue to massage
your body and touch your skin, progressing all the way down to
your feet. If you prefer, just massage your face, neck, and shoulders.
Notice how much pleasure you derive from this simple act.

You have just completed your second body connection. Move on
to breakfast and showering and dressing. As you shower, continue to
be aware of your body and to enjoy your physical presence.

If you see fat on your body that you don't like, remind yourself
that the body fat is historical. It means that you consumed more
calories than your body needed at that time. Part of accepting yourself is honoring that, in the past, for the level of skill you had at that
time, you needed that food and it's good that you got what you
needed. However, now you are pumping up these skills so that more
and more of the time, you won't need the food. You can push away
from the table with relative ease. Accept that extra weight as part of
your personal history that is already fading during these three days.

Again, groom and dress in ways that support your body pride.
When you are done, go on to have your Great-start breakfast.

Great-Start Breakfast:
Cheese, Tomato, and Basil Omelet

Cheese, Tomato, and Basil Omelet

Cheese, Tomato, and Basil Omelet (see recipe on page 264)

Water, decaffeinated coffee or tea, or herbal tea, with 1 percent
low-fat or nonfat milk and sugar substitute, if desired

White Stuff: 1 cup of coffee or whatever you really need

Eat a Great-Start Breakfast

This breakfast is also based on using Light Eggs but has the variety of including vegetables. If you don't like omelets in the morning, scramble two whole eggs plus an extra egg white. Although you can use refrigerated egg whites instead of whole eggs, I suggest using whole fresh eggs for better flavor.

This breakfast is a 1-2-3 Meal, including at least one food from each group:

1. The Fiber Group	Tomato
2. Healthy Fats	Canola margarine
3. The Protein Group	Light Eggs and reduced-fat cheese

After enjoying your breakfast, go on to morning meaningful pursuits.

Morning Meaningful Pursuits: Emotional Housecleaning

Your Morning Plan

- Use checking in at least three times. If you are below the line, use emotional housecleaning. Record your results on your day 2 Solution pocket reminder.
- Work with intensity and purpose for no fewer than three hours and no more than four hours.
- Drink at least two 8-ounce glasses of water.
- If you are hungry, snack on a handful of baby carrots.
- Relax and reflect: say one positive thing about your morning.

Use Solution Skills

Begin checking in with yourself regularly—on the hour every hour, if that works for you. Check in at least three times this morning and record your findings on your day 2 pocket reminder.

This is your second day of retraining your feeling brain to stay above the line. What you did yesterday was intensive. Whatever progress you made yesterday will strengthen today. Each time you go inside, you are disrupting the internal party that's below the line and lifting yourself up above the line. It's the layering of the skills, the repetition, that enables them not only to go deeper and be more revealing and helpful but also to bring you one step closer to rewiring your feeling brain.

Take out your day 2 pocket reminder and be sure that your way of reminding yourself to check in is in place. Again, check in hourly or use other prompts to remind you to check in—being in the car, going to the restroom, turning on your computer, whatever works for you. However, please keep in mind that without these prompts, it is very easy, in what seems like the blink of an eye, for a whole morning or afternoon to go by. Both today and tomorrow, be sure to use those reminders.

When you do emotional housecleaning, be sure to try to access these four feelings: anger, sadness, fear, and guilt. If any of them is hard to access, that's fine. You'll access it in time. But for now, when you use emotional housecleaning and a feeling does not arise, pause for a moment. Just wait. If it doesn't arise, simply go on to the next feeling.

Work with Intensity and Purpose

With respect to morning meaningful pursuits, do something this morning that matters to you and is intense, for no fewer than three hours and no more than four hours. Work with passion and intensity, stopping short of losing yourself in your work. Keep your fingers on the pulse of your inner life, check in hourly, and keep in the back of your mind your basic expectation, the one you crafted this morning.

If you are hungry, snack; otherwise, do not. Either way, have at least two full glasses of water or another calorie-free, caffeine-free beverage.

After four hours at the most, stop working, even if there is more to do.

Pause and Reflect

Instead of rushing to lunch, stop for just a couple of moments. Your dopamine levels are up, and the flood of serotonin you can create by pausing and reflecting will stop the drain of that dopamine and stave off an appetite that can appear in the evening.

Pause for one minute to take a big, deep breath and reflect on your morning. Even though there were upsets, stresses, or boredom, say one positive thing to yourself about the morning. Say one thing that you did well or that you appreciate about what you accomplished. Then take an extra minute—one minute!—and feel that surge of satisfaction that your positive thoughts created.

You have completed your second morning on your 3-Day Solution Plan!

Balancing Lunch: Steak and Salad

Steak and Salad

Teriyaki Flank Steak Salad (see recipe on page 275)

Water, decaffeinated coffee or tea, or herbal tea, with 1 percent low-fat or nonfat milk and sugar substitute, if desired

White Stuff: diet soda or whatever you really need

Eat a Balancing Lunch

Consider checking in right as you take your lunch break, finding out how you feel and what you need. If you aren't hungry, get some fresh air, relax, or do something that is a change of pace from the morning activities.

This is an easy lunch because you can use leftovers from the evening before. This is also an easy meal to order from a restaurant. When you go to a restaurant, don't take the menu too seriously. Instead, know what food you need and request it. As long as the ingredients are on hand, most restaurants will accommodate. Continue to check in with yourself and record your findings on your day 2 pocket reminder.

This salad is a 1-2-3 Food:

1. The Fiber Group:	Lettuce, jicama, carrots, and snow peas
2. Healthy Fats:	Olive oil
3. The Protein Group:	Sliced teriyaki flank steak

Prepare for Your Afternoon

Before you begin your afternoon, bring to mind your most basic expectation, the intention that goes a long way toward creating your day: *I expect myself to do the best I can to stay above the line and ...* [*your purpose*].

Having the intention to create life above the line today weakens the neural networks in our brains that contradict that intention, such as "I expect myself to be perfect. I expect everything to go my way. I expect nobody to irritate me. I expect to be in complete control"—and thousands of other below-the-line expectations. You can't focus on staying above the line *and* on any of these things. It simply does not work.

That focus may begin to affect some of the neural networks in your feeling brain, so you might notice yourself thinking, "I wouldn't do that. That's below the line." By this afternoon, you may begin to be aware of small but important changes you are making that are not conscious!

Take a moment during this lunch break to consider the pace of your afternoon and whether you need to increase or decrease it. Your priority is to work with intensity and purpose without abandoning your own needs.

You have eaten a balancing lunch. Continue with afternoon meaningful pursuits.

Afternoon Meaningful Pursuits: Emotional Housecleaning

Your Afternoon Plan

- Use checking in every hour on the hour or at least three times. If you are below the line, use emotional housecleaning. If you have not used emotional housecleaning yet today, use it at least once this afternoon, even if you are above the line. Record your findings on your day 2 Solution pocket reminder.
- Work with intensity and purpose for no fewer than three hours and no more than four hours.
- Drink at least two 8-ounce glasses of water.
- If you are hungry, snack on some Cottage Snack (see recipe on page 292).
- Pause and reflect: say one positive thing about your afternoon.

Use Solution Skills

Continue to check in with yourself regularly. Use emotional housecleaning at least once, even if you are above the line all afternoon. If there is a feeling that is particularly difficult for you to feel, such as anger or guilt, look for even a wisp of that feeling. Try to dig it up! Assessing each feeling is a different skill. Some people find it so easy to feel sadness, for instance, but can't find the anger within. Many people find it difficult to access guilt. Guilt is so important, because it leads to change. Shame just stays stuck. Being ashamed about something gives you ample reason to wallow in it. However, if you feel the above-the-line feeling of guilt, it will fade and you will say "Oh, yeah, that's right. I feel guilty that I didn't pay my credit-card bill on time. I need to pay it early so I won't forget." Or "I feel guilty that I was nasty to my son. I need to say I'm sorry." No shame—it's such a relief! And it creates the climate for positive changes.

Work with Intensity and Purpose

Take it easy this afternoon. Don't work too hard, if possible, because you have a full afternoon and evening ahead. In the work you do, be sure to stay above the line, doing what matters and letting the rest go. Notice how other people in your workplace may be below the line, doing unnecessary tasks, getting into control struggles, working slowly, or not putting their heart into what they do.

You can notice this without judgment, but recognize that you are on a different pathway. You are holding yourself accountable to yourself. You care about doing your best to stay above the line and engage in activities that matter. You are focused and doing the best job you can do. The reward is not just that the boss may notice or that your company may stay in business so you keep your job—both of which are important—but that you have the earned reward of personal integrity. You take both your time and yourself seriously. You take pride in your craft, whether it is brain surgery or cleaning homes. That is an intrinsic reward that turns off the drive to overeat.

Have Water and a Snack

This afternoon, drink plenty of water and have a snack if you are hungry. You may be more likely to need a snack in the afternoon than in the morning.

Pause and Reflect

After three to four hours, when you stop working, pause and reflect again. This is not an affirmation or just any positive, powerful statement. It is the statement you make after reflecting on the afternoon and how that afternoon was for you. It is seeing yourself for who you are, living the afternoon you just lived. It's a statement that rings with authenticity and depth. Say one positive thing to yourself about your afternoon.

Notice that, once again, you have created that surge of serotonin that turns off the drive to overeat. You may have four or more check-ins yet to do. That's fine. Just do them, approximately one per hour, until you have checked off 10 for the day.

Afternoon Body Work: Connect with Yourself

Connect with Yourself

For 45 to 60 minutes:

- Go on a solo walk, take a hike by yourself, or light a candle and do yoga.
- Lock the door and turn on an exercise video, lift weights, or shoot hoops alone.

Exercise for 45 to 60 Minutes

This afternoon, engage in one hour of physical activity that enhances your connection to yourself, your awareness of your body, your feelings, your mind, and your spirit. This kind of intense intimacy with ourselves is the foundation upon which intimacy with others rests. This can involve going for a walk or run alone or doing yoga. Perhaps it's going for a walk someplace that is inspiring to you or doing something else that brings you a sense of peace or vibrancy yet also involves physical activity.

The balancing effect of your first day's exercise will have worn off by now. The change in neurotransmitters lasts 24 hours. This evening's activities are pleasurable, and exercising this afternoon will enhance your energy and mood so that you enter into the evening's activities in the most promising way.

During this time, continue checking in regularly. When you have completed your body work, please check it off on your pocket reminder and continue with your evening.

Time to Restore: Relaxation

Relaxation

Spend one hour of uninterrupted time doing whatever relaxes you.

Take Time to Restore

This evening, you will have intimacy time and an intimate encounter for dinner. The foundation of intimacy with others is intimacy with ourselves, so please take an hour to relax, shower, bathe, commune with nature, enjoy soft music, and rest. You don't need to do this perfectly. Just do whatever is most restoring and refreshing to you. If you want to take a bath by candlelight or want to soothe your senses with bath oils and your body with lotions, aftershave, or a brisk towel dry, then do. If you prefer to keep it simple, curl up on a chair or in bed and take a nap. This is not a time to numb out, so television and computers are off-limits. Relax within yourself.

This evening is a very important part of your 3-Day Solution. Regardless of your plans for the evening, and whether you will be with yourself or with others, prepare for romance, intimacy, and sensuality. Bring up body-pride thoughts, allowing yourself to see your body as good. Notice what you appreciate, like, and enjoy about your body and about how you look.

Dress in clothes that bring out the best in your appearance and enjoy putting them on, taking your time in doing so, and paying attention to any adornments, from a watch to jewelry to a scent or lotion. Bring up a nurturing, supportive inner voice as you dress and notice that you are not dressing to have an "effect" on another person but to please yourself. You are grooming, dressing, and adorning in order to feel desirable to yourself. Your sexual and sensual side is based on your own joy in life and in your body. Take all the time you need, then begin an evening in which food is likely to be the least of your pleasures.

Healthy Dinner:
Grilled Salmon with Mango Avocado Salsa

Grilled Salmon with Mango Avocado Salsa

Grilled Salmon with Mango Avocado Salsa (see recipe on page 282)
Asparagus
Mixed Greens with Roasted Pine Nuts (see recipe on page 284)

Water, decaffeinated coffee or tea, or herbal tea, with 1 percent low-fat or nonfat milk and sugar substitute, if desired

White Stuff: 1 large chocolate-dipped strawberry, 5-ounce glass of white wine, or whatever you really need

---

Eat a Healthy Dinner

Create a healthy but decadent dinner, doing many things to make the event memorable, such as lighting candles, turning on music you enjoy, setting the table with care, or perhaps arranging flowers on the table. Of course, be sure to turn off the television, radio, and computer. If you have children at home, get a babysitter or a very absorbing video for them.

Consider making the evening meal more intimate by using one of the activities shown below. The "Feeding Each Other" activity is particularly powerful, but if that doesn't feel comfortable to you, there are several other activities from which to choose. Regardless of whether you are alone or with a partner, this dinner's pleasures will not center on the food.

You may be eating dinner by yourself. The earned reward is that you can have it exactly the way you want it! Turn on sensual music. Enjoy every luscious bite of your food and celebrate your own sensuality in any way that pleases you. Even if you normally have a partner but don't right now, creating a solo sensual evening is worthwhile. It can offer special pleasures that you don't have when you are partnered.

Intimacy Activity Option 1: Feeding Each Other

Each time you want a bite of food, ask your dinner partner to feed it to you.

This activity involves enjoying your dinner and nourishing yourself with food *and* with sensuality, nurturing, or eroticism.

Here is how to do it: Sit down at the table with the plates of food before you. When you want a bite, just say, "I would like a bite of ..." and say what you want. You cannot feed yourself. Notice the way that each bite satisfies you.

You notice that being fed and telling someone exactly what you need is satisfying, too. Perhaps the other person asks for a bite and you do the same for him or her, noticing how rewarding it is for you to feed someone else. This is a sensuous experience, but it can also be quite fun. Don't be surprised if you find yourself laughing and being playful. Notice how you find it to ask for food and how it is for you to be fed. Also, notice how it is for you to be asked for food and to feed another.

When you feel satisfied—that is, when the hunger has gone away—stop eating. Notice how much food is left on your plate! Be aware of how much of your appetite has nothing to do with body hunger but is a way for you to fill up emotionally, to balance your neurotransmitters. Notice how much more you enjoyed the meal by nourishing your spirit and balancing your neurotransmitters rather than simply by eating food.

Intimacy Activity Option 2: Other Pleasures

Choose one of the following:

- Give neck, back, or foot rubs.
- Hug or hold hands.
- Put on music and dance.
- Tenderly rub your own shoulders.
- Dance alone and relish it.
- Create a lush meal with candles and music.

Enjoy the tenderness and fun of the evening and notice that food is one of the least of your pleasures.

Intimacy Time: Sensual Intimacy

Sensual Intimacy

Engage in an activity that honors your sensuality or sexuality.

Take Time for Intimacy

In planning for this time, ask yourself, "What are my needs? How could I meet my needs of sensuality, sexuality, eroticism, and passion within the limits of my circumstances and beliefs? How could I honor them so fully that the drive to overeat would not just fade— but turn off?"

If you are experiencing this time with yourself and not sharing it with another person, that's the only question you need to ask. However, if you have a partner with whom you share sexual pleasures, consider speaking to your partner about his or her needs for sensuality, sexuality, eroticism, and passion. If your tendency is to focus only on fulfilling your partner and not yourself, move that tendency above the line and keep your focus on yourself. It is your responsibility to do your best to honor your sexual needs. If your tendency is to focus only on meeting your own needs, be particularly responsive to your partner's needs. Notice the gratification and fulfillment that can bring.

The following paragraph presents some ideas for either solo or couple intimacy time. There are more ideas on page 139. These ideas may not be right for you, and the listing of them is not meant to imply that you would feel they are acceptable to you, given the limits you put on your own relationships or life. They are meant to be an offering of possibilities, so if any offend you, please simply discount them and identify those that are acceptable and gratifying to you. Also, safety is our first priority, so if you are having any genital contact with another person, double-check that you are protected from diseases. Also, take into consideration your need to prevent unplanned pregnancy.

Here are several ideas: Go get a massage for a full hour and a half. It makes such a difference! Enjoy the sensuous, soothing touch. Read erotica or watch sex videos by yourself or with your partner. Call your partner and have sex by telephone, with each person using images and words to stimulate the other. Take a platonic friend or your partner to a Jacuzzi or hot tub. Be playful in the water and celebrate and enjoy your body. Remember your most scintillating, tender, or outrageous sexual experience. That's all, just remember it and savor that memory. Put on dance music and dance sensually with yourself or ask your partner to join in or to watch. Have good old-fashioned sex just the way you like it.

Take all the time for this that you desire, and then go on to the last element of the day. Consider checking in as you conclude intimacy time, seeing how you feel and what you need.

Evening Check-in: Earned Rewards

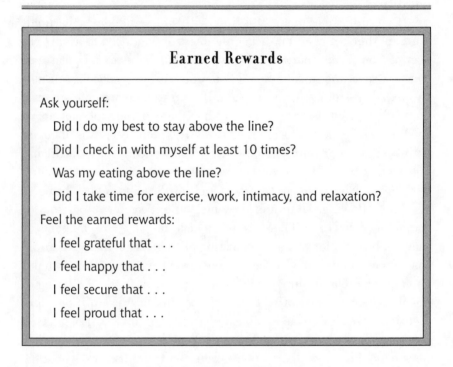

Earned Rewards

Ask yourself:

Did I do my best to stay above the line?

Did I check in with myself at least 10 times?

Was my eating above the line?

Did I take time for exercise, work, intimacy, and relaxation?

Feel the earned rewards:

I feel grateful that . . .

I feel happy that . . .

I feel secure that . . .

I feel proud that . . .

Reap Your Rewards

You are now completing your second day of the 3-Day Solution Plan. You may have enjoyed the day, but you also may have found it unsettling. It's a change, and change is not easy. You might even fear that you can't tolerate all this connection and intimacy. You may be itching to get back to life as usual.

Tomorrow you will be creating your third day above the line and using the most powerful of the three skills, doing cycles. Your body will feel more relaxed, balanced, and vibrant.

For now, it's important to get plenty of sleep and rest. Please conclude the day by completing your pocket reminder, asking yourself:

Did I do my best to stay above the line?
Did I check in with myself at least 10 times?
Was my eating above the line?
Did I take time for exercise, work, intimacy, and
relaxation?

Then give yourself some earned rewards, by completing the sentences for the positive feelings of emotional housecleaning:

I feel grateful that . . .
I feel happy that . . .
I feel secure that . . .
I feel proud that . . .

And turn off the light.

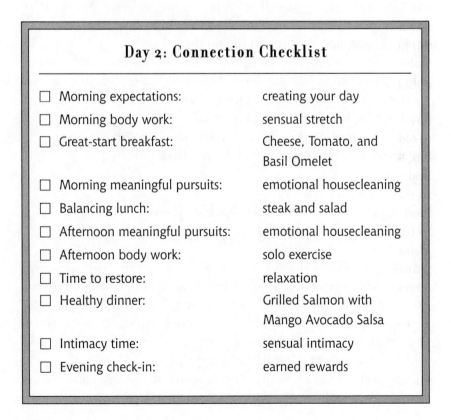

Day 2: Connection Checklist

☐ Morning expectations:	creating your day
☐ Morning body work:	sensual stretch
☐ Great-start breakfast:	Cheese, Tomato, and Basil Omelet
☐ Morning meaningful pursuits:	emotional housecleaning
☐ Balancing lunch:	steak and salad
☐ Afternoon meaningful pursuits:	emotional housecleaning
☐ Afternoon body work:	solo exercise
☐ Time to restore:	relaxation
☐ Healthy dinner:	Grilled Salmon with Mango Avocado Salsa
☐ Intimacy time:	sensual intimacy
☐ Evening check-in:	earned rewards

15

Day 3: Vibrancy

Introduction: The Third Day

THIS IS YOUR third and final day of the 3-Day Solution Plan. Tomorrow morning, if you like, you can start a less intense version of the plan, and at the end of two weeks, you can decide on your next step. Perhaps you will want to use the skills on your own, or perhaps you will want to get on the pathway to a solution, accessing more support and training in the method.

You may be tired of using this plan, but this is not the time to let up! Your body and mind have started to change, but this day will be the *most rewarding* of the three. Just stay with it for one more day, and by tomorrow morning, you will awaken and sense that these three days have changed your life. You can also weigh in tomorrow to see how much weight you have lost.

What You Will Do Today

Solution Skills

Today, you will do cycles! You will use the Solution day 3 pocket reminder, and when you are below the line, you will do a cycle. If you are only a little below the line or right at the line heading south, you can choose to use emotional housekeeping. It is powerful enough to lift you above the line, but at least twice today, you will use the more powerful skill, doing a cycle.

If the prospect of doing a cycle seems daunting, don't worry! Just jump in and do one, without expecting to do it perfectly. The more often you use the skill—and the more effectively you use it—the sooner you will get what will become a very familiar sensation: that pop above the line! You feel that relaxation in your body, that "presto" sense of clarity, vibrancy, peace, hope, and most of all, power! Best of all, that satisfying, intensely pleasurable increase in feel-good neurochemicals is completely calorie-free.

You will begin your day today by creating an expectation that gives you a clear picture of your purpose in life and in the day. That expectation starts with: *"I expect myself to do my best to stay above the line and . . ."* You complete the sentence not with what you want from life but with *what you want to bring to the world,* why your life matters beyond yourself. Again, keeping that expectation in the back of your mind all day, bringing it to consciousness now and then, will trigger small but riveting surprises in your day. You'll notice that you respond to others differently and that the skills are beginning to take hold inside you in exciting and even beautiful ways.

You will check in with yourself 10 times today, as you have been, either at regular natural intervals or hourly with a reminder from a computer, a watch, or another person.

After breakfast and your morning body work, you will check in with yourself, but this time, at least twice today when you are below the line, you will do a cycle. Here is how:

- *Step 1:* Have your Solution day 3 pocket reminder in hand.
- *Step 2:* Ask yourself, "How do I feel?" and record your findings.
- *Step 3:* Ask yourself, "Am I above or below the line?" and record your findings.
- *Step 4:* Take appropriate action, depending on your findings:

  If you're above the line, identify your need, record it, and do your best to meet it.

  If you're below the line, your need is to get above the line. Do emotional housecleaning if you are only slightly below the line. Otherwise, do a cycle. The questions for cycles are on the back of the day 3 Solution pocket reminder. For more about doing a cycle, see page 117.

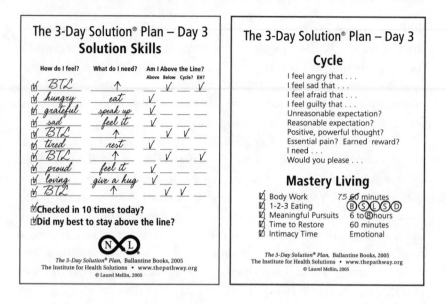

Mastery Living

Today, you will be living a masterful life! You will take pride in your body, allow yourself to "play" when it comes to exercise, and take time to restore what brings you vibrancy. The root word of *vibrancy* is *spirit.* With vibrancy, your body and your essence are in harmony, and your vitality and personal energy come through in everything you do. You glow. You radiate a sense of clarity, peace, and benevolence.

Intimacy time today involves using emotional housecleaning with another person, taking time to listen to the other person's feelings and to share your feelings with him or her. This natural flow of feelings between two people opens the emotional pipeline between them. Imagine two people sitting in chairs opposite each other. They are knee to knee, eyeball to eyeball and bending forward in their chairs slightly, wanting to connect with each other. One of them sits in the chair, being a loving presence for the other, not saying anything at all. Just being. The other feels safe. They use emotional housecleaning, expressing their anger, sadness, fear, and guilt as well as their gratitude, happiness, security, and pride. The listener makes a positive, supportive comment. Then, they exchange roles. The expresser becomes the listener, and the listener becomes the expresser.

The whole activity takes no more than 15 minutes, but the real story is that the emotional pipeline between their two feeling brains has opened. All those below-the-line barriers to that sacred process have fallen away. There is no control struggle, no rampant thinking or judgments to get in the way. There is just a natural flow of feelings, and when the activity concludes, chances are you'll notice that the drive to overeat disappeared. Who wants an extra cookie when they have an emotional connection?

How You Will Feel Today

In some ways, this is a day like any other, in that there could be upsets and challenges that make your day hard. You are not in Tahiti in those grass shacks perched over the water or on some soft, white-sand crescent of a hidden beach. You are right in the middle of messy, demanding, feeling-pulled-in-all-directions *life*.

Yet, chances are, it will be a great day. There is a new party forming in the neural networks in your feeling brain, and even though you are continuing to detox your body and rebalance your neurotransmitters, you will feel far better today than you have during the last two days.

You may find that you have some fears about concluding the three days. Did you do it right? Will it work? Where do you go from here? My suggestion is that you set aside those fears for now. Chapter 17, "The Solution Plan for Days 4 to 14," and Chapter 20, "Day 15 and Beyond," will give you clear choices and options.

My suggestion is that you focus on this one day. Just follow the plan and complete your day. And because this day is full of vibrancy, connection, and play, I hope you pay special attention to enjoying it. *You have earned it.*

The Rewards You Will Reap Today

By this evening, you will notice that your drives to overeat will have faded, your body is releasing weight rather than storing it, and you have more clarity, vibrancy, and peace than you can remember. You will also have in your personal tool kit three basic Solution Skills and a mental template of the five elements of living a masterful life.

You will have a jump-start on the pathway to lasting weight loss.

Morning Expectations: Creating Your Day

Creating Your Day

Create a basic expectation for your day.

Awaken

As you wake up, again take time to relax and prepare for your day.

Connect Inside

Shift your focus to within, breathing deeply and becoming conscious of the sanctuary within that is growing warmer and stronger as you use these skills, day by day.

Create Your Day

When you are ready, begin to consider your day. Instead of feeling as if you are in a tight box, notice that you can think in more spacious and magnificent ways. That's how life above the line is. On the first day, your intention was to stay above the line. On the second day, your intention was to stay above the line and bring yourself what matters most to you. On this third day, you will think about what you want to bring of yourself to the world. How will you give back? What is the larger purpose of your day and your life?

Today, please create a basic expectation that expresses what you want to give back to the world:

I expect myself to do the best I can to stay above the line and . . .

. . . use my talents to give back to the world.

. . . create a happy, healthy family life.
. . . follow my spiritual path, wherever that leads me.
. . . be a source of love in this world.
. . . give back to my community.
. . . or whatever is true for you.

As you move through this day, keep that basic expectation in the back of your mind, bringing it to conscious awareness when a stress, upset, or loss occurs. Make it your personal source of strength for the day. You are creating a day in which you stay above the line and give back to the world in the way that matters most to you.

Please take one moment to state that expectation to yourself:

I expect myself to do the best I can to stay above the line and . . .
[what you want to give back].

Morning Body Work: Body Pride

Body Pride

- *Shower and dress:* As you wash, be conscious of each part of your body, appreciating what it does for you, how it feels, how it smells, and how it looks.
- *Create three thoughts:* As you towel dry or as you dress, come up with three things that you like about your body, how it looks, smells, feels, or what it does.
- *Feel body pride:* Take one more moment just to feel pride in your body and and gratitude for your life, even if that is difficult to do.

Begin Your Day with Body-Pride Thoughts

After stretching and getting out of bed, begin washing and dressing for your day. As you wash each part of your body and as you slip into your clothes, be aware of your body. Enjoy touching it. Appreciate how it looks. Notice any gratitude you feel for what each part of your body enables you to do. Bring to mind at least three body-pride thoughts that reflect your pride in your body and your gratitude for it. As you do these things, notice yourself filling up with a renewed respect for your body and for yourself.

Examples include arms that hug, smooth skin, thick hair, legs that carry me places, strong shoulders, nice teeth, a great smile, scars that reveal my past, large calf muscles, meaty thighs, strong bones, great ankles, fingers that type, hair that is wild, big biceps for lifting things, a big heart that loves.

When you are done, go on to have your great-start breakfast.

Great-Start Breakfast: Solution Cereal

Solution Cereal

Solution Cereal (see recipe on page 267)

Water, decaffeinated coffee or tea, or herbal tea, with 1 percent low-fat or nonfat milk and sugar substitute, if desired

White Stuff: 1 cup of coffee or whatever you really need

Eat a Great-Start Breakfast

This third breakfast is cereal-based. Choose a cereal that has at least 5 grams of fiber per one hundred calories and at least 10 grams of protein. It's important to read the labels. Several cereals that meet these criteria are listed in the recipe; however, products change, so reading nutritional labels is essential. Also, with respect to the fruit in Solution Cereal, blueberries are a particularly good choice because of their high levels of antioxidants. So are dried cranberries.

Since breakfast is such an important determinant of whether your appetite revs up or fades, be sure to be careful about the proportions of each part of this recipe. The more you eat according to these menus and use these recipes, the more you will see subtle but important differences in how you combine foods to make for healthy eating. You won't have to buy so many special products, because with the 1-2-3 Food Lists and a sense of how to combine these foods in ways similar to those shown, you can feel assured that your nutrition will be balanced and optimal.

Some people don't have to be as careful about their breakfast as others. However, if you have any of the following conditions, it might be particularly important to have a 1-2-3 breakfast: carry weight in the middle or have diabetes or metabolic syndrome, a tendency toward emotional ups and downs, premenstrual syndrome (PMS), or seasonal affective disorder (SAD). Also, it's more important to have a 1-2-3 breakfast if you are menopausal or postmenopausal or if you seem to overrespond to stress. Some people secrete more cortisol than others in response to stress, and that cortisol increases insulin. There are no clinically available tests to indicate whether you secrete higher levels of cortisol under stress.

Since most people have one or more of these characteristics, you may want to stick with a 1-2-3 breakfast. If you don't, then try eating a breakfast with less fiber, fewer Healthy Fats, and less lean protein— a good example would be eating two slices of white toast with jam and coffee—and see how that affects your mood and weight. If there is no difference, then continue eating as you please. Chances are, however, that there will be a significant difference in your appetite and your weight.

This breakfast is a 1-2-3 Meal, including at least one food from each group:

1. The Fiber Group	Cereal and berries
2. Healthy Fats	Nuts
3. The Protein Group	Milk

After breakfast, go on to morning meaningful pursuits.

Morning Meaningful Pursuits: Doing Cycles

Your Morning Plan

- Use checking in once per hour or at least three times. If you are below the line, do a cycle or emotional housecleaning. Record your results on your day 3 Solution pocket reminder.
- Work with intensity and purpose for no fewer than three hours and no more than four hours.
- Drink at least two 8-ounce glasses of water.
- If you are hungry, snack on: Grapefruit and Cinnamon Snack (see recipe on page 292).
- Relax and reflect: say one positive thing about your morning.

Use Solution Skills

Continue checking in with yourself and using your day 3 Solution pocket reminder. If you are only a little below the line, use emotional housecleaning. If you are substantially below the line, do a cycle.

It takes 10 to 20 minutes to do a cycle. If you do not have that much time at work to do a cycle, do your cycles during your lunch break and right after work. You can write down your cycle as you do it or call a Solution buddy or friend and ask him or her to listen to you do the cycle. (See page 148 for information on how to ask someone to do a cycle with you.)

As you continue using the skills, they will deepen, and you will experience deeper and more powerful cycles. Right now, however, don't put pressure on yourself to do this perfectly. Just use the skill, learn whatever you can from it, and move along. Simply do your best to express the first four feelings, the natural flow of feelings: anger, sadness, fear, and guilt. Then see what expectation that could be unreasonable is suggested by those feelings. Bring that awareness to your consciousness. Now it's in your frontal lobe, where you have the power to fiddle with that expectation and craft one that is reasonable for who you are in this moment.

Create a new reasonable expectation. It can be easy and effective to start the sentence *"I expect myself to do the best I can to . . ."* and see what words appear in your mind. Fortify that reasonable expectation with some positive, powerful thoughts, the ones you most need to hear right now; for example, "I can do that!" These are encouraging words, not a statement of the payoff of following through. Again, they are the words you most need to hear so that you will continue to follow through.

Then move to the culminating moment of the cycle, when you face the essential pain, the hard part of following through. That essential pain is usually developmental. It's a life lesson that has been difficult to learn, such as:

Life is difficult.
I can't always have it my way.
I'm not perfect.
I'm not in complete control.
Some people may reject me.

Say what the hard part is for you, the essential pain of the human condition you would have to face in order to follow through with ease with that new reasonable expectation. State it and then pause. Allow the feelings that arise from the statement to fade, and chances are, right in front of you—right in your lap—will be the earned reward, the payoff of following through. You might glide above the line (which is likely when you first use cycles), or you might pop above the line. But either way, you will feel much, much better.

The earned reward will logically follow the essential pain. For example:

The Essential Pain	The Earned Reward of Accepting That Pain
Life is difficult.	I won't sweat the small stuff. My life will be better.

I can't always have it my way.	I won't get into control struggles. I can focus on the things that do go my way.
I'm not perfect.	I don't have to be perfect to be wonderful. I am just human. I can finally relax!
I'm not in complete control.	I can stop the control struggles. I can be grateful that I don't have to manage everything!
Some people may reject me.	I won't reject myself. I'll stop being a people-pleaser and learn to find security within myself.

Once you're above the line, you have clarity! You can identify what you need and ask for the support you require to meet that need.

Right now, please take out your day 3 pocket reminder so that you have it on hand, then double-check that you have in place a way to remind yourself to check in at least three times this morning.

Work with Intensity and Purpose

Again, work with intensity and passion and bring to mind often your most basic expectation, the source of strength for the day you are creating for yourself: *I expect myself to do my best to stay above the line and . . . [what you give back to the world].*

Have Water and a Snack

If you are hungry, snack; otherwise, do not. Either way, have at least two 8-ounce glasses of water or another calorie-free, caffeine-free beverage. If you do have the snack suggested for this morning, note that grapefruit has a very low glycemic index and will be likely to stabilize your blood sugar. Cinnamon can have a stabilizing effect on blood glucose, too, so you might want to sprinkle on your grapefruit a little cinnamon plus some sugar substitute, preferably

Splenda or stevia, as they are less likely than other sweeteners to have a negative impact on insulin and blood sugar.

After at least three hours and not more than four hours, stop working, even if you feel like doing more.

Pause and Reflect

Again, take a moment to stop that surge of dopamine and drain of serotonin, and reflect on your morning.

Take a big, deep breath and say to yourself one positive thing about the morning. Say one thing that you did well or that you appreciate about what you accomplished. When you are done, take an extra moment to feel that swelling of satisfaction that follows your personal recognition of yourself and your life this morning.

You have completed your third morning on your 3-Day Solution Plan!

Balancing Lunch: Shrimp Salad Platter

Shrimp Salad Platter

Shrimp Salad Platter (see recipe on page 286)

Water, decaffeinated coffee or tea, or herbal tea, with 1 percent low-fat or nonfat milk and sugar substitute, if desired

White Stuff: diet soda, 1 cup of coffee, or whatever you really need

Eat a Balancing Lunch

This lunch is one that will keep you alert all afternoon. You're probably noticing by now that you are hungry and that the food you're eating affects your mood. Having slightly more fiber and protein but not too much food at lunch sets you up to think better all afternoon. By including some fat in the meal, it will give you more staying power all afternoon. You'll avoid the after-lunch sleepiness that follows overeating or eating too much sugar and refined carbohydrates.

This salad platter is a 1-2-3 Meal:

1. The Fiber Group: Lettuce, tomato, and cucumber
2. Healthy Fats: Olive oil
3. The Protein Group: Shrimp and egg

Take time for some fresh air or a change of pace before or after you eat. Continue to check in with yourself and record your findings on your day 3 pocket reminder.

Prepare for Your Afternoon

Before you begin your afternoon, bring to mind your most basic expectation, the intention that goes a long way toward creating your day: *I expect myself to do the best I can to stay above the line and . . . [whatever you want to give back]*. Prepare yourself to notice all afternoon the small signs that your intention to give back is being seen. It matters. Expect to notice signs that what you have inside is spilling out into the world, that the universe, or the spiritual forces as you see them, are cooperating with your intention.

Pause for a moment to make any adjustments in the pace of your afternoon. If you need to slow it down a bit, consider that. If you need more intensity, by all means, increase it. You are trying to get that second dopamine surge so that the serotonin flush nourishes you the way food never could.

Afternoon Meaningful Pursuits: Doing Cycles

Your Afternoon Plan

- Use checking in at least three times. If you are below the line, do a cycle or use emotional housecleaning. Record your finding on your day 3 Solution pocket reminder.
- Work with intensity and purpose for no fewer than three hours and no more than four hours.
- Drink at least two 8-ounce glasses of water.
- If you are hungry, snack on Veggies and Dip Snack (see recipe on page 293).
- Pause and reflect: say one positive thing about your afternoon.

Use Solution Skills

Continue to check in with yourself regularly all afternoon. It's important not to let up. The party below the line is breaking up, and the one above the line is forming. It's practice and repetition—not personal brilliance—that changes the feeling brain. If you do not have the flexibility to do a cycle at work, do one right after work. Don't worry if you don't pop above the line. For now, enjoy the slide above the line. That sensation of popping above the line will come in time.

Work with Intensity and Purpose

Move through your afternoon, enjoying seeing yourself live life above the line. Notice that you move through some of the unavoidable pain of life rather than getting stuck in it. Even if you do get stuck in it, you don't stay there for as long. Be sure to use emotional housecleaning if you cannot pause to do a cycle. It will nudge you above the line. Then, you can do a cycle after work that will have an even greater effect.

Have Water and a Snack

This afternoon, drink at least two 8-ounce glasses of water or some other no-sugar, no-caffeine beverage. Snack if you are hungry. If you eat dinner after 7:00 p.m., you may need a late-afternoon snack to avoid being ravenous at dinner. If you carry weight on the lower part of your body, not the middle, it's more important that you have a snack if you're at all hungry at this time. It's more difficult to mobilize fat tissue into the blood and raise blood sugar if you have a lower-body weight pattern than an upper-body one.

Pause and Reflect

After three to four hours, when you stop working, pause and reflect again. Envision yourself moving through your afternoon. See how it was for you and to what extent you stayed with your most basic expectation—staying above the line and giving back to the world in ways that matter most to you. Say one positive thing to yourself about your afternoon. Enjoy that surge of serotonin and relax.

Notice how many check-ins you have left to do in order to complete 10 for the day. Continue with afternoon body work.

Afternoon Body Work: Play!

Play!

For 45 to 60 minutes:

Enjoy baseball, soccer, squash, tennis, golf, jumping rope, or horseback riding.

Exercise for 45 to 60 minutes

It's time to play. When you play, have fun, express yourself, or do things you used to do as a kid, the drive to overeat turns off. When we play as our form of physical activity, we don't have to express our need to play by overeating.

Here are some ideas for the day: Go to a dance class, such as ballet, folk dancing, or swing dancing. Go to a gym and play basketball, squash, racquetball, or volleyball. Go to a gym with a rock wall and go rock climbing. Ask some kids in the neighborhood to shoot hoops with you. Go to a special place in nature and run, jump, skip, or hike. Go out in nature and find rocks for your "collection." Go to the batting cages and hit balls. Put on a flowing dress or leotard, turn on music at home, and dance! Go fishing, skip stones across the lake, walk, or jog. Go ice-skating, roller-skating, snowboarding, or skateboarding. Go horseback riding and bring your horse carrots. Take a bicycle ride all by yourself or with a friend. Go to the driving range and hit a large bucket of balls or play nine holes. Go to the garden with your shovel or clippers and make a huge mess. Rent a kayak, rowboat, or rowing shell and row, row, row. Get wet! Swim laps, dive, and play in the water. Have a party. Invite friends who are doing the 3-Day Solution and complete your 3-Day Solution (satisfying dinner, time to restore, and intimacy time) with them.

If you're tempted not to play but to "exercise as usual," resist it. Playing means not being in complete control and not obsessively thinking. It's *so* above the line! Finding a Solution means having fun, whether you like it or not. Just think of those serotonin and dopamine levels rising and that drive to overeat turning off!

Do something playful that involves moving your body for one hour. Then proceed to the evening's activities.

Healthy Dinner: Pasta Bolognese

Pasta Bolognese

Pasta Bolognese (see recipe on page 284)
Mixed greens with Mandarin Orange Slices (see recipe on page 284)

Water, decaffeinated coffee or tea, or herbal tea, with 1 percent low-fat or nonfat milk and sugar substitute, if desired

White Stuff: grated parmesan, 5 ounces of fine red wine, 1 sumptuous bite of fine dark chocolate, or whatever you really need

---

Eat a Healthy Dinner

Enjoy a pleasurable dinner, including pasta. Relax at dinner, slow your pace of eating, and enjoy every bite. This is the last of the three days, and there is a lot to celebrate! This pasta dinner includes as much protein as you'd have in a chicken meal. You're using whole-grain pasta—my family's favorite is spelt, which has a light, fresh flavor but is whole-grain—and you can choose from a variety of whole-grain pastas that are available.

Amounts count with grains, as does whether they really are whole-grain or just look brown! Having a meal with lots of greens, meat, oil, and a small amount of whole-grain pasta affects insulin and blood sugar differently than a sugary pasta sauce with white pasta and white bread. Just a reminder: amounts count not only with grains but also with oils.

That is true especially for oils, nuts, and grains: they are nutritionally fabulous, but the amounts matter. About three-quarters of a cup of cooked pasta is a serving, but if you're still hungry after having that much, consider serving yourself more salad. If you're still hungry after eating another half plateful of salad, have a spoonful more pasta. You are more important than your food, and if you really need it, by all means, have it.

This is a 1-2-3 Meal:

1. The Fiber Group: Whole-grain pasta, tomato
                         sauce, greens, oranges, onion
2. Healthy Fats: Olive oil
3. The Protein Group: Meat

Continue with time to restore and intimacy time. You have almost completed your third day of the plan!

Time to Restore: Inspiration

> ## Inspiration
>
> Spend one hour of uninterrupted time doing whatever inspires you.

Take Time to Restore

Take this time to restore yourself and do something that inspires you. Make it a time of repose, contemplation, and renewal.

During this last time to restore, consider activities such as meditation, prayer, inspirational reading, being in nature, lighting a candle, listening to the beauty of the quiet, or even watching a sunset. Ask yourself, "Where do I want to be that is most inspiring to me?" or "What can I do that will nourish my spirit and inspire me to stay above the line, experience my life more fully, and give back to the world what I want to give?"

What matters the most is that you commit this time to experiencing something that deeply restores you, that nourishes your spirit and makes you more aware of the grace and mystery of life.

Intimacy Time: Emotional Intimacy

Emotional Intimacy

Take time for emotional intimacy, sharing your feelings and listening to the feelings of another person.

Emotional Intimacy Activity Option 1: A Community Connection

Call or meet with someone who is reasonably above the line. Ask this person if he or she will listen to you do some emotional housecleaning. Say that it will take ten minutes and that his or her job is not to give advice or to interrupt but to be a loving presence, just listening. When you are done, the other person is to make a short, positive statement starting with the word *I* that reflects what it was like for him or her to listen. Examples: "I appreciate what you said. Thank you for sharing." "I feel grateful to know you better." "I learned a lot from what you said."

When you are both ready, begin. Do emotional housecleaning, receive your kind remark, and notice how it is to have your feelings honored by another person.

I feel angry that . . .

I fee sad that . . .

I feel afraid that . . .

I feel guilty that . . .

I fee grateful that . . .

I feel happy that . . .

I feel secure that . . .

I feel proud that . . .

Take Time for Intimacy

This last activity of your 3-Day Solution enhances the emotional intimacy of your day. Each moment of emotional intimacy nudges you just a little further out of the toxic spiral and above the line. You may need only half an hour of intimacy a day, not an hour, but making it a point to have some intimacy time with emotional depth is key to turning off the drive to overeat.

Choose one of the following two activities: Community Connection or Two Chairs. If your relationship is difficult, it's safer to choose the first option, Community Connection. Community Connection enhances your skill at creating emotional intimacy, so even if there is not another person around or the person who is around is not skilled in creating intimacy connections, at least you have done your part. The second option, Two Chairs, encourages an even exchange of sharing between two people. The first priority is safety, so use Two Chairs only if you feel secure that it would be reasonably safe for you to do so.

Emotional Intimacy Activity Option 2: Two Chairs

1. *Position two chairs.* Move them so they are facing each other, about four feet apart. Each person sits in one of the chairs. Use connecting body language: put knees to knees, look eyeball to eyeball, and lean forward toward each other.
2. *Take turns speaking.* Decide who will go first. If it is your turn to speak, do emotional housecleaning. If it is your turn to listen, do not speak. Listen with empathy and compassion.
3. *Offer tender morsels.* After completing this exercise, do something to show your appreciation for the other person's sharing, either by giving each other a tender morsel (that is, a nurturing comment), a hug, holding hands, or doing something to recognize this moment of caring.

When you are done, move along to the last element of the 3-Day Solution Plan, reaping your rewards.

Evening Check-in: Reaping Your Rewards!

Reaping Your Rewards!

Ask yourself:

> Did I do my best to stay above the line?
>
> Did I check in with myself at least 10 times?
>
> Was my eating above the line?
>
> Did I take time for exercise, work, intimacy, and relaxation?

Feel the earned rewards:

> I feel grateful that . . .
>
> I feel happy that . . .
>
> I feel secure that . . .
>
> I feel proud that . . .

You have completed the 3-Day Solution Plan!

You have spent three days living a more masterful life. You have pumped up your skills and have experienced more clarity, vibrancy, and peace. The drive to overeat is fading, and you are beginning to step out of the toxic spiral.

Consider what you learned from these three days. What are the rewards of having taken three days away from the stress, isolation, and temptations of modern life? What has it been like to draw a line in the sand around yourself and to have lived—inside and out—in a way that turns off the drive to overeat? Check to see if you have even an inkling of a feeling that you are complete, that on the day you were born, you had all the inherent strength, and goodness that you would ever need to be free of common excesses, to live life to the fullest, and to do what you came to Earth to do. All you required were the tools to access them. If you have even an inkling of that, regardless of whether or not you are aware of it, you are on the pathway to finding your Solution.

Tomorrow, you can begin the second phase of the program, which is far less intense but extremely important. After two weeks of life above the line, you will consider your next step, including accessing the training to rewire your feeling brain. It is only with repeated practice of these skills and others that the neural networks in the feeling brain spontaneously favor life above the line and the drive to overeat fades.

For now, it's important to get plenty of sleep and rest. Please conclude the day by completing your pocket reminder and asking yourself:

> Did I do my best to stay above the line?
> Did I check in with myself at least 10 times?
> Was my eating above the line?
> Did I take time for exercise, work, intimacy, and
>   relaxation?

Then give yourself some earned rewards by completing the sentences for the positive feelings of emotional housecleaning:

> I feel grateful that . . .
> I feel happy that . . .
> I feel secure that . . .
> I feel proud that . . .

Congratulations for having completed the 3-Day Solution Plan! And turn off the light.

Day 3: Vibrancy Checklist

☐ Morning expectations: creating your day

☐ Morning body work: body pride

☐ Great-start breakfast: Solution Cereal

☐ Morning meaningful pursuits: doing cycles

☐ Balancing lunch: Shrimp Salad Platter

☐ Afternoon meaningful pursuits: doing cycles

☐ Afternoon body work: play!

☐ Healthy dinner: Pasta Bolognese

☐ Time to restore: inspiration

☐ Intimacy time: emotional intimacy

☐ Evening check-in: reaping your rewards!

16

Menus for the 3-Day Solution Plan

Day 1

Great-Start Breakfast: Light Eggs and Fresh Strawberries
Light Eggs (see recipe on page 265)
1 cup of fresh strawberries

Water, decaffeinated coffee or tea, or herbal tea, with
   1 percent low-fat or nonfat milk and sugar substitute, if desired

White Stuff: 1 cup of coffee, cook eggs in 1 teaspoon of butter, or
   whatever you really need

Restaurant request: Ask for a bowl of strawberries and three eggs
   over easy; don't eat all the yolks.

Morning Snack
1 fresh apricot, 2 dried apricot halves, or 2 large stalks of celery

Balancing Lunch: California Chicken Salad
California Chicken Salad (see recipe on page 269)

Water, decaffeinated coffee or tea, or herbal tea, with
   1 percent low-fat or nonfat milk and sugar substitute, if desired

White Stuff: diet soda, 1 cup of coffee, or whatever you really need

Restaurant request: Ask for tossed greens, chicken breast with
   tomatoes, and olive oil vinaigrette on the side.

Afternoon Snack
1 small apple and 5 cashews or almonds

Healthy Dinner: Grilled Flank Steak and Green Beans

Grilled Flank Steak Teriyaki (see recipe on page 280)
Spicy Garlic Green Beans (see recipe on page 288)
Butter Lettuce with Feta and Cucumber (see recipe on page 277)
Cantaloupe slices topped with raspberries

Water, decaffeinated coffee or tea, or herbal tea, with 1 percent low-fat or nonfat milk and sugar substitute, if desired

White Stuff: 5 ounces of fine red wine, whipped cream on dessert, or whatever you really need

Restaurant request: Ask for grilled flank steak or top sirloin, steamed green vegetables, and fresh greens with olive oil vinaigrette on the side.

Day 2

Great-Start Breakfast: Cheese, Tomato, and Basil Omelet

Cheese, Tomato, and Basil Omelet (see recipe on page 264)

Water, decaffeinated coffee or tea, or herbal tea, with 1 percent low-fat or nonfat milk and sugar substitute, if desired

White Stuff: 1 cup of coffee or whatever you really need

Restaurant request: Ask for egg substitute or egg-white omelet with cheese, tomato and basil. Request "light on the cheese."

Morning Snack

A handful of baby carrots

Balancing Lunch: Teriyaki Flank Steak Salad

Teriyaki Flank Steak Salad (see recipe page 275)

Water, decaffeinated coffee or tea, or herbal tea, with 1 percent low-fat or nonfat milk and sugar substitute, if desired

White Stuff: diet soda, 1 cup of coffee, or whatever you really need

Restaurant request: Ask for baby greens, sliced grilled top sirloin, and vegetables with oil and vinegar dressing.

Afternoon Snack

Cottage Snack (see recipe on page 291)

Healthy Dinner: Grilled Salmon with Mango Avocado Salsa

Grilled Salmon with Mango Avocado Salsa (see recipe on page 282)
Asparagus
Mixed Greens with Roasted Pine Nuts (see recipe on page 295)

Water, decaffeinated coffee or tea, or herbal tea, with
1 percent low-fat or nonfat milk and sugar substitute, if desired

White Stuff: 1 large chocolate-dipped strawberry, 5-ounce glass of
white wine, or whatever you really need

Restaurant request: Ask for grilled salmon and asparagus or other
steamed vegetables with "no added butter." Order fresh baby
greens sprinkled with walnuts and olive oil vinaigrette on the side.

Day 3

Great-Start Breakfast: Solution Cereal

Solution Cereal (see recipe on page 267)

Water, decaffeinated coffee or tea, or herbal tea, with 1 percent low-
fat or nonfat milk and sugar substitute, if desired

White Stuff: 1 cup of coffee or whatever you really need

Restaurant request: Ask for bran cereal with nonfat milk and
berries; request almonds on the side or bring your own.

Morning Snack

Grapefruit and Cinnamon Snack (see recipe on page 292)

Balancing Lunch: Shrimp Salad Platter

Shrimp Salad Platter (see recipe on page 286)

Water, decaffeinated coffee or tea, or herbal tea, with
1 percent low-fat or nonfat milk and sugar substitute, if desired

White Stuff: diet soda, 1 cup of coffee, or whatever you really need

Restaurant request: Ask for a shrimp salad with egg and vegetables and dressing on the side.

Afternoon Snack

Veggies and Dip Snack (see recipe on page 293)

Healthy Dinner: Pasta Bolognese

Pasta Bolognese (see recipe on page 284)
Mixed Greens with Mandarin Orange Slices (see recipe on page 284)

Water, decaffeinated coffee or tea, or herbal tea, with 1 percent low-fat or nonfat milk and sugar substitute, if desired

White Stuff: grated parmesan, 5 ounces of fine red wine,
1 sumptuous bite of fine dark chocolate, or whatever you really need

Restaurant request: Ask for whole-grain pasta with marinara meat sauce. If whole-grain pasta is not available, request pasta with marinara sauce, topped with grilled chicken breast. Order mixed greens with olive oil vinaigrette on the side. In either case, eat half the pasta served.

Part 4

THE SECOND
PHASE OF
THE PLAN

17

The Solution Plan for Days 4 to 14

YOU HAVE JUMP-STARTED your way to lasting weight loss with the 3-Day Solution Plan. However, to begin to reap the longer-term rewards of these three days, it's important to move right into the second phase of the plan. This second phase will complete your first two weeks of using the method.

This phase of the plan will involve the same Solution Skills and the same elements of Mastery Living but applied in a less intense, more flexible way. You do something for exercise, meaningful pursuits, time to restore, and intimacy each day. You continue your 1-2-3 Eating, but the calorie levels of the meals are slightly higher and at a level of intake that is sustainable for most people while still producing weight loss at the rate of about a pound or so per week. This is the rate that encourages lasting weight loss.

This phase of the plan will also be easier because you have already built some Solution Skills and are accustomed to checking for all five elements of Mastery Living. Also, your body has changed. You have detoxed, and the drive to overeat has started to fade. Your body is releasing weight rather than storing it.

By staying with this plan for days 4 to 14, you can expect to:

• *Avoid dieter's rebound and keep losing weight:* Following all the intensity of the 3-Day Solution Plan, there is a natural tendency to relax, let go, and return to your old ways. It's not just psychological but physical. Before the plan, your body was at a "set-point" weight, and there are multiple mechanisms in place to enable your body to defend that weight. If you don't continue with the plan, it's likely that your appetite will increase and you'll regain whatever weight you lost within a week. But if you do continue with the plan, you will keep that weight off and lose more.

• *Continue rewiring your feeling brain:* The feeling brain changes only by repeated experience; even three days of intensive Solution training is only the start of rewiring your feeling brain. You built a good base of the skills during those three days, but having any lasting effect takes continuing to use the skills often and well.

• *Become comfortable with a new lifestyle:* You used Mastery Living intensively for three days. In order for this plan to work for you in the longer term, you must find a way to weave it into your life. During this second phase of the plan, you'll learn to use Solution Skills and create a masterful life while still dealing with life's realities. This plan is constructed to be flexible, so you can adapt it to the changing demands of your life and the ongoing stresses you encounter.

• *Recheck for health-care needs:* Some people who use the 3-Day Solution Plan become aware that they need more medical or emotional support. It may become more important to them to take care of that knee or back problem, those allergies, or those hormone issues. Using the skills and tapping into feelings may have triggered their awareness that they are more depressed or anxious than they realized. Before proceeding with the plan, it's important to meet your self-care and health-care needs in order to make this method safe and effective.

Although the next step is to focus on the second phase of the plan so you can complete two weeks of using this method, there is support after that time, if you want a solution in your life. You are on your way to rewiring your feeling brain, but you will not be finished in two weeks. Even if you are in a honeymoon phase in which it seems that you have a Solution, rewiring the brain takes far longer. Even if you wish you could snap your fingers and have a Solution, you need to keep at it to see lasting results. So in phase 3 (discussed in Chapter 20), you will acquire more skills in 1-2-3 Eating. You will also learn about options for using these basic skills on your own or for obtaining Solution training.

Right now, the focus is to build on the foundation of those first three days and extend them into two weeks of using the method. After that time, you will have much more clarity about what is the right next step for you. In the following chapters, there is more help for this second phase of the plan, including menus for days 4 to 14 (Chapter 18, "More Menus from Solution Providers") and recipes (Chapter 19, "Recipes from the Solution Community"). There is also a Solution phase 2 pocket reminder at the end of the appendix, which can serve as a handy reference for what you should focus on to get the best results.

The Solution Plan

- *Phase 1—the 3-day plan:* Spend three days detoxing and learning the basics of the method.
- *Phase 2—the plan for days 4 to 14:* Complete two weeks of using the method and enhance the benefits of the first three days.
- *Phase 3—the plan for day 15 and beyond:* Continue using the method on your own or become more involved in Solution training, getting on the pathway to finding your Solution.

Solution Skills

Continue with your morning check-in and then do your best to stay above the line during the day. When you go to sleep in the evening, be sure to check in with yourself to review the day and reap your rewards: grateful, happy, secure, and proud.

Morning Expectations

When you awaken in the morning, continue to take time to create your day in your mind. Consider the day ahead and establish a basic expectation that you will do your best to reach for the skills and stay above the line. Bring to mind why this matters and what your purpose is in terms of the rewards for yourself or the force you want to be in this world. You need not stay with the same expectation but may want to consider several.

You will probably notice that your basic expectation evolves during these two weeks. What is it like for you to go through a day with a clear expectation that you will stay above the line and give unconditional love to others? How does that experience differ from going through the day with the purpose of staying above the line to create a fulfilling family life, to turn off the drive to overeat, or to experience every moment with the greatest possible vibrancy?

This is not a time to be contained, perfectionistic, or controlled but rather to allow your mind to travel in spacious, even magnificent ways. You have done the hard work of the 3-Day Solution Plan, and you have even more internal skills than you had before. Now, you can begin to play with them and enjoy them in new ways. Who knows what could happen?!

Staying Above the Line

Continue to check in with yourself regularly. Begin to have a sense that you are keeping your fingers on the pulse of your inner life, checking in and reaching for the tools to move yourself above the line.

You are likely to be below the line often. You may completely forget to check in for an afternoon or an evening. That's the power of the "party" of neural networks below the line. Just catch yourself and start using the skills again. If you go way below the line and are having a difficult time getting back above, try one or more of these tools:

- *Bring up a supportive inner voice.* Just put your right hand on your left shoulder and stroke your arm. Say to yourself with a nurturing inner voice, "Oh, well. I'm a bit below the line. That's okay. I can tell I'm below the line, and that's progress. I am mastering these skills, and eventually, I will be above the line more of the time."
- *Get one cell above the line.* Understand that you don't have to get your entire being above the line to make your life better. When you check in with yourself, if you can

bring even one cell of your consciousness above the line, everything changes. You can *see* yourself more accurately from that perspective. You stop feeling lost or abandoned. You have yourself, so even if things are not perfect, they are far better.

- *Reach for your basic expectation.* Hold on to that basic expectation that expresses what you intend to manifest in your own life and what you want to give to the world. It can have a tremendously stabilizing effect.

- *Feel your feelings and allow them to fade.* Feeling your feelings and allowing them to fade is such a powerful skill! Just allow the feeling to rise up in your belly and burn in your throat, saturating your being. Devote your full attention to the feeling. Do not stuff it, control it, or analyze it. Just *feel* it and allow it to fade, which it will do. Unless you are way, way below the line to start with, you'll find that, quite miraculously, you're now above the line!

- *Appreciate each check-in.* Each and every time that you check in with yourself and bring to consciousness the emotions at your core, you become your own agent for change. You open up the possibility of rewiring the neural networks in your feeling brain so that more often you will spontaneously live life above the line. It will take far less effort!

Each day that you continue to use your Solution Skills, watch for subtle but profound changes that come with life above the line. Expect wonderful things to occur, because they will. By shifting that basic expectation and drawing upon these skills, we tap into the immense power of the feeling brain. It is our emotional, relational, and spiritual core, so the results that follow these changes in the feeling brain are developmental. The world begins to look different, and as we develop, there is no going back. Even during these first two weeks of using the method, you may begin to notice small signs of these changes that seem of a different dimension and appear when you least expect them.

Over time, food will recede in importance. As much as this might sound impossible to you at the moment, losing weight will feel *good.* Having small wisps of hunger throughout the day and reaching for a beautiful, ripe peach instead of cookies will seem rewarding. Your attention will focus on shedding extra weight so that you can live with more gusto—climb mountains, eat strawberries in bed, and generally, live life to the hilt. You will feel passion and creativity that you have not felt in years, and the source of that spirit will not be a pill. You will have done it yourself. You will have had the courage to master these skills, rewire your feeling brain, and live life above the line.

At the conclusion of each day, be sure to do one last check-in. . . .

Evening Check-in

Just as you did during the three-day plan, as you go to sleep at night, check in with yourself and ask:

Did I do my best to stay above the line?
Was my eating above the line?
Did I take time for exercise, work, intimacy, and
     relaxation?

Then go inside, bring up a supportive inner voice, and complete the following sentences:

I feel grateful that . . .
I feel happy that . . .
I feel secure that . . .
I feel proud that . . .

And turn out the light.

Mastery Living

This is a time to treat yourself very well, buying the freshest food and double-checking that you continue to take time for yourself rather than feeling pulled in all directions. As you begin to change, you will observe positive and negative reactions from those around you. It's not unusual for people close to us to be ambivalent about our changes, because often those changes are unsettling, even if they make us happier and healthier.

What you are doing is not "normal." Most people are resigned to going on and off diets their whole lives and watching their waistlines continue to expand. You are doing something different, even revolutionary. Revolutionaries need support. They require focus, and this is your time to focus on jump-starting a new way of living—inside and out.

Body Work

As much as you may have to rearrange your lifestyle to do this, it's essential that you exercise. The impact on neurotransmitters lasts 24 hours. That's it! So each day, you start fresh, and you engage in some activity that you love. Drudgery for 45 minutes to an hour will not do. The value of taking even a few moments to stretch in the morning and feel that sense of integration in mind, body, and spirit goes a long way toward lifting you above the line.

You tried several activities during the 3-Day Solution Plan. Although you may have a tendency to regress to avoiding exercise, set the bar higher. Expect yourself to do something daily that you love and that involves exercise. Pair exercise with nature, expression, music, or play. If you love competing with yourself, set goals for lifting weights, improving your heart rate, or expending more calories on the treadmill. If the physical activities you choose don't feel like recreation or fun, they won't last.

Use these 11 days to continue to explore and experiment, so that by the end of this time, you have an activity plan to which you look forward each day.

Solution 1-2-3 Eating

Do not diet. Focus on turning off the drive to overeat. You might say to yourself, "What that does not involve food would gratify me right now?" The menus during these 11 days are high in protein, fiber, and healthy fat. They taste delicious. However, there are no unlimited choices or unlimited amounts, except for vegetables.

Compared to the first three days of the plan, you will have

slightly more flexibility with food, but I suggest that you stick with the menus that are high in protein, fiber, and healthy fat rather than those containing sugar, alcohol, and less healthy fat. If it is really important to you to have White Stuff, then you should definitely have it and savor every mouthful.

When you do have White Stuff, though, favor foods high in Healthy Fat rather than those high in sugar. The quickest way to stop the process of shedding weight is to overload on sweets, so eat them if you need them, but if you can satisfy yourself with some cashews or a few chocolate-covered almonds instead of sugar cookies, that's probably smarter.

There are times when you need to eat for enjoyment and not for health. Use the skills, pop yourself above the line, and see with 20-20 vision what you need. If you need to eat for pure pleasure, then have a Self-Acceptance Meal (discussed further on page 274). That's a meal at which you accept that you are human and you need to eat for pleasure at times. However, because you're above the line, instead of eating a chicken breast and salad plus a chocolate sundae, you just have the chocolate sundae. Calories do count, so with the Self-Acceptance Meal, there are no limits whatsoever on what you eat. Instead, stop eating after you've consumed 350 calories.

It's a good idea to have one Self-Acceptance Meal during phase 2 of the plan, because part of having a weight Solution is muscling up the skill to eat for pure pleasure and then immediately returning to eating 1-2-3 Meals. All cultures have feasts, but those feasts do not prompt weight gain if, immediately afterward, we snap back to 1-2-3 Eating.

Otherwise, stay with 1-2-3 Eating for the full 14 days. It's only 14 days! After 14 days, food may begin to look different to you, and you can reconsider what food plan is right for you. It takes most people the full 14 days, though, to adjust to this new way of eating.

Meaningful Pursuits

Continuing to engage in meaningful pursuits with intensity and purpose may be one of the most challenging parts of this plan. However, for the remainder of the first two weeks of the plan, please engage in meaningful pursuits for no fewer than six hours per day and no more than eight.

If you are accustomed to overworking, cutting back on your hours may be very difficult for you. It's really common for work, family, and love to become mixed up with one another. Often, it's easy to displace the need for personal loving relationships onto striving for money, success, or acceptance at work. Overworking can be a socially acceptable way to avoid disappointments at home. In fact, after three days of working for only eight hours, it's common to be itching to get back to overworking. There are a million reasons why you "must."

If your basic expectation in life is, for example, to stay above the line and give back through your work, *and* you limit your work to eight hours, then things are going to change. The combination of this limit and checking in hourly will bring some revelations. You will probably notice that you are less patient than you were before about spending time in control struggles, mindless activities, procrastination, and busywork. Also, the more you're above the line, the more you will notice that some of your colleagues and coworkers are below the line. All these observations are likely to nudge you toward functioning at work in ways that are better for you and better for your organization's bottom line.

If you are accustomed to underworking, then you may be relieved that the intensity of the three-day plan is over and you are anxious to get back to having lots of unstructured time or engaging in activities at a slower pace. This is not a good idea. Although you may have opportunities to live a low-intensity lifestyle, it is not necessarily in your best interest nor conducive to turning off the drive to overeat.

Your genetic destiny requires you to have challenge and intensity, that is, trying to do something you don't know that you can do, pushing the envelope, doing something at which you could fail if you didn't call on all your energies and faculties. Only with the dopamine rise that comes with pain can you get that serotonin flush that turns off the drive to overeat.

Many people who underwork feel as if they've earned their leisure because they are retired or are still looking for their true purpose in life. Some are just lazy. However, underworking is a form of personal deprivation from that ennobling sense of having accomplished something in the world. You don't have to do the perfect thing. Just do *something* that gives back, makes a difference, and gets you out of the house.

If you are underworking because you are in a job that doesn't tax you, look for another job or create "bookends" on your day that increase your intensity. I recall being in an undergratifying job once, so I volunteered at Nazareth House down the street at lunchtimes, visiting with older people in the infirmary. My close friend Emily, who was in a similar situation, spent her lunch hours once a week teaching English to a woman who had recently immigrated to the United States. Our jobs were not fulfilling, but we found other "work" that was. It makes such a difference in stopping the drive to overeat!

During these 11 days, continue using the technique of relaxing and reflecting. Work with passion and intensity for three or four hours, then take a moment to state to yourself one positive thing about those hours and allow the sense of satisfaction to flow through your body. Take a break at lunch, both to eat and to leave your workplace for at least ten minutes to get a change of pace and scenery.

Time to Restore

During the second phase of the training, do not let up on taking your one hour per day of time for pure pleasure, relaxation, or inspiration. It would be so easy—and so ungratifying—to slip back into watching television and spending hours and hours engaged in activities that really don't satisfy you. You may still want to watch television, but limit your screen time to no more than two hours total after 5:00 p.m. The rest of the time, find some activity that has a better payoff. Keep in mind that one way of looking at the drive to overeat is that it's a natural consequence of "reward-deficiency syndrome," not getting enough real gratification in life. So rather than "chewing-gum" activities, just lying around and doing nothing, get up off the couch and do something so rewarding that it will turn off your drive to overeat. What makes you laugh, sigh, cry, scream, or swoon?

If you live with others, they may not like the fact that you are taking one hour for yourself. In order to make this request—for them to honor your need for one hour of time to restore daily—you may have to face the essential pain that they may be angry. The earned reward? Life above the line. Turning off the drive to overeat. Stepping out of the toxic spiral.

You may need to come to some agreements, such as "trading." For example, "I get 6:00 p.m. to 7:00 p.m. for time to restore while you take care of the kids, and you get 9:00 p.m. to 10:00 p.m. for time to restore while I do the dishes." Reach agreements so that this can be a two-way street. Arranging for even half an hour of time to restore is important. If you have difficulty taking this time, consider doing some cycles about it. Often, for those who have the external solution of being busy-busy-busy, it comes down to facing the essential pain of "I can't avoid my feelings" or "I can't avoid my problems at home," which leads to earned rewards such as "I can feel!" and "I can deal with my problems. My life will get better."

Others can't take time to restore because of the external Solution of people-pleasing or rescuing others. They have absolutely no time left to please or rescue themselves! Decreasing the drive to people-please often takes facing the essential pain that "others may reject me" and receiving the earned reward that "I won't reject myself," together with a new sense of security. Decreasing the drive to rescue others is very difficult because we have to face our aloneness. The essential pain is often that "they may hurt," and the earned reward is that "they will learn from that pain" and "I will stop blocking their development."

Intimacy Time

One of life's sweetest rewards is intimacy. It is also often furthest from our grasp. Being close to someone and authentic takes a great deal of skill. You may find it easy to be intimate with people with whom you do not have a committed relationship and harder when the stakes are higher and the relationship involves more interdependency.

If you already have solid, loving relationships in your life, great sex, and a deep spiritual connection, then lasting weight loss will be easier for you. If your relationships are disengaged or fraught with power struggles, it's easy to identify the fact that you don't have all the intimacy you'd like. On the other hand, if your relationships are merged—that is, overly close, so that you know how the other person feels and what he or she needs but lose sight of your own feelings and needs—it's harder. Because you feel the emotion of love for the person, you assume that you have intimacy, but intimacy requires two people who are authentic and separate, yet who are close.

During the 3-Day Solution Plan, you had three kinds of intimacy: social, emotional, and sensual/sexual. During phase 2 of the plan, touch on one of these kinds of intimacy each day. If your life is abundant with intimacy already, this means getting more of the good that is already there. If your intimacy in one of these areas is quite limited or nonexistent, emphasize the other two. Our genes are flexible in this regard! We don't need all three kinds of intimacy dished up in perfect proportions in order to have a weight Solution.

Also, as you continue to use the skills, chances are that the intimacy in your life will be enhanced. You will also clarify the extent to which each kind of intimacy is essential to your weight Solution.

If you have a spouse or partner but did not do the intimacy activities on days two and three of the plan with him or her, consider why. If there is more dissatisfaction in your relationship than you would like to have, consider getting support from a counselor or even going yourself if your partner is not willing to go with you.

If your partner did do one or both of these activities with you, consider the possibility of both of you being involved in this work. Improved intimacy is one of the predictable rewards of mastering the skills. In a couple in which only one partner is using the method, the skills can be infectious. However, the method is far more effective when both partners use it, and often, those who continue with the method without their partners' involvement look back and regret that they didn't include them. By that time, the developmental divide between them is too wide and sometimes relationships that could have been saved through Solution training end. For more support in how to bring up Solution training to your spouse or partner, order the Pathway Partners Program CD on our website.

These skills are not gender-specific. They are not male or female skills but human skills. When we began disseminating the method, mainly women with weight issues came into our groups. Now there are men and women who want to turn off the drive for various common external solutions or who just want to have more of life's rewards. Interestingly, the most common goals for women using the method are losing weight and acquiring more emotional balance. For men, it is quite different. They may use the method for a range of external solutions, but the reward they want most is intimacy. Both men and women are motivated to use the method to create an environment in which their children master these skills early on so as to prevent problems from being transmitted from one generation to the next.

After two weeks of using the method, chances are that you will have continued to lose weight, deepened the skills, and explored life above the line enough to determine whether you have what you need from this plan or you'd like to become more involved in using the method. For now, it's best to focus on the next 11 days.

18

More Menus from Solution Providers

AFTER YOU COMPLETE your 3-Day Solution Plan, the 11 days of menus in this chapter will give you ideas for meals and snacks based on 1-2-3 Eating. These menus are followed, in Chapter 19, by recipes for preparing selected dishes.

If no recipe is mentioned in the menu, it's fine to purchase that menu item. This is not a diet, and you are more important than your food. As you approach each meal, if you *really need* White Stuff, you should definitely have it and thoroughly enjoy it. But if you don't really need it, then skip it. Do what is right for you.

Day 4

Great-Start Breakfast: Fruit, Yogurt, and Nut
> Fruit, Yogurt, and Nut Breakfast (see recipe on page 265)
> Water, decaffeinated coffee or tea, or herbal tea, with 1 percent low-
> fat or nonfat milk and sugar substitute, if desired

Morning Snack
> Baby carrots

Balancing Lunch: Grilled Chicken and Spinach Salad
> Grilled Chicken and Spinach Salad (see recipe on page 271)
> Water, decaffeinated coffee or tea, or herbal tea, with 1 percent low-
> fat or nonfat milk and sugar substitute, if desired

Afternoon Snack

Fruit and More Snack (see recipe on page 292)

Healthy Dinner: Halibut with Ginger Glaze

Halibut with Ginger Glaze (see recipe on page 283)
Arugula and Spinach Salad (see recipe on page 277)
Seedless red flame grapes, small cluster
Water, decaffeinated coffee or tea, or herbal tea, with 1 percent low-
fat or nonfat milk and sugar substitute, if desired

Day 5

Great-Start Breakfast: Light Eggs and Grapefruit

Light Eggs (see recipe on page 265)
Grapefruit half, sprinkled with cinnamon and sugar substitute, if
desired
Water, decaffeinated coffee or tea, or herbal tea, with 1 percent low-
fat or nonfat milk and sugar substitute, if desired

Morning Snack

Celery and Nut Butter Snack (see recipe on page 291)

Balancing Lunch: Roasted Turkey Sandwich

Roasted Turkey Sandwich (see recipe on page 273)
Water, decaffeinated coffee or tea, or herbal tea, with 1 percent low-
fat or nonfat milk and sugar substitute, if desired

Afternoon Snack

Yogurt and More Snack (see recipe on page 293)

Healthy Dinner: Pork Tenderloin and Spinach and
Strawberry Salad

Grilled Marinated Pork Tenderloin (see recipe on page 281)
Spinach and Strawberry Salad (see recipe on page 288)
Water, decaffeinated coffee or tea, or herbal tea, with 1 percent low-
fat or nonfat milk and sugar substitute, if desired

Day 6

Great-Start Breakfast: Light Scrambled Eggs and Cheese
Light Scrambled Eggs and Cheese (see recipe on page 266)
Bowl of blueberries
Water, decaffeinated coffee or tea, or herbal tea, with 1 percent low-
fat or nonfat milk and sugar substitute, if desired

Morning Snack
4 ounces of sugar-free vanilla or fruit yogurt

Balancing Lunch: Grilled Salmon Salad
Grilled Salmon Salad (see recipe on page 281)
Water, decaffeinated coffee or tea, or herbal tea, with 1 percent low-
fat or nonfat milk and sugar substitute, if desired

Afternoon Snack
Fresh sliced strawberries, 1 cup

Healthy Dinner: Salata with Grilled Chicken
Salata with Grilled Chicken (see recipe on page 271)
Water, decaffeinated coffee or tea, or herbal tea, with 1 percent low-
fat or nonfat milk and sugar substitute, if desired

Day 7

Great-Start Breakfast: Solution Cereal
Solution Cereal (see recipe on page 267)
Water, decaffeinated coffee or tea, or herbal tea, with 1 percent low-
fat or nonfat milk and sugar substitute, if desired

Morning Snack
1 hard-boiled egg

Balancing Lunch: Roast Beef Sandwich
Roast Beef Sandwich (see recipe on page 272)

Water, decaffeinated coffee or tea, or herbal tea, with 1 percent low-
fat or nonfat milk and sugar substitute, if desired

White Stuff: diet soda or 1 cup of coffee, if you need it

Afternoon Snack

Fruit and More Snack (see recipe on page 292)

Healthy Dinner: Shrimp Tostada

Shrimp Tostada (see recipe on page 287)

Water, decaffeinated coffee or tea, or herbal tea, with 1 percent low-
fat or nonfat milk and sugar substitute, if desired

Day 8

Great-Start Breakfast: Sausage and Eggs

Sausage and Eggs (see recipe on page 267)

Bowl of blackberries

Water, decaffeinated coffee or tea, or herbal tea, with 1 percent low-
fat or nonfat milk and sugar substitute, if desired

Morning Snack

1 small apple

Balancing Lunch: Chicken Curry Pita

Chicken Curry Pita (see recipe on page 270)

Water, decaffeinated coffee or tea, or herbal tea, with 1 percent low-
fat or nonfat milk and sugar substitute, if desired

Afternoon Snack

6 cashews and a tall glass of iced tea

Healthy Dinner: Farmer's Market Fish

Farmer's Market Fish (see recipe on page 279)

Orange slices topped with fresh mint

Water, decaffeinated coffee or tea, or herbal tea, with 1 percent low-
fat or nonfat milk and sugar substitute, if desired

Day 9

Great-Start Breakfast: Light Eggs and Fresh Strawberries
Light Eggs (see recipe on page 265)
Sprinkling of salt and freshly ground pepper
1 cup of fresh strawberries
Water, decaffeinated coffee or tea, or herbal tea, with 1 percent low-fat or nonfat milk and sugar substitute, if desired

Morning Snack
4 ounces of sugar-free yogurt

Balancing Lunch: Farmer's Market Fish Salad
Leftover Farmer's Market Fish, heated and placed on a bed of spring greens
Water, decaffeinated coffee or tea, or herbal tea, with 1 percent low-fat or nonfat milk and sugar substitute, if desired

Afternoon Snack
Veggies and Dip Snack (see recipe on page 293)

Healthy Dinner: Creamy Vegetable Soup and Hot Bread
Creamy Vegetable Soup (see recipe on page 278)
Toasted Whole-Grain Slices (see recipe on page 289)
Water, decaffeinated coffee or tea, or herbal tea, with 1 percent low-fat or nonfat milk and sugar substitute, if desired

Day 10

Great-Start Breakfast: Blueberry-Pecan Pancakes
Blueberry-Pecan Pancakes (see recipe on page 264)
Water, decaffeinated coffee or tea, or herbal tea, with 1 percent low-fat or nonfat milk and sugar substitute, if desired

Morning Snack
1 hard-boiled egg

Balancing Lunch: Turkey Caesar Salad
Turkey Caesar Salad (see recipe on page 276)
Water, decaffeinated coffee or tea, or herbal tea, with 1 percent low-
  fat or nonfat milk and sugar substitute, if desired

Afternoon Snack
1 slice low-fat mozzarella

Healthy Dinner: Grilled Sirloin Roast and Twice-Cooked Potatoes
Grilled Sirloin Roast (see recipe on page 282)
Twice-Cooked Potatoes (see recipe on page 290)
Spring greens with vinaigrette
Water, decaffeinated coffee or tea, or herbal tea, with 1 percent low-
  fat or nonfat milk and sugar substitute, if desired

Day 11

Great-Start Breakfast: Cheese, Tomato, and Basil Omelet
Cheese, Tomato, and Basil Omelet (see recipe on page 264)
½ cup mixed fresh fruit
Water, decaffeinated coffee or tea, or herbal tea, with 1 percent low-
  fat or nonfat milk and sugar substitute, if desired

Morning Snack
Celery and Nut Butter Snack (see recipe on page 291)

Balancing Lunch: Sirloin Steak Salad
Leftover sirloin steak, thinly sliced, on bed of spring greens, with
  sliced red onion, red peppers, and carrots
Olive oil and balsamic vinaigrette
Water, decaffeinated coffee or tea, or herbal tea, with 1 percent low-
  fat or nonfat milk and sugar substitute, if desired

Afternoon Snack
Yogurt and More Snack (see recipe on page 293)

Healthy Dinner: Garlic-Ginger Chicken and Broccoli Florets

Garlic-Ginger Chicken (see recipe on page 279)

Steamed Broccoli Florets (see recipe on page 289)

1 orange, sliced

Water, decaffeinated coffee or tea, or herbal tea, with 1 percent low-
fat or nonfat milk and sugar substitute, if desired

Day 12

Great-Start Breakfast: Whole-Grain Toast and Almond Butter

1 slice of 100 percent whole-grain bread, toasted, topped with
2 teaspoons of almond (or other nut) butter

2 slices of Canadian bacon

½ cup ruby red grapefruit

Water, decaffeinated coffee or tea, or herbal tea, with 1 percent low-
fat or nonfat milk and sugar substitute, if desired

Morning Snack

1 small apple

Balancing Lunch: Self-Acceptance Meal

Self-Acceptance Meal (see recipe on page 274)

Afternoon Snack

Mineral water or seltzer with a slice of lemon or lime

Healthy Dinner: Chef Salad

Chef Salad (see recipe on page 278)

Water, decaffeinated coffee or tea, or herbal tea, with 1 percent low-
fat or nonfat milk and sugar substitute, if desired

Day 13

Great-Start Breakfast: Light Eggs and Grapefruit

Light Eggs (see recipe on page 265)

Ruby red grapefruit, sprinkled with cinnamon and sugar substitute, if
  desired
Water, decaffeinated coffee or tea, or herbal tea, with 1 percent low-
  fat or nonfat milk and sugar substitute, if desired

Morning Snack
  2 large stalks of celery

Balancing Lunch: Yogurt and Nuts Lunch
  Yogurt and Nuts Lunch (see recipe on page 276)
  Water, decaffeinated coffee or tea, or herbal tea, with 1 percent low-
    fat or nonfat milk and sugar substitute, if desired

Afternoon Snack
  Sliced yellow and red peppers

**Healthy Dinner: Roasted Winter Vegetables and Pork
Tenderloin**
  Grilled Marinated Pork Tenderloin (see recipe on page 281)
  Roasted Winter Vegetables (see recipe on page 285)
  Olive oil and balsamic vinegar
  Water, decaffeinated coffee or tea, or herbal tea, with 1 percent low-
    fat or nonfat milk and sugar substitute, if desired

Day 14

Great-Start Breakfast: Solution Cereal
  Solution Cereal (see recipe on page 267)
  Water, decaffeinated coffee or tea, or herbal tea, with 1 percent low-
    fat or nonfat milk and sugar substitute, if desired

Morning Snack
  Veggies and Dip Snack (see recipe on page 293)

Balancing Lunch: Cheesy Roasted Vegetables
  Cheesy Roasted Vegetables (see recipe on page 270)

Water, decaffeinated coffee or tea, or herbal tea, with 1 percent low-fat or nonfat milk and sugar substitute, f desired

Afternoon Snack
1 hard-boiled egg with salt and cracked pepper

Healthy Dinner: Grilled Salmon with Mango Avocado Salsa
Grilled Salmon with Mango Avocado Salsa (see recipe on page 282)
Asparagus
Mixed greens with cherry tomatoes and vinaigrette
Water, decaffeinated coffee or tea, or herbal tea, with 1 percent low-fat or nonfat milk and sugar substitute, if desired
White Stuff: 1 large chocolate-covered strawberry or 5-ounce glass of white wine, if desired

19

Recipes from the Solution Community

MANY OF THE recipes in this chapter were inspired by members of our community, and one, Salata with Grilled Chicken, submitted by Najwa, a program participant, was chosen as the Grand Prize winner. All recipes serve one unless otherwise noted. A few recipes came from our Solution providers, including those on our nutrition team who tested the recipes: Jill Shafer, R.D.; Carra Richling-Knox, R.D.; Donna Accosta, R.D.; and Sylvia Cramer, Ph.D., R.D. Also, Alia Witt, M.F.T., R.D.; and Eve Lowry, R.D., contributed to the recipes in this chapter. (See more about our nutrition team in the acknowledgments.) The names of other Solution community members who submitted recipes for the plan are included in the acknowledgments.

These recipes were chosen with an eye toward ease of preparation. Some are so simple that you'd think there was no need for a recipe at all. We've included these recipes because proportions of ingredients and size of servings matter tremendously. By using them, you'll quickly get the idea of the proportions of foods and portion sizes that make it easier to turn off the drive to overeat and achieve lasting weight loss.

Breakfasts

BLUEBERRY-PECAN PANCAKES

Blueberries and pecans make these pancakes special! Cool, creamy, sweet vanilla yogurt is such a delicious accompaniment to whole-grain pancakes.

⅓ cup whole-grain, high-protein pancake mix
Low-fat milk
1 tablespoon bran or wheat germ
1 tablespoon chopped pecans
½ cup blueberries
Cooking spray
½ cup sugar-free vanilla yogurt

Choose a pancake mix that is whole-grain and make the pancake batter, replacing the water called for in the mix's preparation instructions with milk and adding the bran. Add the pecans and ¼ cup of the blueberries to the mixture. Coat a grill or frying pan with cooking spray and cook the pancakes on both sides. Remove from heat and serve warm, topped with yogurt and the remaining blueberries.

CHEESE, TOMATO, AND BASIL OMELET

I love this omelet because it's so quick and simple to make. The basil gives it a delicious fresh flavor.

1 whole egg, plus 2 egg whites
¼ cup tomato, chopped
1 tablespoon white onion, finely chopped
¼ cup shredded low-fat mozzarella
Cooking spray
1 teaspoon canola margarine
1 tablespoon chopped fresh basil

Combine the egg and egg whites in a small bowl, using a fork. Set aside.

Chop the tomato, onion, and basil, and set them aside. Shred the mozzarella.

Lightly coat a nonstick pan with cooking spray and add the canola margarine. Heat the pan over medium heat until hot. Add the eggs to the pan. When the eggs begin to set around the edges of the pan, start shaking the pan back and forth while stirring the eggs with a fork using a circular motion. Be sure not to scrape the pan with the fork. Continue shaking and stirring until the eggs are still moist but almost set.

Place the tomato, onion, cheese, and basil across the center of the omelet. Using a spatula, fold the omelet in half and serve warm.

Variation: Use ¾ cup egg substitute instead of fresh eggs.

FRUIT, YOGURT, AND NUT BREAKFAST

Here's another breakfast staple that's worth fine-tuning to your tastes. In the summer, fold in fresh peaches, apricots, or blackberries, and during the winter, try apples, raisins, and dried cranberries or blueberries.

1 cup lowfat yogurt, without sugar
2 tablespoons coarsely chopped walnuts or sliced almonds
1 cup blueberries or other fresh fruit or 2 tablespoons dried fruit

Use sugar-free yogurt, fruit-flavored, vanilla, or plain. If you prefer to avoid the aspartame in those foods, purchase low-fat or nonfat plain yogurt and, if you like, add Splenda or stevia to taste.

Place the yogurt in a bowl and top with the nuts and fruit.

LIGHT EGGS

Light Eggs are standard fare in my home. If you prefer egg substitute, that's fine, but if your cholesterol levels are low and you don't have heart disease, this recipe is quick and easy and will give you staying power.

Cooking spray
1 teaspoon canola margarine or butter, if you really need it
2 whole eggs, plus 1 extra egg white
Salt
Freshly ground pepper

Spray a frying pan with cooking spray and heat it over medium heat. Add either canola margarine or butter. Although I don't usually recommend cooking with butter because other good options are so readily available—such as olive oil, canola margarine, and cooking spray—in this recipe, it can add significantly to the tastiness of the dish.

Place the eggs in the pan and sprinkle them with salt and pepper. Turn over briefly and serve warm with fruit.

The dab of canola margarine or butter, plus the sprinkling of salt and freshly ground pepper add to the flavor. The flavor of the eggs will come through in this recipe, so use the freshest eggs available.

Variation: If you prefer, substitute for the fresh whole eggs and egg white ¾ cup egg substitute and increase the margarine to 2 teaspoons.

LIGHT SCRAMBLED EGGS AND CHEESE

This quick and easy recipe is very good with egg substitute as well as real eggs.

2 whole eggs, plus 1 extra egg white, scrambled; or ¾ cup egg substitute
1 ounce low-fat cheese of your choice
Salt
Freshly ground pepper
Cooking spray
1 teaspoon canola margarine

Place the eggs and egg white in a small bowl. Grate the cheese. Add the cheese, salt, and pepper to the egg mixture and stir.

Spray a frying pan or grill with cooking spray, heat it over medium heat, and add a dab of canola margarine. Pour the egg mixture into the pan and cook, stirring until the eggs reach the desired doneness. Serve warm.

Variations: Sprinkle cinnamon sugar (3 parts sugar to 1 part cinnamon) on cooked eggs or add your favorite herbs to the egg mixture before cooking.

SAUSAGE AND EGGS

2 low-fat sausages or tofu links
½ cup egg substitute
Salt and freshly gound pepper to taste
½ whole grain English muffin
1 teaspoon canola margarine

Spray a frying pan with cooking spray and heat it over medium heat. Add the links and cook until golden brown, turning as needed. Remove from pan.

Wash pan, spray with cooking spray, and place on medium heat. Add the egg substitute, stirring with a wooden spoon until cooked. Meanwhile, toast the muffin. Place on a plate and top with margarine, egg, and sausages.

Variation: Use 1 fresh egg instead of egg substitute.

SOLUTION CEREAL

It's so easy for a cereal breakfast to trigger a blood-sugar low by midmorning. Adding nuts and fruit and using high-fiber cereal curb that tendency. After trying this recipe, if you still get a midmorning blood-sugar low, skip the fruit.

½ cup high-fiber breakfast cereal
2 tablespoons sliced almonds or other nuts
1 cup fresh berries or 2 tablespoons dried fruit
1 cup 1 percent low-fat or nonfat milk
Sugar substitute, if desired

Much of the success of this recipe lies in the shopping. Peruse the grocery-store shelves to find a whole-grain cereal that is high in fiber and protein and low in sugar. The manufacturers change the formulas of their brands often, so there's no substitute for reading the labels and tasting the products. Some are wonderful . . . and some are not.

If you like cereal and Solution Cereal is going to be one of your staple breakfasts, then it's worth trying out various brands. My favorite is Kellogg's Special K Low Carb Lifestyle, with 10 grams of protein, 5 of grams fiber, and 2 grams of sugar in 100 calories. Another good choice is Kashi's Go Lean, with 7 grams of fiber, 9 grams of protein, and 4 grams of sugar per 100 calories.

Oddly, it's difficult to find a cereal that is high in fiber, low in sugar, and high in protein and doesn't contain aspartame. Even General Mills' Total Protein cereal, with 11 grams of protein and 2 grams of sugar has only 3 grams of fiber per 100 calories. If you aren't sensitive to aspartame, there are more high-protein, high-fiber, low-sugar cereals available, such as Kellogg's Morning Start, which is high in protein and fiber and low in sugar. Interestingly, all industry-sponsored studies show that aspartame is 100 percent safe, yet 89 percent of independent studies show one or more side effects. Sugar and obesity have risks, too, so how much aspartame you consume is an individual decision.

As for the nuts, walnuts are high in omega-3 and omega-6 fatty acids and are popular, but use any nut that you enjoy. Watch the amount of nuts you include closely, though, because of their high caloric density.

Use fresh berries—strawberries, blueberries, blackberries—or if none are available, add two tablespoons of dried fruit. Raisins are a good choice, as are dried cranberries, blueberries, strawberries, apricots, and peaches.

If you like nonfat milk, then use it. If you don't, use 1 percent low-fat milk. In our home, we use nonfat milk for drinking—it's more refreshing and lower in calories—and 1 percent milk for cereal and coffee and to pour over fruit.

You may not need to add sweeteners, but if you do, try Splenda or stevia.

Place the cereal in a bowl, top with the fruit and nuts, and cover with milk. Add sugar substitute, if desired.

Lunches

CALIFORNIA CHICKEN SALAD

The classic flavors of California cuisine work beautifully in this salad. Enjoy the addition of smooth, creamy avocado chunks and crunchy sunflower seeds.

1 skinless chicken breast
Salt
Pepper
Cooking spray
1 teaspoon olive oil
¼ avocado
2 green onions
½ tomato
1 tablespoon sunflower seeds
1 teaspoon mustard
2 teaspoons light mayonnaise
Romaine

Cook the chicken breast with care. (Cook more if you would like leftovers.) This step makes a tremendous difference in the taste of the salad. Rinse the chicken breast and pat it dry. Sprinkle with salt and pepper. Coat a frying pan or grill with cooking spray and place it over medium-high heat, stopping just short of being so high it would burn the chicken. Add the olive oil. Place the chicken breast in the pan and sauté for exactly 4 minutes with the temperature as hot as possible without burning. Turn the chicken and cook another 3 to 5 minutes just until it is firm to the touch. Remove from the heat and shred or chop.

For a quicker version, purchase cooked chicken breasts.

Slice and dice the avocado and place it in a small bowl. Slice the green onions and dice the tomato and add them to the bowl along with the chicken, sunflower seeds, mustard, and mayonnaise. Mix and serve on a bed of romaine.

CHEESY ROASTED VEGETABLES

These roasted vegetables are even better the second day, and topped with melted mozzarella, they make a lunch that is savory and delicious.

1 ½ cups leftover Roasted Winter Vegetables (see recipe on
    page 285)
2 ounces low-fat mozzarella cheese
Freshly ground pepper or red pepper flakes

This dish can easily be microwaved at work, but if you have a broiler on hand, it's even better. Place the roasted vegetables in a nonplastic container and microwave until steaming hot. Meanwhile, grate the mozzarella cheese. Top the hot roasted vegetables with the cheese and pepper and slip them under the broiler briefly until the cheese melts and turns golden brown. Serve hot.

CHICKEN CURRY PITA

Enjoy the contrasts in this quick lunch entrée—hot curry, cool chopped grapes, and hearty whole-wheat pita.

4 ounces cooked chicken
1 teaspoon curry powder
⅛ teaspoon mustard powder
2 tablespoons low-fat plain yogurt
½ cup chopped grapes
1 whole-wheat pita

Shred the cooked chicken (the California Chicken Salad recipe, on page 269, provides directions for cooking chicken). In a bowl combine the curry powder, mustard powder, and yogurt, add the chicken, and grapes and mix to coat. Fill the pita with the chicken mixture and serve.

Variation: If you prefer, substitute ½ cup chopped apple for the grapes.

GRILLED CHICKEN AND SPINACH SALAD

This flavorful salad is enlivened by the flavors of feta cheese and mango and brought together by the addition of a balsamic vinegar–based dressing.

4 ounces grilled chicken
2 cups baby spinach
4 thin slices red onion
¼ mango
2 tablespoons balsamic vinegar
1 teaspoon olive oil
1 tablespoon sliced almonds
2 tablespoons feta cheese
Freshly ground pepper

Grill a chicken breast for 4 minutes on each side or sauté it (the California Chicken Salad recipe, on page 269, provides directions for cooking chicken). Wash and dry the spinach, slice the red onion, and peel and thinly slice the mango. Combine the balsamic vinegar and olive oil. Place chicken, onion, mango, almonds, cheese, and oil and vinegar in a bowl and toss to combine. Add the spinach to the bowl. Toss and serve.

GRILLED SALMON SALAD

Creamy, salty salmon with a crust that hints of teriyaki on top of bitter mixed greens is delicious and elegant.

One 5-ounce salmon fillet
½ cup teriyaki marinade, purchased
½ cup cucumber, peeled and sliced
½ cup red pepper, sliced
Spring greens
Olive oil and balsamic vinaigrette
Freshly ground pepper

Marinate the salmon fillet in purchased teriyaki marinade for at least 15 minutes.

Prepare a bed of spring greens on a plate. Wash, peel, and slice the cucumber and wash and slice the red peppers and place both on top of the greens.

Heat a grill or barbecue until it is very hot, so it will sear the outside of the salmon and create a subtle crispy sweet crust. Cook the salmon for 3 to 5 minutes on each side, or until it reaches the desired doneness. Do not overcook. The flesh should be slightly translucent in the middle when done.

Remove the salmon from the heat and place it on top of the greens and vegetables. Add olive oil and balsamic vinaigrette and freshly ground pepper to taste and serve.

ROAST BEEF SANDWICH

A hearty roast beef sandwich brings back memories for me of lunches in downtown San Francisco when women still wore hats and gloves! The old roast beef sandwiches weren't very healthful, but this one is—and it's even more delicious.

5 ounces sirloin tip roast
Salt
Freshly cracked pepper
2 slices tomato
1 thin slice red onion
Lettuce
Mustard
Whole-grain bread (see Note)
2 teaspoons vinaigrette

Use purchased thinly sliced roast beef or cook a sirloin tip roast and slice it. Bring uncooked meat to room temperature, then sprinkle liberally with salt and freshly cracked pepper and cook for 1 hour per pound at 300° F. Cool and slice.

Slice the tomato and red onion. Wash the lettuce and break it apart. Spread mustard on the bread, then add the meat. Top with the vegetables, vinaigrette, and salt and pepper. Serve.

Note: You can be flexible about your choice of bread in this sandwich. If you're not really hungry or want to lose weight more rapidly, use 1 slice of whole-grain bread that provides 100 calories per slice or 2 slices of high-fiber bread that contains 50 calories per slice. If you are very hungry or not as concerned about rapid weight loss, have the sandwich on 2 pieces of whole-grain bread. This sandwich is great on 100 percent stone-ground whole-wheat bread or sprouted organic whole-wheat berry bread. If you are ordering this sandwich at a deli, this is equivalent to half a large deli sandwich, so just order half.

ROASTED TURKEY SANDWICH

Use leftover turkey breast to make this light, delicious sandwich or purchase fresh roasted turkey slices at the deli counter of your grocery store. Crisp lettuce and a dollop of cranberry sauce make this a special treat.

5 ounces turkey breast
Lettuce
Whole-grain bread
1 teaspoon low-fat mayonnaise
1 tablespoon cranberry sauce
Salt
Freshly cracked pepper

Use purchased or leftover turkey breast (the Turkey Caesar Salad recipe, on page 276, provides instructions for cooking a turkey breast).

Select bread based on your needs (see the Note that discusses bread choices above).

If you are ordering this sandwich at a deli, this is equivalent to half a large deli sandwich, so just order half.

Slice the turkey and wash the lettuce and break it apart. Spread mayonnaise on the bread, then add the turkey. Top with lettuce, cranberry sauce, and a sprinkling of salt and pepper. Serve.

Self-Acceptance Meal

When we're below the line about food, it's so easy to become either compulsive about nutrition or oblivious to it—not fully aware that what we eat affects our health and happiness in profound and immediate ways. With The Solution Method, we pay really close attention to how much we eat and what we eat, so we feel our best but stop short of depriving ourselves. It's a moment-to-moment process, always checking in with ourselves about how we feel and what we really need.

When we're above the line, we are not lost in the moment. We can see the consequences of our actions, and even when we plan to behave in ways that are not good for us, we focus on getting the most satisfaction for the damage done. We focus on minimizing the negative effects of our behavior. We also don't judge ourselves. The last thing we would feel is shame or even guilt.

When you really need to eat nutritional-garbage food, then by all means have it. However, don't eat all the healthy stuff and then the garbage. You'll gain weight! Eat precisely what you want but limit the calories to 350. A supersized Big Mac meal can contain 1,000 or more calories, so this doesn't mean eating whatever you want in whatever amounts you want. You could do that, but it wouldn't be a Self-Acceptance Meal. It would be a binge or nutritional overload and, for some of us, it might take several days to return to balance physically from one of those.

If you're not aware of the calories in foods, then here are some examples of Self-Acceptance Meals that add up to about 350 calories: 1 large 3 Musketeers candy bar, 1 large scoop of designer ice cream on a sugar cone, 2 Krispy Kreme doughnuts, 1 glass of red wine and 1 large (3" diameter) chocolate-chip cookie, or 1 small bag (1 serving) of potato chips and a regular non-diet Coke. Be picky as you select foods for this meal and consume the foods that give high "pleasure density," the most satisfaction per calorie.

After your Self-Acceptance Meal, you may want to take a walk or go to the gym. Also, for the next 24 hours, eat in a particularly healthy way to rebalance your neurotransmitters and hormones. Avoid going below the line, denigrating yourself for having eaten that food or feeling cleansed or overly virtuous for having snapped back to healthy living. The teeter-totter of devil and angel or being too bad then too good can become its own external solution. The menus for days 12 and 13 of the plan (pages 260 and 261) show how you can make subtle changes in your food to help rebalance your body.

If you are a binge eater or have an eating disorder, this is not a good meal for you to have. If, for any reason, it seems counter-productive to you, then don't have it. However, this meal is *not* a binge, because you are not eating rapidly and you have no self-deprecating thoughts afterward. In fact, you are savoring and thoroughly enjoying your food. This is part of life above the line. There are times when eating nutritional garbage can be seen as one of life's pleasures.

The most important thing about a Self-Acceptance Meal is that it is always there for you. At any moment, you could choose it because you are not on a diet. You have the means of getting your needs met for sugary, fatty foods without excessive negative effects on your weight and on the balance of your neurotransmitters and hormones.

TERIYAKI FLANK STEAK SALAD

Use leftover flank steak—briefly heated—to top cool crisp greens.

5 ounces of leftover Grilled Flank Steak Teriyaki (see recipe on page 280)
¼ cup carrots, peeled and sliced
¼ cup jicama, peeled and sliced
¼ cup snow peas, ends cut and sliced
Several leaves romaine lettuce
Olive oil and balsamic vinegar
Freshly ground pepper

Prepare a bed of romaine leaves on a plate. Wash, peel, and slice carrots, jicama, and snow peas and place on top of greens.

Slice leftover steak and heat briefly in microwave, about 30 to 45 seconds on high. Do not overcook.

Remove the steak from the microwave and place it on top of the greens and vegetables. Add olive oil, balsamic vinegar, and freshly ground pepper to taste and serve.

TURKEY CAESAR SALAD

This salad can be prepared at the last minute using sliced deli natural turkey breast, but it is even better if you bake a turkey breast to use for sandwiches and salads all week.

5 ounces of turkey breast broken into bite-size pieces
4 asparagus spears
Spring greens
Shavings of parmesan
2 tablespoons low-calorie Caesar salad dressing

Either purchase a turkey breast or cook your own. I often cook a turkey breast after dinner in the evening to have it ready to make lunches the next morning. It usually lasts all week. Most turkey breasts come with a "pop-up" temperature indicator so you can tell when they are done. For a moist, flavorful breast, leave the skin on and brush generously with olive oil, then sprinkle with salt and pepper. Cook at 325° F. It will take longer than cooking at higher heat, but the turkey will be far moister.

Microwave the asparagus briefly, then plunge it into cold water so it will retain its color and crispness. Cut on the diagonal. Wash and dry the spring greens and place them on a plate. Top with turkey, asparagus, shavings of parmesan, and Caesar salad dressing.

YOGURT AND NUTS LUNCH

When you have nothing in the house to eat or you are doing errands during your lunch hour at work and don't have time to stop to pick something up, this lunch works well. You can keep nuts, raisins, yogurt, and apples on hand for quite a while.

1 cup yogurt, any flavor but without sugar
3 tablespoons chopped walnuts or sliced almonds
½ cup chopped green apple or 1 tablespoon raisins

Use sugar-free yogurt, either fruit-flavored or vanilla, or use low-fat or nonfat plain yogurt and add Splenda or stevia, if you like. Place the yogurt in a bowl and top with the nuts and fruit.

Dinners

BUTTER LETTUCE WITH FETA AND CUCUMBER

Enjoy feta, English cucumber, and green onions atop soft cups of butter lettuce.

MAKES 2 SERVINGS.

2 cups butter lettuce
¼ cup thinly sliced peeled English cucumber
1 tablespoon thinly sliced green onion
1 tablespoon crumbled feta cheese
2 tablespoons vinaigrette (store-bought)
Freshly ground pepper

Wash lettuce and tear leaves in half. Place in a large bowl. Peel and slice cucumber and slice green onion. Place both on lettuce and top with crumbled feta. Sprinkle with vinaigrette and freshly ground pepper. Toss and serve.

ARUGULA AND SPINACH SALAD

This is a colorful salad that offers a complex blend of tastes and textures.

1 cup arugula
1 cup baby spinach leaves
1 tablespoon chopped walnuts
1 tablespoon dried cranberries
1 tablespoon feta, crumbled
2 thin slices red onion
1 tablespoon olive oil
Freshly ground black pepper
Balsamic vinaigrette

Wash the arugula and spinach and place them in a bowl. Add the remaining ingredients, including a splash of balsamic vinaigrette. Toss and serve.

CHEF SALAD

Chef Salad is a last-minute healthy answer to dinner. It calls for ingredients that you would typically have on hand, and the ham can be a welcome change from fish and poultry.

1 egg
Spring greens
1 ounce low-fat mozzarella
2 thin slices red onion
Juice from ½ lemon
4 ounces ham and turkey deli meat, thinly sliced
1 tablespoon capers
1 tablespoon olive oil
Freshly ground pepper

Hard-boil the egg. Peel and quarter it, then set it aside. Wash and prepare the greens and grate the mozzarella. Slice the onion and wash and quarter the lemon.

Place the ham and turkey, onion slices, capers and egg on a bed of spring greens and top with juice from the lemon and olive oil. Season with freshly ground pepper and serve.

CREAMY VEGETABLE SOUP

This soup is easy and fun to prepare, and you can use a variety of vegetables or just your favorite one.

MAKES 3 SERVINGS.

1 onion
4 cups favorite vegetables, sliced (for example, broccoli or leeks are great)
1 tablespoon olive oil
2 cups chicken broth
1 can evaporated low-fat milk
1 teaspoon sugar
White pepper

Slice the onion and vegetables. Sauté the onion in a large pan in olive oil until golden. Add the vegetables and chicken broth and simmer until the vegetables are soft. Cool slightly, then purée in a blender or food processor. Return the vegetable mixture to the large pan. Add evaporated milk, sugar, and a pinch of pepper. Heat and serve.

FARMER'S MARKET FISH

This delicious and colorful dish was one of the favorites of our nutrition team of Solution providers. Make extra to have for the next day's salad lunch.

MAKES 4 SERVINGS.

2 cups onion, chopped
2 cups red bell pepper, chopped
1 cup zucchini, chopped
1 cup tomato, chopped
2 tablespoons fresh basil, chopped
1 garlic clove
2 teaspoons olive oil
Salt
Freshly ground pepper
1 pound halibut or salmon, cut into ¼-pound portions
½ cup feta cheese or ¼ cup grated Parmesan cheese

Chop the vegetables and peel and mince the garlic. Heat the oil in a large skillet over medium-high heat. Add the onion, garlic, bell pepper, and zucchini and cook, stirring occasionally, for 3 to 5 minutes. Add the tomato, basil, salt, and pepper and cook for an additional 3 minutes. Reduce heat to medium-low. Place the fish on top of the vegetables, cover, and simmer for 5 minutes. Sprinkle with cheese, cover, and cook an additional 5 minutes, or until the fish flakes easily when tested with a fork.

GARLIC-GINGER CHICKEN

The flavor of this delicious and easy Asian-inspired chicken is enlivened by fresh ginger and green onions. Other than the ginger, the ingredients are ones you're apt to have on hand.

MAKES 4 SERVINGS.

1 pound boneless, skinless chicken breasts or thighs, well trimmed of fat

Salt

Pepper

Paprika

1 tablespoon canola or olive oil

1 cup scallion whites, minced, plus 1 cup scallion greens, sliced and kept
    separate

3 cloves garlic, crushed

1 tablespoon ginger, minced

1 cup chicken broth

⅓ cup rice wine vinegar

2 tablespoons soy sauce or hoisin sauce

1 teaspoon sugar

Sprinkle the chicken with salt, pepper, and paprika to taste. Heat 2 teaspoons of the oil in a large, heavy skillet over medium-high heat. Add the chicken and cook until well browned on each side, about 3 minutes per side. Remove the chicken from the pan and keep it warm.

Add the remaining teaspoon of oil to the pan. Add the scallion whites, garlic, and ginger and cook, stirring frequently, for 1 minute. Add the broth, vinegar, soy sauce, and sugar. Bring to a simmer and cook until slightly thickened, about 3 minutes.

Return the chicken and the juices to the pan. Reduce heat to low. Simmer until the chicken is cooked through, about 4 minutes. Transfer the chicken to a platter. Season the sauce with additional soy sauce, if desired, and spoon it over the chicken. Garnish with scallion greens.

GRILLED FLANK STEAK TERIYAKI

A few special touches with flank steak make this sweet, lean cut of beef an elegant satisfier. Plan to prepare enough steak for dinner tonight and for tomorrow's lunch. If you have time to marinate the meat at room temperature for 1 to 2 hours, the outside "crust" will be crispy.

MAKES 4 SERVINGS.

⅔ cup teriyaki marinade, purchased
2 large garlic cloves, minced
1 tablespoon toasted sesame seeds
2 tablespoons honey
Flank steak, 1½ pounds

Combine teriyaki marinade, garlic, sesame seeds, and honey in a large bowl. Add the flank steak and marinate it for 15 minutes or more. Heat a barbecue, grill, or broiler on high. Grill the steak briefly on each side, basting with additional marinade. Remove from the grill, slice thinly on the diagonal, and serve.

GRILLED MARINATED PORK TENDERLOIN

For a quick meal, use purchased marinated pork tenderloin. If you want leftovers, double the recipe and slice and heat the pork to top greens for the next day's lunch or dinner.

MAKES 2 SERVINGS.

4 tablespoons green onion, minced
2 large garlic cloves, minced
2 tablespoons dried rosemary
1 tablespoon honey
½ cup olive oil
2 tablespoons balsamic vinaigrette
Salt
Fresh ground pepper
1 pork tenderloin, 8 to 10 ounces

Mix all the ingredients except the pork tenderloin in a small bowl, including salt and pepper to taste, and pour over the pork tenderloin. Marinate for 30 to 60 minutes. Grill or broil on very high heat until done, usually 15 minutes on each side. Do not overcook and do not cook at a lower temperature or the pork will not be moist. Slice and serve.

GRILLED SALMON WITH MANGO AVOCADO SALSA

This entrée was a favorite of our Nutrition Team who tested the recipes. Elegant, quick, and stylish!

MAKES 2 SERVINGS.

2 salmon steaks, 5 ounces each or 1 10-oz salmon fillet
1 ripe mango, cut from the pit, peeled, and chopped
2 red bell peppers, finely chopped
¼ cup avocado, chopped
2 red onions, finely chopped
⅓ cup lime juice
1 serrano chile, minced
2 tablespoons fresh cilantro, minced
Pinch of salt
Freshly ground pepper

To prepare salmon, heat grill on high. Sprinkle salmon with salt and pepper. Grill 4 minutes on each side. Meanwhile, prepare salsa by combining remaining ingredients in a small bowl and tossing gently. Remove salmon from grill and top immediately with the salsa and serve.

Variations: The mango avocado salsa is also tasty when spooned over grilled chicken or mahimahi.

Note: You can make the salsa up to two days in advance; it will keep well for that long in an airtight container in the refrigerator.

GARLIC MUSTARD SIRLOIN ROAST

Lean, spicy, and satisfying, this roast takes one hour to prepare. While it's cooking, consider going for a walk or soaking in a hot tub.

MAKES 6–8 SERVINGS.

3 fresh garlic cloves, minced
Mustard, spicy, sweet, or Dijon
2 pounds sirloin tip roast
Salt
Freshly ground pepper

Preheat the oven to 550° F. Place the garlic and mustard in a small bowl and mix until they form a paste. Rub the paste on the roast, sprinkle with salt and pepper. Place the roast on a rack in a pan in the oven. Reduce the temperature immediately to 325° F. Cook for 30 minutes per pound. Cook at higher temperatures or for longer to preferred doneness. Serve 4- to 5-ounce portions for dinner—about the size of the palm of your hand—and use the rest for a lunch salad the next day.

HALIBUT WITH GINGER GLAZE

This sweet-tart ginger glaze is a perfect complement to the mild-flavored halibut.

MAKES 4 SERVINGS.

¼ cup red miso (soybean paste)
2 tablespoons brown sugar
2 tablespoons sweet rice wine (mirin)
4 halibut fillets (1½ pounds total)
⅓ cup honey
⅓ cup fresh lime juice
2 tablespoons fresh ginger, peeled and minced
Cooking spray
1 tablespoon black or white sesame seeds, toasted

Combine the miso, brown sugar, and mirin in a small bowl. Brush the fish with the miso mixture. Cover and refrigerate for 30 minutes.

Meanwhile, combine the honey, lime juice, and ginger in a small saucepan over medium heat. Bring to a boil and cook, stirring often, for 10 minutes or until the mixture thinly coats the back of a spoon. Set it aside.

Preheat the broiler. Place the halibut on a broiler rack coated with cooking spray. Broil for 3 minutes on each side, or until the fish flakes easily when tested with a fork.

To serve, drizzle the honey mixture over the fish and sprinkle with the sesame seeds.

MIXED GREENS WITH ROASTED PINE NUTS

Roast several batches of pine nuts to have on hand for snacking. Add a few to the salad to boost its flavor and fiber.

MAKES 2 SERVINGS.

½ cup pine nuts
2 cups mixed greens
½ cup cherry tomatoes, halved
2 tablespoons balsamic vinaigrette (prepared)

Spread pine nuts on a cookie sheet and place in 400° F oven. Roast for 3 to 4 minutes or until lightly browned. Place mixed greens in a bowl, add pine nuts, sliced tomatoes, and vinaigrette. Toss and serve.

MIXED GREENS WITH MANDARIN ORANGE SLICES

This quick side salad is light and fresh.

MAKES 2 SERVINGS.

2 cups spring greens
¼ small red onion
½ cup mandarin orange slices
1 tablespoon chopped pecans
2 tablespoons vinaigrette (prepared)

Place washed greens in a bowl. Thinly slice and quarter onion. Top greens with onion, orange slices, and pecans. Add vinaigrette, toss and serve.

PASTA BOLOGNESE

Delicious flavors and seasonings typical of Italian cooking—red wine, fennel, tomatoes—come together beautifully to make this delicious meat sauce. It's quick and easy to prepare, too. Try pairing it with spelt, a very tasty whole-grain pasta, or with another whole-grain pasta of your choice.

MAKES 4 SERVINGS.

1 cup onion, chopped
1 cup carrots, chopped
1 pound ground sirloin
3 garlic cloves, minced
½ cup red wine
1 teaspoon fennel seeds
1 teaspoon freshly ground pepper
One 28-ounce can crushed tomatoes
5 ounces whole-grain pasta

Cook the onion, carrots, sirloin, and garlic in a large skillet over medium-high heat, occasionally breaking up the sirloin. When the sirloin is browned, add the wine and cook for 1 minute.

Add the fennel seeds, pepper, and tomatoes. Turn heat to high and bring to a boil. Reduce heat to a simmer, cover, and cook for 40 minutes.

Cook pasta according to package directions, omitting salt. Drain and serve topped with sauce.

ROASTED WINTER VEGETABLES

Roasting vegetables brings out their natural sweetness. Make enough to have leftovers for the next day's lunch.

MAKES 8 SERVINGS.

1 whole shallot, peeled and separated
2 pounds carrots, peeled and cut into pieces
2 pounds parsnips, peeled and cut into pieces
2 pounds sweet potatoes, peeled and cut into pieces
2 pounds Brussels sprouts, trimmed
2 tablespoons olive oil
2 teaspoons fresh thyme
2 teaspoons fresh sage
Salt
Freshly cracked pepper

Preheat the oven to 450° F.

Combine the shallot, carrots, parsnips, sweet potatoes, and Brussels sprouts in a large bowl. Combine the olive oil, thyme, and sage in a small bowl. Drizzle the oil over the vegetables. Add salt and pepper and toss well to coat the vegetables.

Arrange the vegetables in a single layer on a shallow roasting pan. Roast the vegetables for 40 minutes, stirring occasionally until they are soft, brown, and sweet.

SALATA WITH GRILLED CHICKEN

This recipe was the Grand Prize winner in our Solution Community Recipe Contest for this book. The Solution providers who tested these recipes—Jill Shaffer, Carra Richling-Knox, Donna Acosta, and Sylvia Cramer—found it hard to keep this salad in the house. It disappeared!

MAKES 4 SERVINGS.

1 head romaine lettuce, chopped
2 cups (about 2 bunches) Italian parsley, chopped
3 to 4 green onions, chopped
¼ cup fresh mint leaves, chopped
1 large cucumber, peeled, halved, and thinly sliced
1 yellow or orange bell pepper, seeded and chopped
2 medium tomatoes, chopped
One 15-ounce can garbanzo beans, drained
4 skinless, boneless chicken breasts, cooked
4 tablespoons olive oil and balsamic vinaigrette

Combine the lettuce, parsley, onions, mint, cucumber, bell pepper, tomatoes, garbanzo beans, and vinaigrette in a large salad bowl and toss to mix well. Top with sliced grilled chicken breast (the California Chicken Salad recipe, on page 269, provides directions for cooking chicken) and serve.

SHRIMP SALAD PLATTER

Solution Provider Jill Shaffer developed this recipe and tested it on a group of friends for supper over the New Year's holiday. Everyone loved it, and it has great eye appeal and flavor!

MAKES 4 SERVINGS.

1 pound large (21–26 count) cooked shrimp
1 cup snow peas
½ cup grape tomatoes, halved
½ cup cashews
4 cups spring greens
Juice of one large lemon
¼ teaspoon of lemon zest
¼ teaspoon salt (optional)
Freshly ground pepper to taste
¼ cup olive oil
2 teaspoons dijon mustard

Wash the shrimp, snow peas, and tomatoes. Trim snow peas and halve the tomatoes. Combine the first 5 ingredients in a large bowl. In a small bowl, place remaining ingredients and mix well. Pour over salad, toss and serve.

SHRIMP TOSTADA

If you love shrimp, this easy, quick, and healthy dish may well turn out to be one of your favorite ways to enjoy it.

Cooking spray
1 whole-wheat tortilla
¼ cup low-fat Monterey Jack cheese, shredded
¼ cup canned black beans, drained
5 ounces tail-off shrimp, cooked
¼ avocado, diced
1 cup romaine lettuce, chopped
1 tablespoon salsa

Coat the grill liberally with cooking spray and place the tortilla on the grill over medium heat. Spread the shredded cheese on the tortilla, then add the black beans. Microwave the shrimp to heat it slightly. Top the tortilla with the shrimp. Heat it briefly, then transfer it to a plate. Top with avocado, lettuce, and salsa.

SPICY GARLIC GREEN BEANS

If you serve this tasty dish to company, be prepared to hand out the recipe!

1 pound fresh green beans
1 tablespoon plus 1 teaspoon bottled minced garlic
1 cup low-sodium soy sauce
1 cup chicken broth
1 teaspoon rice wine vinegar
1 tablespoon sesame oil
1 teaspoon chili oil
2 teaspoons sugar

Place the green beans (see Note) in a large saucepan and add 1 inch of water to the bottom of the pan. Cover and steam briefly until just tender, 4 to 6 minutes. Meanwhile, place the garlic, soy sauce, broth, vinegar, oils, and sugar in a small bowl and combine with a whisk.

Place the beans in a serving dish and drizzle with the dressing. Serve immediately.

Note: Frozen green beans may be used if you prefer, but fresh green beans have a much better flavor.

SPINACH AND STRAWBERRY SALAD

Serve this dish with pork tenderloin or another lean protein food and it's an entire meal. It's simple and visually stunning!

MAKES 4 SERVINGS.

8 cups baby spinach leaves
1 pint strawberries, hulled and sliced
¼ cup sliced almonds
¼ small red onion, thinly sliced
4 tablespoons olive oil
4 tablespoons raspberry vinegar
1 teaspoon Dijon mustard
Freshly ground black pepper

If necessary, tear spinach leaves into bite-size pieces. Place the spinach, strawberries, almonds, and onion in a large salad bowl. Combine the remaining ingredients, including freshly ground black pepper to taste, in a small bowl, stirring with a fork or a whisk. To serve, drizzle the dressing on the salad and toss gently to combine the ingredients and coat the salad with dressing.

STEAMED BROCCOLI FLORETS

Broccoli is very rich in antioxidants and phytochemicals. In this recipe, garlic, pepper, and sugar enhance its naturally mustardy flavor and crunchy texture. Buy florets to make preparation faster.

1 cup broccoli florets
1 tablespoon olive oil
1 garlic clove, minced
Red pepper flakes
½ teaspoon sugar
Salt
Ground black pepper

Wash the florets and place them in a steaming basket over 1 to 2 inches of boiling water. Cover and steam for 3 minutes or until tender but crisp. If you don't have a steaming basket handy, cook them in an inch of water, then drain. Place the olive oil in a pan and heat on medium-high. Add the garlic, then the steamed florets, a pinch of red pepper, sugar, and salt and ground black pepper to taste. Serve immediately.

TOASTED WHOLE-GRAIN SLICES

These toasty fresh bread slices complement a hearty soup. Don't skimp on the oil and be sure to use whole-grain bread.

MAKES 8 SERVINGS.

Small loaf of 100 percent whole-grain bread
Cooking spray

¼ cup olive oil
2 fresh garlic cloves, minced

Cut the bread on the diagonal into approximately ⅜-inch-thick slices. Coat the grill with cooking spray and heat it. Place the slices on the grill over medium heat and toast one side until brown. Combine the oil and garlic in a small bowl. Turn the slices over and brush with the olive oil and garlic mixture. When the second side is toasted, remove from the grill and serve two small slices with each bowl of soup.

TWICE-COOKED POTATOES

This recipe is a favorite of mine from friends Andrea and Daniel Sharp, whose amazing cooking always astonishes me. I couldn't write a weight-loss book without including it.

MAKES 4 SERVINGS.

1½ pounds small creamer potatoes
Salt
2 tablespoons extra virgin olive oil
¼ cup chopped garlic
¼ cup canola oil
2 teaspoons lemon zest
¼ cup fresh Italian flat-leaf parsley, chopped
Freshly ground pepper

Put the unpeeled potatoes in a large pot with enough generously salted water to cover them. Bring to a boil and cook until a knife slips into the potatoes easily, about 20 minutes. Drain the potatoes and cool sufficiently so you won't burn your hands. Press each potato with the heel of your hand until it is about ½ inch thick. The skin will split, but don't press so hard that it completely falls apart. The skin should hold the potato together.

Place the olive oil in a separate small frying pan and heat. Add garlic and sauté until lightly browned. Set aside.

Heat the canola oil over moderately high heat in a large skillet. Add the potatoes and cook them, turning gently, on both sides until crisp and browned, about 10 minutes. There will be some crumbling of the potatoes, but don't worry, the crispy, small particles just add to the experience. Place the potatoes in a bowl and top with the sautéed garlic, lemon zest, parsley, and salt and freshly ground pepper to taste. Serve immediately.

Note: Use creamer potatoes, Yukon Gold preferred, but reds work well, too.

Snacks

When you are hungry between meals—just a little bit hungry, not starving—a handful of veggies and some liquids will stave off hunger until your next meal. You might have some herbal tea, a glass of seltzer with a squeeze of lime or lemon, some mineral water, or a cup of decaf coffee with a splash of milk. Or try a piece of fruit.

If you are hungrier and sense you need something with greater staying power, choose one of these heartier, more substantial snacks, which will more effectively hold off body hunger until your next meal. Keep the amounts modest, though. You don't want to disrupt your normal hunger cycle for breakfast, lunch, and dinner.

The thought, smell, or sight of food has a strong influence on the brain and stimulates hunger. So being able to focus on food three times daily, eat until satisfied, then not think about food at all encourages lasting weight loss. When you shift your focus from food to what you are building in your own life or in the lives of others, hunger fades.

CELERY AND NUT BUTTER SNACK

The celery is cool and crisp, the butter, salty and satisfying.

1 stalk of celery
1 tablespoon almond or peanut butter

Wash and dry the celery and spread it with almond or peanut butter. Slice diagonally into smaller pieces.

COTTAGE SNACK

Cottage cheese works well for quieting late-afternoon appetites. Just a little bit of cottage cheese and 8 ounces of a favorite beverage and you won't be hungry until dinner.

½ cup nonfat or low-fat cottage cheese

Accent of your choice:

- Cinnamon and sugar substitute
- 1 teaspoon toasted wheat germ and sugar substitute
- 1 tablespoon chopped dried fruit (such as apricots)
- ¼ cup fresh fruit (such as peaches or apples)

Cinnamon has a balancing effect on blood sugar and insulin levels, but any of these toppings will flavor the cottage cheese and boost nutrition.

FRUIT AND MORE SNACK

When you add some nuts or a milk product to fruit, you give it more staying power.
   Here are some popular combinations:

- ½ pear and 5 walnuts
- 1 small apple and a slice of low-fat mozzarella cheese
- 1 fresh peach with ½ cup 1 percent low-fat milk and a sprinkling of nutmeg
- 1 orange and a tablespoon of pecans
- ½ banana and 3 walnuts
- 1 cup blueberries, ½ cup 1 percent low-fat milk, and sugar substitute
- 1 cup strawberries and 4 almonds

GRAPEFRUIT AND CINNAMON SNACK

Grapefruit has a low glycemic index and a satisfying sweet-sour taste. Choose the best-quality ruby red grapefruit. Have half a grapefruit or a whole one for a snack. Combine the grapefruit with one of the following:

- Cinnamon sugar (3 parts sugar to 1 part cinnamon or a sprinkling of sugar substitute and cinnamon)
- Toasted wheat germ and sugar substitute
- Dollop of sugar-free yogurt

VEGGIES AND DIP SNACK

Veggies are the number one snack choice, as they are high in fiber, low in calories, and have a low glycemic index. However, when you are really hungry, adding something to veggies that heightens their appeal and satisfaction is a good idea. Boost healthy fats in combination with veggies by relying on small amounts of humus or guacamole (about 2 tablespoons) to accompany as many veggies as you like. Another option for an easy, healthy dip for veggies is canned spicy refried black beans (heat in the microwave until soft enough for a dip). All three are readily available at most grocery stores. Here are some favorite combinations:

- Jicama and humus
- Red peppers and guacamole
- Sliced cucumbers and humus
- Celery dipped in refried black beans
- Endive spears and humus
- Baby carrots and guacamole

YOGURT AND MORE SNACK

Yogurt is high in protein; tryptophan, the precursor of serotonin; and calcium, a natural relaxant; plus bacteria that are beneficial to the gut. Yogurt already contains carbohydrates in the form of lactose, which is a problem only for those who lack enough of the enzyme needed to break it down. However, commercial flavored yogurts are high in sugar syrup, which is a refined carbohydrate.

Yogurt can mimic a comfort food for many people, leading them to eat large quantities when they are not hungry. If it stimulates your appetite rather than quieting it, yogurt may not be a good snack for you. For a snack, 4 to 6 ounces of yogurt and ½ cup of fruit should be plenty. If you want nuts or wheat germ, add a tablespoon. If you like yogurt that much, consider having larger amounts and enjoying it for a meal. As a snack, stick with a few spoonfuls, just enough to tide you over until the next meal.

A great way to get the benefits of yogurt is to buy unflavored yogurt and flavor it with a sugar substitute and/or fruits. Also, you can choose sugar-free yogurts that are presweetened with a sugar substitute. Even better, enjoy one of the following combinations:

- Vanilla yogurt and 1 tablespoon pecans
- Strawberry yogurt topped with 1 tablespoon sliced almonds
- Cantaloupe topped with raspberry yogurt
- Blueberry yogurt with blueberries and almonds
- Plain yogurt and kiwi slices, with sugar substitute, if desired
- Tangerine yogurt, chopped cashews, and fresh mint

Part 5

A TRUE

SOLUTION

20

Day 15 and Beyond

AFTER TWO WEEKS of using the method, you are ready for phase 3.

In phase 3 of the training, there are no menus and no recipes as you have used the 1-2-3 Eating enough so that you're aware of portion sizes and how to combine foods. However, in Chapters 21 and 22, there are more ideas about how to choose foods for lasting weight loss and the Solution 1-2-3 Food Lists guide your choices. Chapter 23 presents the stories of nine people who have been involved in Solution training.

In terms of rewiring the feeling brain so that you have a Solution, at this point you probably know if you want or need more training in the method. We have no long-term research that describes the results people experience after using the 3-Day Solution Plan without continuing their training. Doubtless, some people will have enough with only this book. All our testing of the method has been done with those who completed the Solution course, which provides advanced skills and deepens and extends the skills. It covers more sophisticated uses of them, including developing a supportive, nurturing inner voice, taking out emotional trash, doing lifestyle surgery, and staying above the line during stressful times.

If you want more information about the training, just visit our website at www.thepathway.org and, if you still have questions, call the institute at (415) 457-3331. The Institute for Health Solutions is a non-profit organization.

You may want to try this next phase on your own. It seems that most people have a sense of what they need at this point. Some people know they want to become involved in Solution training, and others prefer to let their efforts from the first two phases of the plan "sink in" and see whether they want or need more.

Although, we do know that retraining the feeling brain to the point that you have a Solution—lasting weight loss, freedom from the whole range of external solutions, and an abundance of life's rewards—is not easy, and that's why we offer the kits and the professional support. We also know that many very resilient people come to this work and almost all find that they need both the kits and some groups' support to find their Solution. You may be different, though.

The next two chapters present more information on the Solution 1-2-3 Eating. With all the food information, my worry is that you'll get caught up with the food and lifestyle part of the program. If you do, the plan has scant chance of bringing lasting change. If you prefer to focus on lifestyle and not the skills, consider checking in with yourself six months from now. If the drive to overeat has not turned off by then with no crossover external solution replacing it, and you don't have an abundance of the rewards of the training—integration, balance, sanctuary, intimacy, vibrancy, and spirituality—then consider whether or not it would be worth your while to become involved in Solution training.

More about Solution Training

The Solution Method was developed at the University of California–San Francisco's School of Medicine in the departments of family and community medicine and pediatrics over the last 25 years. In a way, it was perfect that the method started with a focus on obesity, because weight is often the toughest excess to resolve. We can't abstain from eating, and more than 70 percent of us have eating or weight issues.

Only in the last 5 years has its use been extended to the whole range of common excesses—smoking, drinking, drugs, overworking, overspending, and the softer excesses such as people-pleasing, rescuing others, putting up walls, and thinking too much. In recent years, we've found that many people enroll in the training not to turn off an emotional appetite but to be happier and healthier, to live life above the line.

Solution training involves completing 6 Solution Kits. Each kit includes a workbook/journal and four CDs, plus three months of membership in our Solution community. The kits are designed to give your brain just the experiences needed to revise the neural networks to favor life above the line at each phase of the journey. However, participants can choose different kinds of support. Some just use the Internet support that is included with the kit. Others join Solution groups, enroll in Solution three-day retreats, or participate in Solution coaching provided by certified Solution providers.

All Solution providers are licensed health professionals with a minimum of 18 months of training in the method. Our providers use the method themselves, as our research has shown that unless therapists or health professionals have a Solution in their own lives, they are unlikely to bring a participant to a Solution.

If there is not a Solution provider in your area, Solution telegroups conducted by Solution providers are available through the institute and on our website. Guidelines are available for how to create a self-help Solution circle in your neighborhood. We also offer Basic Solution Support, a four-week telephone group, or two private sessions with a Solution provider, for those who want to get off to a good start and complete the kits with community support. There is a Solution buddy list on our website for those who successfully complete this basic support. Getting on that list will enable you to contact others around the country and the world who have demonstrated mastery of the basic skills and have met our safety guidelines with the method. These skills grow best in a warm, safe community, and our community is growing rapidly.

The Institute for Health Solutions, the nonprofit organization that provides this training, has been approved to offer Continuing Education by the American Psychological Association, the Board of Behavioral Medicine, and the American Dietetic Association. Our mission is to support the development, evaluation, and dissemination of developmental skills training (The Solution Method) for the prevention and treatment of common problems and the promotion of health and happiness. For program research or for group locations near you, please visit our website.

For more information about The Solution Method, contact the Institute for Health Solutions, (415) 457-3331, or visit www.the pathway.org.

The application of this method to children and adolescents is available as The Shapedown Program. For information about The Shapedown Program, visit www.childobesity.org.

21

Eating for Lasting Weight Loss

THE BASIC PRINCIPLES of the Solution 1-2-3 Eating are to eat regularly throughout the day—breakfast, lunch, and dinner. If you are hungry at midmorning or midafternoon, have a snack. It's fine to snack after dinner if you're hungry, but most late-evening hunger is emotionally driven. It's appetite, and instead of reaching for something to eat, it's best to obtain pleasure, relaxation, or inspiration from something other than food.

Only eat when you are hungry, that is, when you feel body hunger. Body hunger is tricky, as you have seen from reading about the toxic spiral. Often we think we're hungry or we even feel body hunger, but our bodies do not need food. As you continue using the method, eating the 1-2-3 way, and living above the line, you'll be able to trust your hunger signals more. An appreciation for reasonable portion sizes can be a helpful guide, although it's not something to stick with when you *really need* more food! If you really need it, then by all means eat something. Making not eating more important than meeting your true needs just triggers feeling abandoned or adolescent rebellion. In my own life, neither has ever helped me lose weight.

The 1-2-3 Eating approach means choosing foods from three groups:

1. *The Fiber Group,* which includes vegetables, fruits, and high-fiber whole grains.
2. *Healthy Fats,* which includes oils and foods high in monounsaturated fats.

3. *The Protein Group,* which includes low-fat and nonfat
   proteins, such as lean meat, chicken, fish, beans, soy
   products, and milk products.

Centering your food intake around foods in these groups helps to turn off the drive to overeat. They are highly nutritious; they balance your serotonin, dopamine, and endorphins; and they keep you above the line, where your drive to overeat fades. It's important to eat for both health and pleasure, so even if a food in this group is very nutritious, don't eat it unless you like it. Please take a moment, when you're ready, and turn to Chapter 22 and check off all the 1-2-3 Foods that you find pleasing. These foods will be the mainstay of your diet.

It's best to eat most of your foods from these groups all the time. However, it becomes even more important to eat these foods if your body is out of balance, either from being overweight, from chronic stress in your life, or from having a difficult temperament—that is, being someone who either tends to think rather than feel or has overwhelmingly strong feelings. Eating these foods is also best when your body is under stress, due to such factors as hormonal changes (premenstrual syndrome or perimenopause, for example) or seasonal changes (seasonal affective disorder, for example). If you carry your weight in the middle—under your ribs, not just under your skin—it's particularly important to have most or nearly all of your foods from these three groups.

Once your weight is within your genetic comfort zone, the difference between the food you eat to lose weight and to maintain it is very subtle, so even then, in order to keep the weight off, you will not eat much differently than you do on this plan. What is the essential pain? You will never be able to eat whatever you what to eat whenever you want to eat without gaining weight. The earned reward? You will feel great. You will live life above the line, and you will never have to go on a diet again.

A fourth group, White Stuff, includes everything that is not on the first three lists. Although all the foods in this group are not necessarily white, they do have low values in terms of health promotion, disease prevention, and weight loss. These are foods high in sugars, refined carbohydrates, trans fats, saturated fats, alcohol, artificial sugar substitutes other than Splenda or stevia, and caffeine.

Many beverages fall into the White Stuff group, including sodas, diet sodas, full-strength juices, coffee, beer, wine, and liquor. This means opting most of the time for water, decaffeinated coffee and tea, herbal tea, half-strength juices, seltzer water, mineral water, nonfat milk, and 1 percent (low-fat) milk. Sugar substitutes other than Splenda or stevia either increase insulin and prompt an increased appetite or are not safe. However, if the earned reward of using them is greater than the essential pain for you, then by all means, use them without guilt and in moderation.

The 1-2-3 Eating plan is clear-cut, inasmuch as the foods that support vibrancy are on the 1-2-3 Food Lists and everything else is White Stuff. We don't differentiate, for example, between white bread and sugar or between hot dogs and bacon. None of these foods are strong contenders for promoting health, nutrition, and vibrancy, so they are all combined in one group. No foods are bad, however, and ultimately, it's how much and how often they are eaten that counts.

For some people, the White Stuff group includes other things they put into their bodies as external solutions, such as recreational drugs, cigarettes, or unneeded over-the-counter or prescription drugs. Feel free to add to the White Stuff category other things that constitute external solutions in your life, if that is helpful to you.

How to Plan Meals and Snacks

The 1-2-3 system of eating helps you make decisions about food that enable you to eat for both health and pleasure. It is not a diet, because you ultimately control the boundaries of what you eat and how much of it you eat. You cannot go "off" this plan; it simply varies depending on how you implement it. Use it in the way that gives you the rewards you most value, whether that be the immediate pleasure of a chocolate candy bar or the feeling of lightness and vibrancy that comes from eating more 1-2-3 Foods.

To plan a meal, choose at least one food from each of the 1-2-3 Food Lists: at least one food from The Fiber Group, one from

Healthy Fats, and one from The Protein Group. You'll have about six servings of fruits and vegetables a day and at least two servings of milk products. You'll get plenty of protein from various sources as well as some Healthy Fats to increase satisfaction and prevent excessive intake of carbohydrates.

After you choose at least one food from each of the 1-2-3 groups, ask yourself, "Do I really need White Stuff?" If you do, have all that you really need; but if you don't really need it, then don't have any. After all, eating White Stuff makes it easier for your body to go below the line. But if you need it, have it guilt-free and enjoy every bite.

The reason you should have it without guilt is because 1-2-3 Eating isn't just about the food—it's also about satisfaction. If you deprive yourself of something you really feel you need, you'll probably make up for it later by overeating. When people are put on low-sugar diets, over time, their fat intake usually increases. When people are put on low-fat diets, their sugar intake increases. When people are kept on extremely high-fiber diets, they often increase the amount of food they are eating to make up for the satisfaction they are missing. In short, any extreme diet is unlikely to prove effective in producing lasting weight loss. Whenever eating a certain way becomes more important than your personal happiness, there is usually a backlash. You are always more important than your food plan. If you really need something, by all means, have it—but do it from above the line, where you accept responsibility for your actions.

A good rule of thumb is that if you really need it and must have it, then have it no matter what. If you really need it, have three bites, then check again after every bite to see whether you really need more. As soon as the answer is "no," stop.

Also, choose the White Stuff that causes the least disruption in your weight loss. If you are highly stressed or if you carry your weight in the middle, you're better off with something high in fat than something high in sugar—say, one bite of chocolate or a chocolate-dipped strawberry, both of which are high in fat, rather than a sugar cookie or a caramel.

It's best to have your White Stuff with meals rather than alone as snacks, because it will cause less havoc with your blood sugar and insulin levels. When you snack, have something with a low emotional payoff. I learned long ago never to ask my children if they were hungry. Their answer was always, "Hungry for what?" If you keep to 1-2-3 Foods when you snack, and even then stick to veggies unless you're so hungry that you need more calories than that, you won't be tempted to check what you're hungry for! Likewise, if you are really hungry and it'll be more than two hours until your next meal, have a small amount of food from two groups, such as a few nuts and a piece of fruit, to keep your blood sugar stable until your next meal.

Be sure to drink plenty of fluids, as thirst is often mistaken for hunger, and a tall glass of iced tea, seltzer water with lime, or lemon water (a thick ring of fresh lemon topped with ice and water) can often wash away hunger. We recommend drinking 6 to 8 glasses of water or other beverages daily.

Perhaps most important is to keep breakfast very healthy. That's the time when cortisol levels are the highest, so eating re-fined carbohydrates and sugars triggers a spike in insulin and blood sugar that leads to a midmorning blood-sugar low. All the break-fasts on the menus in this book include at least 15 grams of protein, foods from each of the 1-2-3 Eating groups, and minimal or no White Stuff. Each is a good way to start a day during which your drive to overeat will stay low.

However, what you need is important, so again, if you really need something, have it and enjoy it!

How Much to Eat?

Some people really need to measure their foods. They simply can't tell the difference between a cup of pasta and three cups. Measuring food and writing it down tend to decrease our intake of calories by 25 percent, so if you want to do that, by all means do. However, con-sider instead being more flexible and using the included menu plans to gain a sense of the amounts we recommend for safe weight loss. Each meal has about 350 calories, so all the meals are interchangeable.

After you have a sense of what is a reasonable amount of food to eat, if you need to, modify it to make it work for you. You don't have to be perfect to be wonderful, and neither does your food. If you're exercising more, you may need to eat more. If it's the second half of your cycle, you may need more. Check with your doctor to determine the right level for you and take into consideration that smaller people do well with slightly less food and larger people with slightly more.

If you stick with a rigid diet, there's a high likelihood that you'll overeat at certain times and undereat at other times, neither of which is good for staying above the line.

You are eating so that you stay above the line, so that you feel vibrant but don't consume any more calories than you really need (in fact, you'll need to consume a few less than you need if you want to lose weight).

If you aren't hungry, do not eat. If you are hungry, eat before you're starving and trigger an eating binge. If you are a little bit hungry, have some water, take a walk around the block, or eat some veggies or fruit. Stop eating as soon as the hunger disappears. In 10 to 20 minutes, you'll feel full. Do not eat until you are full or you will feel stuffed, which takes you below the line and also hampers your weight loss. Your liver can only process a five hundred–calorie meal. Above that, it preferentially shunts your dinner into your fat cells. Bear in mind that most restaurant meals contain a thousand or more calories.

If you're below the line, it's easy to confuse body hunger with emotional hunger. When you feel pain and stress, that's your feeling brain calling out to you, signaling that all is not well. Don't assume that because you want food, your body needs it. If you have the urge to eat (feeling brain) and you think (thinking brain) that you may not be hungry, then consider what you really need: to get above the line. Don't eat. Instead, do a cycle! See whether you can pop yourself above the line to where you will know whether it's body hunger or emotional hunger, and you can make the decision that is right for you about whether to eat.

Most of us have a few "problem foods," those that trigger us to overeat. Usually, these are White Stuff—one spoonful of ice cream leads to another—but even foods with plenty of nutritional power can have this effect. Variety is important, but if you know you have a problem food, either skip that food altogether or put big, thick limits around it. For example, nuts are often problem foods, so we recommend snacking on only 15 small nuts or 10 large ones. But if eating nuts immediately makes you think of having them sprinkled over an ice cream sundae, then avoid them altogether.

There are times when you will have little control over the kind of food you are eating, perhaps at a dinner party or a lunch meeting or when the boss rewards everyone at work by ordering pizza. In those situations, instead of controlling what you eat, focus more on how much you're eating, and eat about one-third less than you normally would. You may be hungrier sooner, but that's not the worst thing—and neither is having a small piece of pizza. In other words, it's important to lighten up and be flexible. The stress of worrying about what you are eating is probably worse than the food itself.

Don't Sweat the Small Stuff

Rather than counting every calorie or calculating every gram, put eating in context. Eating is a behavior that is soothing and comforting. If your weight is greater than the weight that is within your genetic comfort zone, you have been soothing and comforting yourself with food more than your body and activity level have required. For the three days of the 3-Day Solution Plan, you will be discovering other ways to soothe and comfort yourself and seeing how doing that works for you. If you don't like it, you won't continue. If you do, you just might!

Food is only one part of the toxic spiral of weight gain, and stepping out of the spiral is easier when you have reasonable expectations and you know what is coming. Although it's extremely important to be above the line and living a masterful life that includes 1-2-3 Eating, there are bigger fish to fry when it comes to weight loss. You need to take the long view.

The long view, lasting weight loss, doesn't mean that you diet, exercise, and live differently so that you lose weight right now. It means that you gain the skills you need to keep that weight off.

That means pumping up your Solutions Skills, which will give you the power, persistence, and tenacity to glide over the bumps in the road to lasting weight loss.

Your 3-Day Solution will give you just the jump start you need, but it's only when weight loss is sustained that you lower your risk of disease and open up more opportunities to enjoy life to the fullest.

The first bump in the road is that you must face the essential pain that if you are not hungry, it's not a good idea to eat. It takes some skill to keep your fingers on the pulse of your inner life, and if you find that you are not hungry, even though you may want food, most of the time, you don't eat. This takes accepting the essential pain that we can't eat in the absence of body hunger just for fun, release, or comfort.

You can do that. It's not so hard, and during your 3-Day Solution, you'll prove that to yourself.

The second bump in the road is that, as you lose weight, there may be times when you feel somewhat uncomfortable, stressed, or in pain. Although you must be careful not to allow yourself to get too hungry, there will be moments now and then when you will feel hungry but will need to go for a walk, drink some water, or eat a vegetable rather than having a milk shake.

That discomfort—even if it's only small wisps of discomfort—will be most acute for the first two weeks and will return in waves now and then. Your appetite signals will adjust to having less food, and you will probably go through a time when it's not hard at all to lose weight. You may even have times when being a little bit hungry feels good. You feel light and free, and your mind is on the earned reward: "I'm hungry, so I must be using body fat for fuel. Wow. It's working!" Or when you dish up a light meal and say to yourself, "The essential pain is that I'm eating less and I'm eating healthy. But the earned reward: feeling great, looking great, being vibrant!"

This may take longer if your weight is high and your neurotransmitters are abnormally elevated, the way they are when people have become hooked on food. Just as with substance abuse, normalizing those neurotransmitters may take longer. However, in time, they will change, and you will slide over this bump.

After the 3-Day Solution, you will feel much stronger and somewhat inspired. That inspiration plus more skills and support can work wonders to keep you on the pathway to your weight Solution until you hit the next bump in the road.

The third bump comes when your body fat is significantly reduced and your body's fat signals, leptin, ghrelin, and insulin, will signal your brain to consume more calories and expend fewer of them. You will find that your appetite has returned and your exercise doesn't sound so appealing—and cheeseburgers and double-crusted pizza never looked so good!

That's when all your hard work at pumping up your Solution Skills, all your diligence in having White Stuff only when you really needed it, and all your progress in creating a masterful life will pay off. You will attend to using all these skills a little bit more often and more effectively, and chances are, before long you'll notice that those fat signals have settled down and you have found a new set point for your body weight. This is your new normal body weight, and from then on, it will be somewhat easier to maintain.

There is a fourth bump in the road, and that comes up when you've lost some extra weight—whether it be 5 pounds or 105 pounds—and people start responding to you differently. Or perhaps you start feeling different about yourself.

Our body size speaks volumes for us—wordlessly—and when we lose weight, we give up whatever our higher weight communicated. It's completely unconscious for most people, but all of a sudden, we are eating when we're not even hungry, and we give up the exercise program, and . . . we gain weight. The key is to identify the message that the extra weight communicates for us and say those words aloud, so we don't need to regain the weight we've lost. What could be the hidden benefit of keeping on extra pounds? There are limitless possibilities, ranging from saying to the world, "I don't feel safe" to "I don't matter."

In the method, we employ a tool called "use words, not weight." This fourth bump doesn't apply to everyone, but if it does apply to you, getting more skills or seeing a therapist to express those words will enable you to lose weight and keep it off.

The bottom line is that it's absolutely essential, if you want a weight Solution, to be gentle but persistent with yourself. Don't fuss about a calorie here or a calorie there. Focus on stepping back from the food and saying, "I want a real Solution, and I'm going to obtain the skills, at my own pace and in my own way, to get one."

What Is Special About 1-2-3 Foods?

In an age when so much nutrition misinformation is available and sugary, fatty ketchup is touted as a "heart-healthy" food (because it contains lycopene), it's helpful to have a list of foods that create the kind of personal balance that's conducive to lasting weight loss.

In order to get on the 1-2-3 Food Lists, a food's nutritional profile must be impressive in terms of nutrient density, phytochemicals, and preventive nutrition. Foods that contain nutrients that promote weight loss, such as milk products and very high-fiber grains, are favorably considered. Nutritional wannabes, such as white bread with added fiber, are not. We also took note of any food that contains nutrients that have a balancing effect on neurotransmitters—for example, those high in omega-3 fatty acids; tryptophan, which is a serotonin precursor; or phenylalanine, a dopamine precursor. Foods high in both tryptophan and phenylalanine are almonds, turkey, chicken, and milk products.

Staying above the line is easier when blood sugar is stable or, at least, avoids peaks and valleys, so healthy fats and lean proteins are emphasized. Although the glycemic index has some merit, 1-2-3 Eating combines foods, so the glycemic index of an individual food has less impact. In fact, when combining a variety of whole foods, most of which have a low glycemic index, there is no scientific basis for calculating it. Even potatoes will not cause spikes in blood sugar for most people when eaten in moderation as part of a meal that includes all three groups.

The foods in The Protein Group—beans, meat, poultry, fish, soy, and milk products—are the choices among those kinds of foods that are low in fat. Eggs are included in this group, but we recommend using Light Eggs (that is, tossing out one of the yolks), eating whole eggs just a couple of times a week, or using egg substitutes. Each egg white provides 10 grams of protein, and 20 grams of protein is recommended for a balancing breakfast. The yolk contains the fat and cholesterol, but the yolk is a concentrated source of other nutrients, including omega-3 fatty acids. Check with your physician about your particular response to dietary cholesterol, as the impact on lipid profiles of eating eggs varies considerably.

Some foods on the list vary in toxic load. Choose organic foods when possible and keep informed about the safety of all foods you eat, especially large fish or fish that is high in fat. For example, farmed salmon and tuna may have unacceptably high levels of toxins; however, even recently, those advisories are changing. Reliable Internet sites are often the best source of information.

We recommend that you take daily one therapeutic-strength vitamin/mineral supplement such as Centrum, 500 milligrams of calcium, and 1 gram of omega-3 fatty acids. The menu plans for 1-2-3 Eating contain approximately twelve hundred to fourteen hundred calories per day, equally split among fat, carbohydrate, and protein. The menus are very low in saturated fat (about 7 percent of calories), moderate in polyunsaturated fat, and high in monounsaturated fat (18 percent). Monounsaturated fat is believed to lower cholesterol and may assist in reducing heart disease and certain cancers, such as cancers of the breast and colon. Like polyunsaturated fat, it provides essential fatty acids for healthy skin and the development of body cells. The menus are typically high in vitamin E, the antioxidant vitamin, which is in short supply in many Western diets. Cold-pressed extra virgin olive oil, if not overheated, provides a range of phytochemicals and phenols, which help you boost immunity and maintain good health.

The fiber level of the menus is 22 grams—in fact, more than the 13 grams per 1,000 calories currently recommended—amounting to about 20 grams daily. Calcium intake from food alone is about 1,000 milligrams and, with the supplementation of 500 milligrams, meets or exceeds recommendations for adults. Although milk and soy products are included in The Protein Group, consumption of soy should be moderate. Some processed soy products, soy isolates, and soy supplements may be less valuable in terms of preventing osteoporosis and breast cancer. All the meals and recipes have been analyzed for nutrient content, and all are approximately the same nutritionally, with each meal providing about 350 calories and must have at least 20 grams of protein.

What About Processed Foods?

Nutrition has never been bigger business, and the corporate way is to make profits off of single nutrient claims and to do everything possible to misrepresent products. Since "new" always increases product sales, there will always be new products rolling out.

How do you figure out what processed foods are really 1-2-3 Foods, not White Stuff? The easiest way is to avoid processed foods. Shop on the perimeter of your grocery store with your 1-2-3 Food Lists in hand, and put in your basket the foods on the lists that you enjoy. Then create meals using those foods.

If you are going to purchase processed foods, then read the labels. Here are a couple of ways to zero in on the information you most need to determine whether a particular product is a 1-2-3 Food.

Look at the ingredients list. This is not the nutrition labeling, but the small-print ingredients. This list may be under a flap or shown in tiny type on a bottom corner of a box. The ingredients are listed in order by weight, with the biggest amount listed first. For breads and cereals, the first ingredient needs to be a whole grain with significant amounts of fiber. For cereal, that is 6 grams of fiber per 100 calories, and for bread, it's 3 grams per 100 calories.

As a general rule, if the first three ingredients are on the 1-2-3 Food Lists, it's probably a 1-2-3 Food, except for one thing: check to be sure that the word *hydrogenated* is nowhere on the ingredients list. Hydrogenated foods contain trans fats, and no amount of trans-fatty acids are considered safe to consume. Trans fats are more potent in increasing the risk of heart disease than saturated fats, so if the word *hydrogenated* appears anywhere on the ingredients list, the food is White Stuff.

Check the nutrition labeling for other pertinent information. The food industry makes this more difficult because it manipulates serving sizes. A can of soda that functionally is one serving can have nutritional labeling based on one serving's being half a can. This requires math skills! To lose weight slowly or maintain weight, most people need about 350 to 450 calories in a meal and about 100 calories in a snack. Eating about 1,200 to 1,400 calories per day enables most people to lose weight at the rate of about one pound per week if they are physically active. It's best to weigh yourself once a week and not take the number seriously for one month, as there can be changes in fat, muscle, or water that affect the number on the scale. A healthy ongoing weight loss involves losing an average of half a pound to one pound per week. Once you've lost weight, the 3-pound rule is smart. If the number on the scale goes up 3 pounds, make adjustments right away to get above the line and lose that weight. It's so much easier to face 3 pounds than 30.

Breakfast, Lunch, and Dinner . . .

Although you are eating for health and pleasure, food will not be the most rewarding part of your day. It tastes good, but other aspects of your day are even better. The primary purpose of eating is to give you the energy and nutrition you need to stay above the line. If you eat too much food or eat when you aren't hungry, it drags you below the line, and you feel sluggish, tired, or stuffed. If you don't eat enough or regularly, you feel irritable, depressed, or numb. Both extremes are reflections of imbalances in neurotransmitters, so feed your body to stay above the line and in balance. That means eating breakfast, lunch, and dinner and snacking only if you are hungry.

In general, having a late-afternoon snack is a good idea, so that you can eat dinner between 6:00 p.m. and 8:00 p.m. and have two hours or more after eating and before going to sleep.

When you finish dinner, there should be a gleam in your eye, as you anticipate the ways you will please and restore yourself in the evening that have nothing to do with eating. Your best dessert should not be edible, which is why you will shortly be planning the other elements of Mastery Living.

22

The Solution 1-2-3 Food List

THIS CHAPTER PRESENTS three lists: The Fiber Group, Healthy Fats, and The Protein Group. If you choose one food from each group at a meal, you're likely to get the balance of nutrition needed to give you an edge in losing weight and feeling great.

Eat only the foods you like, so consider checking off the foods that bring you pleasure. All the foods not listed are White Stuff. Have them when you really need them, and don't feel guilty about doing so. If you don't really need them, then don't have them. These 1-2-3 Foods will bring you more of the earned rewards of optimal vitality and lasting weight loss.

The Solution® 1-2-3 Food List

1. The Fiber Group

Fruit
- ☐ Apples
- ☐ Apricots
- ☐ Bananas
- ☐ Blackberries
- ☐ Blueberries
- ☐ Cantaloupe*
- ☐ Cranberries
- ☐ Cherries
- ☐ Grapefruit
- ☐ Grapes*
- ☐ Guavas
- ☐ Figs
- ☐ Honeydew melon
- ☐ Kiwis
- ☐ Lemons
- ☐ Limes
- ☐ Mangoes
- ☐ Melons
- ☐ Nectarines
- ☐ Oranges
- ☐ Papayas
- ☐ Peaches
- ☐ Pears
- ☐ Persimmons
- ☐ Pineapples
- ☐ Pomegranates
- ☐ Plums
- ☐ Prunes
- ☐ Raisins*
- ☐ Raspberries
- ☐ Strawberries
- ☐ Tangelos
- ☐ Tangerines
- ☐ Watermelon*

Vegetables
- ☐ Acorn squash
- ☐ Artichokes
- ☐ Arugula
- ☐ Asparagus
- ☐ Bamboo shoots
- ☐ Banana squash
- ☐ Bean sprouts
- ☐ Beets
- ☐ Bok choy
- ☐ Broccoli
- ☐ Brussels sprouts
- ☐ Butternut squash
- ☐ Cabbage
- ☐ Carrots
- ☐ Cauliflower
- ☐ Celery
- ☐ Chard
- ☐ Chayote
- ☐ Corn
- ☐ Cucumbers
- ☐ Eggplant
- ☐ Endives
- ☐ Fennel
- ☐ Green beans
- ☐ Green onions/scallions
- ☐ Hubbard squash
- ☐ Jicama
- ☐ Kale
- ☐ Leafy greens
- ☐ Leeks
- ☐ Lettuce
- ☐ Mushrooms
- ☐ Okra
- ☐ Onions
- ☐ Parsnips
- ☐ Pea pods
- ☐ Peppers
- ☐ Potatoes*
- ☐ Pumpkin
- ☐ Radishes
- ☐ Snap peas
- ☐ Snow peas
- ☐ Spaghetti squash
- ☐ Spinach
- ☐ Sprouts
- ☐ Sweet potatoes
- ☐ Tomatillos
- ☐ Tomatoes
- ☐ Tomato juice*
- ☐ Vegetable juices, 100%*
- ☐ Water chestnuts
- ☐ Yams
- ☐ Yellow summer squash
- ☐ Zucchini

Grains
- ☐ Barley
- ☐ Bread, 100% whole-grain
- ☐ Bread, high-protein wheat
- ☐ Bread, sprouted whole-wheat berry
- ☐ Brown rice*
- ☐ Bulgur
- ☐ Cereal, high-fiber
- ☐ Cereal, whole-grain, high-fiber
- ☐ Couscous, whole-wheat
- ☐ Crackers, whole-grain, high-fiber
- ☐ English muffins, whole-grain
- ☐ Kasha (buckwheat)
- ☐ Matzos, whole-wheat
- ☐ Oatmeal
- ☐ Pancakes, whole-grain*
- ☐ Pasta, protein-enriched
- ☐ Pasta, whole-wheat
- ☐ Pita, whole-grain
- ☐ Polenta*
- ☐ Popcorn
- ☐ Potatoes
- ☐ Pretzels, whole-grain
- ☐ Quinoa*
- ☐ Rice bran
- ☐ Rye berries
- ☐ Spelt
- ☐ Tortillas, 100% whole-grain
- ☐ Waffles, whole-grain*
- ☐ Wheat berries
- ☐ Wheat bran
- ☐ Wheat germ
- ☐ Wild rice*

2. Healthy Fats

Nuts, Seeds, & More
- ☐ Almond butter
- ☐ Almonds
- ☐ Avocados
- ☐ Brazil nuts
- ☐ Cashew butter
- ☐ Cashews
- ☐ Flax seeds
- ☐ Guacamole
- ☐ Hazelnut butter
- ☐ Hazelnuts
- ☐ Macadamia nuts
- ☐ Olives
- ☐ Peanut butter
- ☐ Peanuts
- ☐ Pecans
- ☐ Pine nuts
- ☐ Pistachios

2. Healthy Fats, continued...

☐ Poppy seeds
☐ Pumpkin seeds*
☐ Sesame seeds
☐ Soy nut butter
☐ Soy nuts
☐ Sunflower seeds*
☐ Tahini
☐ Walnuts

Oils
☐ Canola mayonnaise
☐ Canola oil
☐ Canola oil margarine
☐ Flaxseed oil
☐ Margarine, trans fat-free
☐ Olive oil

☐ Olive oil, extra virgin
☐ Peanut oil
☐ Safflower oil, high-oleic
☐ Sesame seed oil
☐ Soy oil
☐ Sunflower oil, high-oleic
☐ Walnut oil

3. The Protein Group

Fish & Shellfish**
☐ Albacore
☐ Anchovies
☐ Bluefish
☐ Calamari
☐ Catfish
☐ Clams
☐ Cod
☐ Crab
☐ Halibut
☐ Herring
☐ Lobster
☐ Mackerel
☐ Mahi-mahi
☐ Ono
☐ Prawns
☐ Red snapper
☐ Salmon (wild)
☐ Sardines
☐ Scallops
☐ Sole
☐ Shrimp
☐ Tilapia
☐ Trout

Poultry & Meat
☐ Beef lunch meat
☐ Beef round steak
☐ Beef round steak, ground
☐ Chateaubriand
☐ Chicken, ground
☐ Chicken breast

☐ Chicken drumsticks, skinless
☐ Chicken lunch meat
☐ Chicken thighs, skinless, visible fat removed
☐ Flank steak
☐ Ham, all fat removed
☐ Ham lunch meat
☐ Pork chops, lean
☐ Pork tenderloin
☐ Sausage links, low-fat
☐ Sirloin tip roast
☐ Turkey, ground
☐ Turkey breast
☐ Turkey lunch meat
☐ Veal cutlets
☐ Veal, ground
☐ Veal scallops
☐ Veal steak

Beans & Soy
☐ Black-eyed peas
☐ Black soybeans
☐ Breakfast patties, soy
☐ Cannelloni beans
☐ Chickpeas (garbanzos)
☐ Edamame
☐ Great Northern beans
☐ Hummus
☐ Kidney beans
☐ Lentils
☐ Lima beans
☐ Navy beans

☐ Pinto beans
☐ Red beans
☐ Refried beans, no fat
☐ Soy burgers
☐ Soy cheese, fat-free
☐ Soy cheese, low-fat
☐ Soy crumbles
☐ Soy milk, calcium-fortified
☐ Split peas
☐ Tempeh
☐ Tofu
☐ Tofu links
☐ Veggie burgers
☐ Veggie franks
☐ Yellow soybeans

Milk & Eggs
☐ Almond cheese
☐ Buttermilk, 1%
☐ Cheese, fat-free
☐ Cheese, reduced-fat
☐ Cottage cheese, fat-free
☐ Cottage cheese, 1%
☐ Eggs, in moderation
☐ Egg substitute
☐ Feta cheese*
☐ Milk, lactose-reduced, 1%
☐ Milk, nonfat
☐ Milk, 1%
☐ Ricotta cheese, fat-free
☐ Ricotta cheese, low-fat
☐ Yogurt, sugar-free, low-fat
☐ Yogurt, sugar-free, nonfat

White Stuff

Everything else!

The 3-Day Solution* Plan, Ballantine Books, 2005
The Institute for Health Solutions • www.thepathway.org
© Laurel Mellin, 2005

* The nutritional value of these foods falls outside the normal criteria for the group, but they are rich in other nutrients and phytochemicals that promote health.
** The amount of mercury and other toxins in these foods vary.

<h1 style="text-align:center">23</h1>

<h1 style="text-align:center">Solution Stories</h1>

THIS CHAPTER PRESENTS stories of participants who have used The Solution Method to turn off the drive to overeat and create lasting weight loss. They are from many walks of life and every region of the country, but what they share is the humility to say that they'd like to have more of these skills and the emotional courage to begin. They also share the passion to stay on the pathway until they have a Solution in their life.

I'm extremely grateful to each person who shared his or her story on these pages. These are their own words, unedited, and they reflect their personal experience in rewiring their feeling brain to naturally favor life above the line.

<h2 style="text-align:center">My Solution—Lise A.:</h2>

Self-Acceptance, Authenticity, and Forty-eight Pounds Lighter

Before The Solution, I was a perfectionistic workaholic—and I didn't even know it. I "gave myself away" in working long hours in volunteer work, donating my time and talents as well as money, and simply giving much more than was reasonable or healthy. Coming to realize the levels of people-pleasing and "control" that had led me into such untenable situations astonished me when I came to see the reality. I had gotten ill from the stress and was just starting to recover and reengage (too much, again) when I found The Solution.

I saw Laurel on television and was excited at the idea that

changing my brain would change my life. As a student of psychology, I had been struck by the concept of early trauma changing the limbic brain. When I watched Laurel working with those young women on the television program, I knew that I must pursue Solution training. It was a decision that has changed my life.

I remember the day I first *felt* my own inner sanctuary. I was in the third kit of the course, and seemingly all of a sudden, it was *there*—a firm, flexible, green shoot growing tall and strong within. I felt the sunshine coming out, warming me as on a fresh spring day. I could *smell* the new growth, like a bed of iris coming to bloom. It was at that tender and exuberant moment that I knew I would have my Solution.

So many other "aha moments" and turning points have been part of this journey for me. I remember my trip to buy some ballet shoes for the exercises I had begun anew after being 15 years (and 150 pounds) away from dance. I intended to purchase some plain slippers and came home with the most glorious red satin pointe shoes I have ever seen! While it is a certainty that I will never dance *en pointe* again, having those shoes in the closet (and sometimes, on my feet) has meant the world to me.

Already, there have been significant changes in my relationships, based mostly in the personal authenticity I am devoted to strengthening. My relationship with my husband, always strong and a powerful force for good in my life, is deepening and becoming more vital and alive. I have found a new respect for my husband as I have developed the same for myself.

I have lost 48 pounds since beginning Solution training a year ago. Now, I manage my volunteer efforts more reasonably, focusing more on taking time for myself and my family, saying "no" to unbalanced amounts of effort.

Where would I be without The Solution? I cannot say, but I know that I would very likely still be stuck and unhappy. Certainly, my health would be at greater risk than it is now, for I doubt I would have lost this much weight or be so devoted to my own life. I am so filled with gratitude that I wish there were a thousand words for appreciation in English!

My Solution—Gary T.:
Amazed That Doing Cycles Is Better Than Eating Lunch

My spouse first started The Solution work about a year ago. Initially, "The Solution" wasn't appealing to me at all, as I felt (not thought) that most of my wife's problems (and my problems) were her fault (ahh, part of my dark side). I think, as a result of my spouse's Solution work, she found it within herself to meet her needs and make it clear to me that she needed me to stop blaming her for my problems.

At first, I was hurt, but my wife is the most perceptive person I have ever met, so I knew there must be more to it. Only at that point did I realize that I did have some things about me I wasn't too proud of and some areas of my life I wanted to change. I told my wife that I would give the book a read and see what it was all about. After reading it, I thought it was too good to be true and was a bit skeptical, but it sounded quite appealing.

My spouse was fairly comfortable in talking to people about her life and looking inward. I have never had any therapy or done much in the way of exploring myself and "what makes me tick" before, so viewing The Solution as "therapy" was a big turnoff for me. Additionally, for the most part, I had a very happy childhood and do quite enjoy life. (But things can always get better, can't they?)

The piece that intrigued me the most was the observation that real change only truly occurs through "feeling the feelings." My wife and I have been together for around 13 years, and it was extremely frustrating to both of us that we kept repeating the same hurtful patterns of behavior over and over. While not superdestructive, these patterns certainly make life unpleasant sometimes, and neither she nor I really wanted this anymore.

After I started doing the kits, she encouraged me to join a Solution group. "Oh, no, that wasn't for me. I don't need that." Well, somehow I managed to join, and it's been great. I feel having my Solution provider, Judy, has made a huge difference in my sticking with this. Being around people doing the same work is very powerful. Also, after doing this work, I have a sincere admiration for others doing this work (especially in my group), as I feel that everybody has something that needs work, but these are the people that are actually doing something about it.

So I started The Solution seeking intimacy about eight months or so ago. I don't find myself thinking "Something's bothering me, but I don't know what" as much. I have found myself much more comfortable with myself both in groups of people and by myself. I do feel more balanced (even though I didn't even expect that I needed more balance), and I do find increased integration and acceptance of myself, and my family life is better. I sometimes get very emotional and moody before lunch (always have). Sometimes, the feeling change I get from doing a cycle is just as effective as eating lunch. I know that sounds odd, but from a physiological point of view, I would have *never* imagined anything besides "blood-sugar" issues could change my state so profoundly.

I know I have further to go. I find The Solution to be an absolutely life-transforming experience. I feel extremely grateful to have stumbled upon it.

My Solution—Mark R.:
The Method Made My Appetite Go Away

Someone once said that most of us spend the first half of our lives learning to shorten the second half of our lives. That was certainly the case with me. I learned at an early age to medicate life's pain with food and later added other bad habits, such as smoking, alcohol, and overworking. Through years of refinement, smoking and alcohol dropped away, but food was always at the core of my excesses.

My food issues were deeply embedded in my psyche. At a very tender age, my father gave me the nickname "Bubbles" because I was so fat. Trying to shame a child into losing weight was counterproductive; it only drove me deeper into the comfort of food. Little did I know that the experience of my parents' divorce was one of the pains I was trying to medicate for.

Embarrassingly, I've ended up in the hospital twice due to food-related issues. Once, when I was a child, when my dad went through his second divorce, I ate too much and got very sick. The second incident occurred while enduring the stress associated with an advanced military leadership school. After about seven weeks of intense training, I just got home on a Friday night and continuously ate for about an hour. Later that night, I woke up so sick that I drove myself to the hospital. About two days later, I awoke from a comatose-like state. My doctor said that they couldn't find anything wrong with me. He then leaned over and whispered in my ear that it appeared my intestinal system was so blocked that nothing was moving. It seemed as though my body had shut itself down.

You'd almost infer from all this that, as an adult, I've been very obese. That is not the case at all: my adult weight has never exceeded 215 pounds on my five-foot ten-inch frame. Why? I learned to purge the food binges with harsh exercise. I guess you could call me an exercise bulimic, because I would comfort myself with a food binge and then purge via exercise.

As life's demands escalated with age and professional responsibilities, so did my weight. In despair, at age 32, I ended up converting my lifestyle to that of a vegetarian, to help maintain the rigid height/weight standards required of a military officer. I usually hovered around the middle range of those standards, but during times of intense stress, I've reached or exceeded the maximum limit.

My real anxiety started to occur with my own children. It wasn't long into their lives that I started to notice that one of my daughters was gaining excess weight. Her mannerisms in that direction really advanced while I was flying missions in the first Gulf War and, shortly thereafter, during my divorce. My daughter was using food to cope. My oldest son, who was about 15 at the time, had one alcohol-related incident and then a second. Determined to stop the cycle, I sought the help of a trained professional who specialized in youth problems. But within a year, a third incident had occurred. In desperation, I started bringing my son to a 12-step program. To show him I cared, I sat in the associated-family-member 12-step meeting next door. It wasn't long before I figured out that I needed to be in a program for food.

As you can see, I've searched for the answer and applied myself to any solution that promised relief. I could probably get a degree in nutrition with my knowledge of food. I've fasted, I've been hypnotized, I've run marathons, and I even gave up meat to try to keep off the weight. I thought I'd really found the answer with a 12-step food program—and then a long, drawn-out real estate transaction caused me to gain 60 pounds! It was hopeless.

Months later, while walking through a bookstore, I spied a book that promised to turn off the drives to overeat, drink, and overwork. Nobody I knew had ever linked those drives together, and I knew from my own experience, they were related.

My skepticism was immense: I've spent a lifetime searching for a solution without avail and here comes another book claiming to have an answer. But I glanced through the book and caught another claim that I knew to be true. How could weight problems be solved? I thought, if I sift through this book and I get just one piece of insight that helps me, the price could be worth it. I bought it, took it home, and read it.

It turned out that the book made no outlandish claims or stated facts that are scientifically untrue. It had supporting data. I read it a second time and found that it incorporated everything I knew to be true about food solutions under one cover. After that second reading, I was more accepting of what it had to say. So I started learning the nurturing and limit-setting skills.

And then it happened, late one day, at the end of several stressful workdays. The drive to eat anything in front of me was starting to come to the surface. I had allowed myself to get out of balance. I could succumb to the drive and eat, white-knuckle it, or do a cycle. I chose the cycle, and the drive *went away*! I popped myself above the line! It was like a switch was turned off or I was given some pill that anesthetized the drive in my brain. Almost as if I had conducted an experiment, and I had a measurable result. Unbelievable! I did it once, and then a week later, I did it again and then again.

I'm convinced that not knowing these skills is at the core of my food issues. Yet, like learning a foreign language, they require immersion and practice. And like that foreign language, you'll have measurable results as you become fluent with practice.

It is a language well worth learning. Today, with just nine months of practice, my weight is well within reason. My family life is much more intimate, and maybe, just maybe, my kids won't have to live for years under the pressure of their own life-threatening external solutions.

My Solution—Susan P.:
The Solution Changed Me and Everyone Around Me

My biggest accomplishment from Solution training is that I can express love for others and feel loved myself. This may seem like an unusual achievement for a person who started the program to lose weight, but in truth, being able to love myself and to feel loved by others is the most important thing I accomplished through The Solution.

When I started Solution training, I felt isolated, angry, and depressed. My relationships with my family were seething with underlying hostility. It seemed to me as though no one cared about me, and I made it my business to make sure I didn't care about anyone else. I was also about 50 pounds overweight and miserable most of the time.

I read about The Solution and intuitively knew that it was for me. I contacted the Institute [for Health Solutions] and asked about getting involved in a Solution group. I was put on a waiting list but soon was sitting in a group in a basement classroom at UCSF. I was scared to death and wondered what in the world I was doing there. But gradually, I began to open up to the other members of the group, to express my true feelings and needs, and to talk about why I was so unhappy.

In time, and with a lot of hard work, I began to see that my unhappiness was not because others didn't love me; it was because I didn't love myself, and I had no idea how to give myself the nurturing and limits I needed. This was to be expected, because of the abusive and neglectful home I grew up in. I was simply reliving my personal past.

As my Solution Skills increased, I found that I not only enjoyed life more but that my life itself changed. I left an abusive job and started my own nonprofit focused on helping adults who can provide nurturing homes for abused and neglected children in the foster-care system. I began to express more love and tenderness to my husband and to my own adult children. Gradually, they also began to express their true feelings and needs (including their angry ones!) to me, and a sense of intimacy began to take root.

This was a difficult time. My family would often comment that

I had somehow "changed," but no one knew quite how or why. I stopped overspending and started to be less compulsive than I had been in the past. I also lost almost 50 pounds. When my husband finally disclosed a personal secret that threw our marriage into a crisis, I was able to set some reasonable limits and told him that I needed him to get into Solution training as well.

Today, I am not a perfect person. I still have struggles with giving myself the nurturing I lacked as a child. I often have difficulties setting limits with my work, my weight, and my relationships. And yet, something profound has changed about me. I can accept and love other people (and my recently acquired cat), and I can experience their love and acceptance of me. My children phone and visit often to talk, and my husband calls me his "sweetie." The Solution changed not only my life but the lives of my entire family. I let go of some relationships and deepened others. I do not know what life holds for me in the future, but because of The Solution, I know that I have the basic skills to accept whatever comes my way.

My Solution—Dave S.:
In Better Shape Than I've Been in Years

When I started Solution training, I had just moved back to my hometown. I recently finished all my coursework for my bachelor's degree and was starting a new job.

I found out about Solution training by seeing Laurel on television and read her book. I was somewhat skeptical but also hopeful and decided to give it a shot. The main reason I decided to get involved was that I wanted to be happier and reap the rewards of the training. I realized that I resorted to the external solutions of thinking too much and people-pleasing, and was also an occasional dabbler in eating and drinking too much.

After two weeks of trying to do the work by myself, I became frustrated and quit because I couldn't feel my feelings. I was always a hard-driven type A personality, and I learned quickly that I couldn't approach this work with that attitude. Six months later, I decided to start up again and get support through a telegroup.

Being in Solution training has definitely been a bumpy road.

There were many times I wanted to quit but was helped along with the support of Community Connections, my telegroup, and some personal coaching sessions. The main reason I have stuck with it so far is that I don't want to return to living life below the line. I still have a long way to go with this training, but there's no doubt in my mind that I will stick with it until I get my Solution.

I didn't come to training to lose weight, but I ended up losing about 12 pounds in the first four months. I attribute this weight loss to better food choices in combination with eating until I was satisfied. Since I didn't want to lose weight, I began drinking a meal-replacement beverage with each meal for the extra calories and have slowly gained most of the weight back. Currently, I am about the same weight I was when I started the training, but my body-fat percentage is lower. I am stronger, more flexible, and in better cardiovascular shape.

Emotionally, I feel more secure and balanced than before starting the training. I love feeling healthier physically, but most of all, I am grateful for the emotional balance. This especially means a lot to me because I was sick and tired of going through so many highs and lows depending on what life threw at me. It just feels so good to be happy again.

My Solution—Kate R.:
I Needed Patience, Prayer, and These Skills

At age 25, I felt hopeless and depressed, having suffered from clinical depression in college. I knew there had to be more to life. I had a good life—a vanilla childhood, wonderful parents, great friends, good job, engaged to my boyfriend of four years. Yet I changed from the optimistic, happy, energetic teenager I was in high school to an adult too scared to live. I rarely socialized, ate constantly and often hid it, and slept far too much. I hated exercise, preferring the company of books and computers.

I'd always heard I should learn to love *myself*, but as my weight ballooned up to 230 pounds on my five-foot six-inch frame, I hated myself more every day. Worse, I learned I was insulin-resistant, with a family history of diabetes and heart disease. Yet the thought of a depriving diet terrified me: I would react violently to the thought of it by eating everything in sight. I was too scared of weight-loss drugs and supplements to try any of them. My spiritual well seemed dry. I was at a loss.

Finally, one night when I was alone in bed, I heaved a sobbing prayer. I prayed to God: "I don't know what to do—I'm so scared! I don't want to be miserable anymore! I want to learn to love myself. I know you want me to love myself, I *know* it. I *feel* it. Please help me. I need you. Give me a sign . . . and please make it obvious!!!"

Three days later, I decided to drive up and have lunch with my grandfather at his lake house. I thought he might be lonely, and I admired the strength of this stern and quiet man. On the way back from lunch, I told him how sad I was that I'd become so heavy and that I was too scared to go on a diet. I also told him that I was afraid I was depressed again. That's when he handed me a book by Laurel Mellin, and on the cover, it said, "Never diet again!" I thought, on any normal day, I would have been downright insulted that he had handed me this book—he thinks I'm fat???—but then I understood that *this* was *the sign.* My grandfather explained that the therapist he was seeing for his own depression gives training groups for The Solution. I just thanked him, and inside of me, I was thanking God.

I began reading the book, and I hadn't gotten three chapters into it before I was calling Dr. Anne Brown to find out how soon I could enroll in her Solution group. I knew that *This was the answer I was looking for.* Within two weeks, I was at orientation, scared and excited and hoping it wasn't too good to be true.

That was two years ago. Now I have completed almost all of the six Solution Kits. I have shed 50 pounds, but that is merely a welcome side effect to the rewards I have been experiencing. I now *love* to exercise. I enjoy planning social engagements around physical activities.

Inside, I am no longer all good or all bad, but a whole, authentic human being. I have strong relationships with my fiancé, parents, friends, and our wonderful Solution community. It is the unexpected moments of intimacy with strangers, animals, and God that are holy moments for me. Amazingly, I don't take things personally anymore; I used to take *everything* personally, which is downright *exhausting.* This is what I've always wanted—to not care what other people think about me, loving myself first and best, and not being so judgmental about myself and everyone else. I thought I would just have to sit around and wait for these qualities until they came with age! I'm amazed I do not have to please other people to feel good about myself. I feel good about myself because I am *real*, I am *me*. I am the person I always wanted to know and always wanted to become. This is *now*. I have 27 years to my name.

It hasn't always been easy or simple, but it has been rewarding and fruitful. If you are just starting out on this pathway, my advice to you is to gather every ounce of *patience* you have and use it liberally with yourself—and others—on this journey. This is about remembering who you were before you became your external solutions. That person is there in you, waiting to meet you and the world with wide-open arms. And this community can't wait to meet you, either!

My Solution—Maria L.:
At Fifteen, I Had Tried Every Diet

In the summer of 1986, I weighed 245 pounds. I had tried every diet under the sun. I had been poked, prodded, and humiliated by physicians (and society) more than I care to remember. I had learned to binge and purge without loved ones finding out. I cried myself to sleep every night. I felt that I had already lived a lifetime of shame and feeling hopeless. Yet I was only 15 years old.

In early 1987, our family physician called my mother and told her that he may have found a solution for me. He recommended a program called Shapedown, which was developed for children and teens dealing with obesity. This program was developed by Laurel Mellin, and participants of this program were experiencing positive results. I decided that I would give it a shot.

At my first appointment with Laurel, she asked me a revolutionary question: "How do you feel?" I was shocked! I had *never* been asked that question in my entire life—especially not by a health-care provider. Prior to 1986, all of the programs/diets that I had attempted focused solely on calorie counting and physical activity. Never did any program deal with my emotional well-being or the social/cultural conditions that I lived in. In my heart, I realized that this program was different. For the first time in a very long time, I began to feel the seed of hope.

All I knew prior to starting the program was that I hated my body, I hated myself and my life, and that living was a painful experience to be endured. Early on, I realized that certain substances could numb the pain that life brought with it. For some folks, these substances include alcohol, drugs, gambling, etcetera. Others of us use something that's easier to access: food. But this became a vicious cycle for me: I was numbing my pain with the very substance that was *causing* the pain.

What I learned from my work with Laurel is to identify what my feelings are, to feel them, and to ask myself what I need. Sounds simple, no? Well, it is and it isn't. It's frightening territory if you're not used to feeling feelings. But feelings are just that—feelings. And the rewards are magnificent. Slowly, the weight started to drop off. I wasn't dieting; I was feeling my feelings and asking myself what I needed. I realized that I had options in life.

Here is an example: I often felt lonely when I arrived home from high school. Usually, no one was home, and that became prime binge time for me. By checking in with my feeling about loneliness, it became clear that perhaps it wasn't best for me to go straight home after school. Perhaps participating in an after-school program or going to the library or going for a walk would be better, healthier options. So that's what I did. I didn't go home to an empty house after school; I would go to the library instead—and as a result of not being home alone, I would not binge.

Changes like this started to become more and more common in my life. I began to make healthier food choices. My home life and relationships with family members began to change. My school life began to shift. I started exploring with art and traveling. I began dating and having relationships. I applied to college, deciding to focus on health education. Wonderful opportunities seemed to continue to find their way to me. And still, the weight continued to drop off.

Through my work with the method, I learned to work with tools that became essential for living a healthy life. My life is not perfect by any means, and I often still make wrong choices, but I learn from those choices and move on. There was a point in my life where I didn't think I would live to see 20. I am now 33, I love myself, I am learning to love the body that I have and have lost close to

100 pounds. Life seems like a wonderful buffet of choices. I am alive and kicking, and can't imagine life any other way.

My Solution—Kerry P.:
I Lost Weight and Have Kept It Off for Ten Years

One day, talking to my friend and colleague, we ventured into our favorite topic of conversation—life and all its questions. It dawned on me that with all the work we had done together and questions we seemed to have answered, I hadn't a clue who I was. I knew the facts. I was 37 years old, married, two kids, and a great job in the technology field.

"Are you happy?" she asked. The question hit me. I started to think, I had everything that society said one needed to be happy and successful. People told me I was full of life. So of course I was happy—society *told* me I was happy. "Yes, I am happy," I responded.

I could sense she wasn't buying it, so I added, "Although I could lose some weight. My clothes feel tighter than I like."

She laughed. I hadn't been thinking about weight before, but look what flyer just came in our interoffice mail. It was an announcement of a study that was being conducted by Laurel Mellin, and it was soliciting volunteers to participate in a pilot program called The Solution, a weight-loss program.

"Well," I said, "let's sign up together!"

Saturday, April 1994, I was sitting in the audience as Laurel was explaining the program. An hour into the presentation, she starts with this questioning process we would each need to go through.

What I feel is . . . What I need is . . . Would you please . . . ?

So she was going around the room having people answer. "Well, I am sorry," I said, as my turn came around. . . .

I thought, "What happens if one doesn't even *know* what they are feeling, or to put it more bluntly, what happens when one doesn't even know *how* to feel?"

I continued thinking, "If I don't know *how* to feel, then I can't know *what* to feel, so I don't know what I even *need*. So in order to ask someone, 'Would you please?' How could I do that? That isn't even on my radar! How am I going to do this program?"

Inside, I was crying as it dawned on me—I had to join this program. Yes, I hoped to lose weight, but something deeper in me was turning.

During the next weeks, I would go through a process that would bring me face-to-face with "me"! I would come to an understanding of feelings, where they came from, and I would learn the underlying reasons I did something—usually, out of habit. With this new information, I learned I had choices.

For example, I love Hydrox cookies. I would eat them and often without even being aware of it. One day, I asked myself as I was holding this morsel of delight in my hands ready to enjoy, "Am I hungry?" "No" came the instant reply. With that new bit of information and awareness of my body, I sat down on the couch and had a conversation with this cookie. I realized that what I really needed was some good old-fashioned nurturing. I realized that at my unconscious level, nothing said sweet, good nurturing better than a Hydrox cookie.

I knew this method worked, and over time, I went from 168 pounds to 128. Don't get me wrong; to this day, I still eat my cookies! Now, however, I give the cookie a mission: go to the hidden feeling and nurture it to come up and out in the open, so I can deal with it in a more healthful manner.

With Solution training, I learned skills that would change my life and the way I interact with it. Today, ten years later, I still use those skills on an integrated level, just like breathing.

My Solution—Julie B.:
More Intimacy and Connection Than I Imagined Possible

When I first read about The Solution in a magazine article, I was a single parent who had just discovered that my daughter had learning difficulties. I was shocked and scared. I comforted myself with desserts, alcohol, spending, and smoking. Most of the time, I was either overly busy with parenting and chores or alone watching TV. I completed the first three months of training with support from The Solution Internet community. When I was finishing up the first journal, I realized that I struggled with depression and that I needed support to get to my Solution. I signed up for a group.

I was very committed to reaching my Solution. I wrote daily

and made Community Connections with others in my group. That was the hardest part for me, finding the boundaries to share my feelings through conversations. But having that support really helped, because I was learning to stay in balance with my daughter while taking out piles of emotional trash from the hurts from my childhood. I actively experimented with setting boundaries in my life and with my daughter.

Weight stopped being an issue almost immediately. By making exercise a regular part of my week, the weight slowly came off with not much effort at all. I never really felt deprived. It took longer to stop wanting a cigarette, and drinking remained an issue now and then. The most important thing for me was that the skills helped me stay in balance with my daughter even when she wasn't able to perform to my expectations. Even though my tendency had been to get into the same patterns of overcontrol and judgment with her that my parents had with me, I didn't.

It is so amazing to know that I stopped that pattern from going to the next generation. My daughter is performing academically above average and motivating herself to do her best work in school. She openly discusses difficult middle-school social situations with me. I feel so much pride that I have taught her to be comfortable with her feelings. I enjoy her as a person with different strengths and interests than my own and have learned not to project my unfinished dreams on her the way my parents did to me.

I have discovered how to take care of my true needs, and now I make relationships a priority instead of waiting to connect with people after every chore and all the work is done. I choose not to spend time with family members with whom I abandon my feelings so I can please them. I enjoy weekends without endless to-do lists and have stopped overworking. I have maintained a weight loss of 45 pounds, and I am credit-card-debt-free and still able to travel internationally for vacations. I haven't struggled with depression since finishing my training. Drinking and overspending habits just fell away. I have a healthy, intimate relationship with a man for the first time in my life. I am at ease with myself and often find myself smiling because I feel happy and content.

Appendix

The 3-Day Solution Plan Pocket Reminders

THESE POCKET REMINDERS help you focus on the most important parts of the plan, and you can take them with you to record your progress. There is one reminder for each of the three days of phase 1, the 3-Day Solution Plan. There is also a reminder for phase 2 of the plan.

The 3-Day Solution® Plan – Day 1
Solution Skills

How do I feel?	What do I need?	Am I Above the Line?	
		Above	Below
☐			
☐			
☐			
☐			
☐			
☐			
☐			
☐			
☐			

☐ Checked in 10 times today?
☐ Did my best to stay above the line?

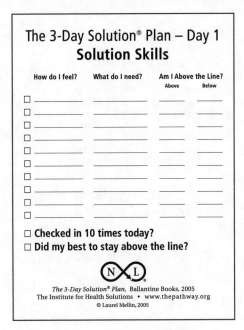

The 3-Day Solution® Plan, Ballantine Books, 2005
The Institute for Health Solutions • www.thepathway.org
© Laurel Mellin, 2005

The 3-Day Solution® Plan – Day 2
Solution Skills

How do I feel?	What do I need?	Am I Above the Line?		
		Above	Below	EH?
☐				
☐				
☐				
☐				
☐				
☐				
☐				
☐				
☐				
☐				

☐ Checked in 10 times today?
☐ Did my best to stay above the line?

The 3-Day Solution® Plan, Ballantine Books, 2005
The Institute for Health Solutions • www.thepathway.org
© Laurel Mellin, 2005

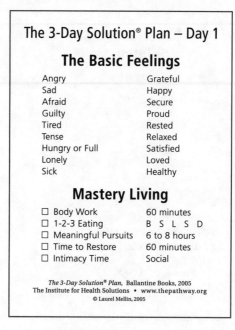

The 3-Day Solution® Plan – Day 1

The Basic Feelings

Angry	Grateful
Sad	Happy
Afraid	Secure
Guilty	Proud
Tired	Rested
Tense	Relaxed
Hungry or Full	Satisfied
Lonely	Loved
Sick	Healthy

Mastery Living

☐ Body Work	60 minutes
☐ 1-2-3 Eating	B S L S D
☐ Meaningful Pursuits	6 to 8 hours
☐ Time to Restore	60 minutes
☐ Intimacy Time	Social

The 3-Day Solution® Plan, Ballantine Books, 2005
The Institute for Health Solutions • www.thepathway.org
© Laurel Mellin, 2005

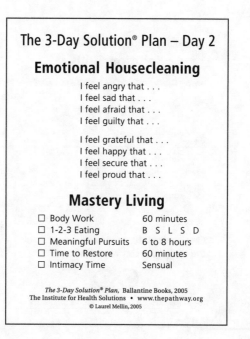

The 3-Day Solution® Plan – Day 2

Emotional Housecleaning

I feel angry that . . .
I feel sad that . . .
I feel afraid that . . .
I feel guilty that . . .

I feel grateful that . . .
I feel happy that . . .
I feel secure that . . .
I feel proud that . . .

Mastery Living

☐ Body Work	60 minutes
☐ 1-2-3 Eating	B S L S D
☐ Meaningful Pursuits	6 to 8 hours
☐ Time to Restore	60 minutes
☐ Intimacy Time	Sensual

The 3-Day Solution® Plan, Ballantine Books, 2005
The Institute for Health Solutions • www.thepathway.org
© Laurel Mellin, 2005

The 3-Day Solution® Plan – Day 3
Solution Skills

How do I feel?	What do I need?	Am I Above the Line?
		Above Below Cycle? EH?

☐ _____ _____ ___ ___ ___ ___
☐ _____ _____ ___ ___ ___ ___
☐ _____ _____ ___ ___ ___ ___
☐ _____ _____ ___ ___ ___ ___
☐ _____ _____ ___ ___ ___ ___
☐ _____ _____ ___ ___ ___ ___
☐ _____ _____ ___ ___ ___ ___
☐ _____ _____ ___ ___ ___ ___
☐ _____ _____ ___ ___ ___ ___
☐ _____ _____ ___ ___ ___ ___

☐ **Checked in 10 times today?**
☐ **Did my best to stay above the line?**

The 3-Day Solution® Plan, Ballantine Books, 2005
The Institute for Health Solutions • www.thepathway.org
© Laurel Mellin, 2005

The 3-Day Solution® Plan – Phase 2
Solution Skills

How do I feel?	What do I need?	Am I Above the Line?
		Above Below Cycle? EH?

☐ _____ _____ ___ ___ ___ ___
☐ _____ _____ ___ ___ ___ ___
☐ _____ _____ ___ ___ ___ ___
☐ _____ _____ ___ ___ ___ ___
☐ _____ _____ ___ ___ ___ ___
☐ _____ _____ ___ ___ ___ ___
☐ _____ _____ ___ ___ ___ ___
☐ _____ _____ ___ ___ ___ ___
☐ _____ _____ ___ ___ ___ ___
☐ _____ _____ ___ ___ ___ ___

☐ **Checked in 10 times today?**
☐ **Did my best to stay above the line?**

The 3-Day Solution® Plan, Ballantine Books, 2005
The Institute for Health Solutions • www.thepathway.org
© Laurel Mellin, 2005

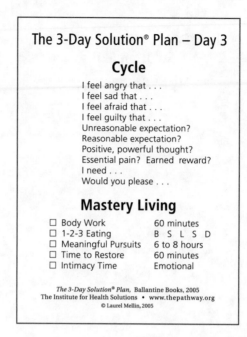

The 3-Day Solution® Plan – Day 3

Cycle

I feel angry that . . .
I feel sad that . . .
I feel afraid that . . .
I feel guilty that . . .
Unreasonable expectation?
Reasonable expectation?
Positive, powerful thought?
Essential pain? Earned reward?
I need . . .
Would you please . . .

Mastery Living

☐ Body Work   60 minutes
☐ 1-2-3 Eating   B S L S D
☐ Meaningful Pursuits   6 to 8 hours
☐ Time to Restore   60 minutes
☐ Intimacy Time   Emotional

The 3-Day Solution® Plan, Ballantine Books, 2005
The Institute for Health Solutions • www.thepathway.org
© Laurel Mellin, 2005

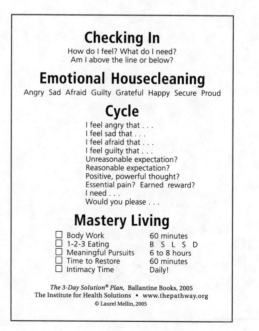

Checking In

How do I feel? What do I need?
Am I above the line or below?

Emotional Housecleaning

Angry Sad Afraid Guilty Grateful Happy Secure Proud

Cycle

I feel angry that . . .
I feel sad that . . .
I feel afraid that . . .
I feel guilty that . . .
Unreasonable expectation?
Reasonable expectation?
Positive, powerful thought?
Essential pain? Earned reward?
I need . . .
Would you please . . .

Mastery Living

☐ Body Work   60 minutes
☐ 1-2-3 Eating   B S L S D
☐ Meaningful Pursuits   6 to 8 hours
☐ Time to Restore   60 minutes
☐ Intimacy Time   Daily!

The 3-Day Solution® Plan, Ballantine Books, 2005
The Institute for Health Solutions • www.thepathway.org
© Laurel Mellin, 2005

Notes

1. Three Days That Will Change Your Life

1. The 3-Day Solution Plan Survey

This plan was inspired by the experience of participants in our three-day Solution Retreats who found that an intense experience using Solution Skills and Mastery Living had remarkable effects. The objective of the survey was to determine the immediate effects of The 3-Day Solution Plan.

We contacted 2,000 people who subscribed to an introductory e-mail course offered on the program's website, describing the plan and offering opportunities to test it. The first 100 people who responded to the notice by returning a signed release were sent a copy of the initial version of the plan. They were also provided with information about how to participate in one of four teleconferencing sessions conducted by the author during the two weeks that followed their receipt of the plan. The objective of the groups was to respond to their questions about the plan and to learn more about their experiences using it. The total number of participants who attended these groups was 60.

Based on these initial evaluations, the plan was revised and, two months later, we contacted 2,000 people who had not tested the plan and had visited our website in the previous three months, announcing the opportunity to test the plan. We accepted into the survey the first 100 people who indicated an interest in testing the plan and returned a signed release. We sent them the revised plan and a brief questionnaire developed by the author, which included basic questions such as their assessment of the plan, their age, gender, race, height, and weight. Of the 100 who responded, 74 returned the completed questionnaire. No compensation was offered to the participants other than a complimentary copy of the book.

The respondants were almost exclusively female and Caucasian, the average age was 45 (range 25 to 64). Additional surveys reflecting the experience of men and minorities would be helpful. Although the first testing of the plan included more men, their responses were based on feedback during a teleconferencing session rather than a questionnaire. The validity of this survey is affected by the sample that may not be representative and by data collection methods—a questionnaire and self-reported weight results. In addition, short-term changes are not necessarily related to long-term outcomes. See note in Chapter 6, Solution Method Research, for data on the impact of long-term use of the method.

The reported weight change after three days on the plan averaged about 3 pounds. The mean weight loss was 2.88 pounds (range 0 to 8 pounds). Some of the participants' responses to general questions regarding the program and physical/emotional state are shown below.

How would you rate the overall plan (percent of responses)?

Excellent	72
Good	27
Fair	1
Poor	0

Would you recommend it to a friend?

Highly recommend	77
Recommend	22
Wouldn't recommend	1

Did your drive to overeat decrease by the end of the third day?

Yes, a lot	51
Yes, somewhat	43
No	6

Did you experience life above the line (clarity, vibrancy, and peace) by the third day?

Yes	78
No	8
Not sure	14

2. Retraining Your Feeling Brain

1. G. F. Koob, "Alcoholism: Allostatis and Beyond, Alcoholism," *Clinical and Experimental Research* 27 (2003): 232–243.

B. S. McEwen, "Protective and Damaging Effects of Stress Mediators," *New England Journal of Medicine* 338 (1009): 171–179.

P. Sterling, J. Eyer, "Allostasis: A New Paradigm to Explain Arousal Pathology, in Handbook of Life Stress," *Cognition and Health* (S. Fisher, J. Reason, eds.), 1988, pp. 629–649, John Wiley.

E. Epel, B. McEwen, J. Ickovics, "Embodying psychological thriving: Physical thriving in response to stress," *Journal of Social Issues* 54 (1998): 301–322.

N. E. Adler, A. C. Snibbe, "The Role of Psychosocial Processes in Explaining the Gradient Between Socioeconomic Status and Health," *Current Directions in Psychological Sciences* 12 (2003): 119–123.

4. Why Diets Don't Work

1. S. C. Wooley and D. M. Garner, "Obesity Treatment: The High Cost of False Hope," *Journal of the American Dietetic Association* 91 (1991): 1248–1251.

S. C. Wooley and D. M. Garner, "Controversies in Management: Should Obesity Be Treated?: Dietary Treatments for Obesity Are Ineffective," *British Medical Journal* 309 (1994): 655–656.

S. Phelan, J. O. Hill, W. Lang, J. R. Dibello, and R. R. Wing, "Recovery from Relapse among Successful Weight Maintainers," *American Journal of Clinical Nutrition* 78 (2003): 1079–1084.

T. Reinehr, K. Brylack, U. Alexy, M. Kersting, and W. Andler, "Predictors in Success in Outpatient Training in Obese Children and Adolescents," *International Journal of Obesity* 27 (2003): 1087–1092.

T. M. Sheperd, "Effective Management of Obesity," *Journal of Family Practice* 52 (2003): 34–42.

Y. D. Miller and D. W. Dunstan, "The Effectiveness of Physical Activity Interventions for the Treatment of Overweight and Obesity and Type 2 Diabetes," *Journal of Science and Medicine in Sport* 7 (2004), suppl. no. 1: 52–59.

H. J. Zunft, D. Friebe, B. Seppelt, K. Widhalm, A. M. Remaut de Winter, M. D. Vaz de Almeida, J. M. Kearney, and M. Gibney, "Perceived Benefits and Barriers to Physical Activity in a Nationally Representative Sample in the European Union," *Public Health Nutrition* 29 (1999): 153–160.

J. P. Foreyt and W. S. Poston II, "The Challenge of Diet, Exercise and Lifestyle Modification in the Management of the Obese Diabetic Patient," *International Journal of Obesity and Related Metabolic Disorders* 23 (1999), suppl. no. 7: S5–S11.

L. M. Delahanty, J. B. Meigs, D. Hayden, D. A. Williamson, and D. M. Nathan, "Diabetes Prevention Program (DPP) Research Group: Psychological and Behavioral Correlates of Baseline BMI in the Diabetes Prevention Program (DPP)," *Diabetes Care* 25 (2002): 1992–1998.

L. Van Horn and R. E. Kavey, "Diet and Cardiovascular Disease Prevention: What Works?" *Annals of Behavioral Medicine* 19 (1997): 197–212.

L. A. Lytle, D. M. Murray, C. L. Perry, M. Story, A. S. Birnbaum, M. Y. Kubik, and S. Varnell, "School-Based Approaches to Affect Adolescents' Diets: Results from the TEENS Study," *Health Education and Behavior* 31 (2004): 270–287.

M. L. Skender, G. K. Goodrick, D. J. Del Junco, R. S. Reeves, L. Darnell, A. M. Gotto, and J. P. Foreyt, "Comparison of 2-Year Weight Loss Trends in Behavioral Treatments of Obesity: Diet, Exercise, and Combination Interventions," *Journal of the American Dietetic Association* 96 (1996): 342–346.

T. A. Wadden, R. A. Vogt, G. D. Foster, and D. A. Anderson, "Exercise and the Maintenance of Weight Loss: 1-Year Follow-up of a Controlled Clinical Trial," *Journal of Consulting and Clinical Psychology* 66 (1998): 429–433.

G. K. Goodrick and J. P. Foreyt, "Why Obesity Treatments Don't Last," *Journal of the American Dietetic Association* 91 (1991): 1243–1247.

M. T. McGuire, R. R. Wing, M. L. Klem, W. Lang, and J. O. Hill, "What Predicts Weight Regain in a Group of Successful Weight Losers?" *Journal of Consulting and Clinical Psychology* 67 (1999): 177–185.

M. M. Clark and T. K. King, "Eating Self-Efficacy and Weight Cycling: A Prospective Clinical Study," *Eating Behaviors* 1 (2000): 47–52.

A. Golay, S. Buclin, J. Ybarra, F. Toti, C. Pichard, N. Picco, N. de Tonnac, and A. F. Allaz, "New Interdisciplinary Cognitive-Behavioral-Nutritional Approach to Obesity Treatment: A 5-Year Follow-up Study," *Eating and Weight Disorders* 9 (2004): 29–34.

A. M. Glenny, S. O'Meara, A. Melville, T. A. Sheldon, and C. Wilson, "The Treatment and Prevention of Obesity: A Systematic Review of the Literature," *International Journal of Obesity and Related Metabolic Disorders* 21 (1997): 715–737.

M. F. Rolland-Cachera, H. Thibault, J. C. Souberbielle, D. Soulie, P. Carbonel, M. Deheeger, D. Roisol, E. Longueville, F. Bellisle, and P. Serog, "Massive Obesity in Adolescents: Dietary Interventions and Behaviours Associated with Regain at 2 Y Follow-up," *International Journal of Obesity and Related Metabolic Disorders* 28 (2004): 514–519.

D. D. Hensrud, "Dietary Treatment and Long-Term Weight Loss and Maintenance in Type 2 Diabetes," *Obesity Research* 9 (2001), suppl. no. 4: 348S–353S.

M. L. Klem, R. R. Wing, W. Lang, M. T. McGuire, and J. O. Hill, "Does Weight Loss Maintenance Become Easier over Time?" *Obesity Research* 8 (2000): 438–444.

M. K. Mattfeldt-Beman, S. A. Corrigan, V. J. Stevens, C. P. Sugars, A. T. Dalcin, M. J. Givi, and K. C. Copeland, "Participants' Evaluation of a Weight-Loss Program," *Journal of the American Dietetic Association* 99 (1999): 66–71.

R. R. Wing, E. Blair, M. Marcus, L. H. Epstein, and J. Harvey, "Year-Long Weight Loss Treatment for Obese Patients with Type II Diabetes: Does Including an Intermittent Very-Low-Calorie Diet Improve Outcome?" *American Journal of Medicine* 97 (1994): 354–362.

L. W. Turner, M. Q. Wang, and R. C. Westerfield, "Preventing Relapse in Weight Control: A Discussion of Cognitive and Behavioral Strategies," *Psychological Reports* 77 (1995): 651–666.

C. Gosselin and G. Cote, "Weight Loss Maintenance in Women Two to Eleven Years after Participating in a Commercial Program: A Survey," *BMC Women's Health* 1 (2001): 2.

F. Grodstein, R. Levine, L. Troy, T. Spencer, G. A. Colditz, and M. J. Stampfer, "Three-Year Follow-up of Participants in a Commercial Weight Loss Program: Can You Keep It Off?" *Archives of Internal Medicine* 156 (1996): 1302–1306.

K. R. Fontaine, I. Barofsky, S. J. Bartlett, S. C. Franckowiak, and R. E. Anderson, "Weight Loss and Health-Related Quality of Life: Results at 1-Year Follow-up," *Eating Behaviors* 5 (2004): 85–88.

R. W. Jeffery, K. M. Kelly, A. J. Rothman, N. E. Aherwood, and K. N. Boutelle, "The Weight Loss Experience: A Descriptive Analysis," *Annals of Behavioral Medicine* 27 (2004): 100–106.

C. Ayyad and T. Anderson, "Long-Term Efficacy of Dietary Treatment of Obesity: A Systematic Review of Studies Published between 1931 and 1999," *Obesity Reviews* 1 (2000): 113–119.

J. D. Latner, A. J. Stunkard, G. T. Wilson, M. L. Jackson, D. S. Zelitch, and E. Labouvie, "Effective Long-Term Treatment of Obesity: A Continuing Care Model," *International Journal of Obesity and Related Metabolic Disorders* 24 (2000): 893–898.

R. W. Jeffrey, A. Drewnowski, L. H. Epstein, A. J. Stunkard, G. T. Wilson, R. R. Wing, and D. R. Hill, "Long-Term Maintenance of Weight Loss: Current Status," *Health Psychology* 19 (2000): 5–16.

2. P. Sahasporn, E. E. York-Crowe, D. A. Williamson, D. H. Ryan, and G. A. Bray, "Americans on Diet: Results from the 1994–1996 Continuing Survey of Food Intakes by Individuals," *Journal of the American Dietetic Association* 102 (2002): 1247–1251.

3. A. A. Hedley, C. L. Ogden, C. L. Johnson, M. D. Carroll, L. R. Curtin, and K. M. Flegal, "Prevalence of Overweight and Obesity Among US Children, Adolescents, and Adults, 1999–2002," *Journal of the American Medical Association* 291 (2004): 2847–2850.

4. Y. C. Chagnon, L. Pérusse, S. J. Weisnagel, T. Rankinen, and C. Bouchard, "The Human Obesity Gene Map: The 1999 Update," *Obesity Research* 8 (2000): 89–117.

5. S. Z. Yanovski, W. H. Dietz, N. J. Goodwin, J. O. Hill, F. X. Pi-Sunyer, B. J. Rolls, J. Stern, R. L. Weinsier, G. T. Wilson, and R. R. Wing, "Long-Term Pharmacotherapy in the Management of Obesity," *Journal of the American Medical Association* 276 (1996): 1907–1915.

6. H. Bays and C. Dujovne, "Pharmacotherapy of Obesity," *American Journal of Cardiovascular Drugs* 2 (2002): 245–253.

7. A. M. Glenny, S. O'Meara, A. Melville, T. A. Sheldon, and C. Wilson, "The Treatment and Prevention of Obesity: A Systematic Review of the Literature," *International Journal of Obesity and Related Metabolic Disorders* 21 (1997): 715–737.

8. T. Martikainen, E. Pirinen, E. Alhava, E. Poikolainene, M. Pääkkönen, M. Uusitupa, and H. Gylling, "Long-Term Results, Late Complications and Quality of Life in a Series of Adjustable Gastric Banding," Obesity Surgery 14 (2004): 648–654.

H. E. Oria, "Outcomes after Bariatric Surgery," *Journal of American College Surgery* 198 (2004): 500–501.

R. E. Brolin, "Bariatric Surgery and Long-term Control of Morbid Obesity," *Journal of the American Medical Association* 288 (2002): 2793–2796.

5. The Crossover Effect

1. F. Contaldo and F. Pasanisi, "Obesity Epidemics: Secular Trend or Globalization Consequences? Beyond the Interaction between Genetic and Environmental Factors," *Clinical Nutrition* 23 (2004): 289–291.

P. Bjorntorp, "Thrifty Genes and Human Obesity: Are We Chasing Ghosts?" *Lancet* 258 (2001): 1006–1008.

2. K. M. Flegal, R. P. Troiano, E. R. Pamuk, R. J. Kuczmarski, and S. M. Campbell, "The Influence of Smoking Cessation on the Prevalence of Overweight in the United States," *New England Journal of Medicine* 333 (1995): 1165–1170.

6. Solution Method Research

1. Solution Method Survey conducted by Nancy Bates, Dr.P.H., R.D., researcher at the University of Illinois–Chicago, 2002, manuscript in preparation; summary published in L. Mellin, *The Pathway* (New York: HarperCollins, 2004).

2. L. M. Mellin, L. A. Slinkard, and C. E. Irwin Jr., "Adolescent Obesity Intervention: Validation of the SHAPEDOWN Program," *Journal of the American Dietetic Association* 878 (1987): 333–338.

3. L. Mellin, M. Croughan-Minihane, and L. Dickey, "The Solution Method: 2-Year Trends in Weight, Blood Pressure, Exercise, Depression, and Functioning of Adults Trained in Developmental Skills," *Journal of the American Dietetic Association* 97 (1997): 1133–1138.

L. M. Mellin, "Developmental Skills Training for the Treatment of Obesity: Integration of Decades of Research" (presented at the annual meeting of the American Dietetic Association, Denver, October 1999).

4. S. Freinkel, "Top Ten Medical Advances of 2000," *Health*, January–February 2001, 152.

8. It's a Toxic World

1. J. E. Seeman, B. H. Singer, J. W. Rowe, R. I. Horowitz, B. S. McEwen, "Price of Adaptation—Allostatic Load and Its Health Consequences: MacArthur Studies of Successful Aging," *Archives of Internal Medicine* 157 (1999): 2259–2268.

B. S. McEwen, "Protective and Damaging Effects of Stress Medications," *New England Journal of Medicine* 338 (1998): 171–179.

2. A. A. Hedley, C. L. Ogden, C. L. Johnson, M. D. Carroll, L. R. Curtin, and K. M. Flegal, "Prevalence of Overweight and Obesity among US Children, Adolescents, and Adults, 1999–2002," *Journal of the American Medical Association* 291 (2004): 2847–2850.

3. B. M. Popkin and C. Doak, "The Obesity Epidemic Is a Worldwide Phenomenon," *Nutrition Reviews* 56 (1998): 106–114.

Y. Wang, C. Monteiro, and B. M. Popkin, "Trends of Obesity and Underweight in Older Children and Adolescents in the United States, Brazil, China, and Russia," *American Journal of Clinical Nutrition* 75 (2002): 971–977.

4. D. Filozof, C. Gonzalez, M. Sereday, C. Mazza, and J. Braguinsky, "Obesity Prevalence and Trends in Latin-American Countries," *Obesity Reviews* 2 (2001): 99–106.

5. J. F. Schumaker, *The Age of Insanity: Modernity and Mental Health* (Westport, CT: Praeger Publishers, 2001).

F. Contaldo and F. Pasanisi, "Obesity Epidemics: Secular Trend or Globalization Consequences? Beyond the Interaction between Genetic and Environmental Factors," *Clinical Nutrition* 23 (2004): 289–291.

J. DeGraaf, D. Wann, and T. H. Naylor, *Affluenza: The All-Consuming Epidemic* (San Francisco: Berrett-Koehler, 2002).

6. Statistical table, "Consumer Credit Outstanding, 1952–2002," *Budget of the United States Government: Economic Report of the President, 2003.*

7. S. T. St. Jeor, B. V. Howard, T. E. Prewitt, V. Bovee, T. Bazzarre, and R. H. Eckel, "Nutrition Committee of the Council on Nutrition, Physical Activity, and Metabolism of the American Heart Association," *Circulation* 104 (2001): 1869–1874.

8. P. R. Amato, "Continuity and Change in Marital Quality between 1980 and 2000," *Journal of Marriage and Family* 65 (2003): 1–22.

9. U.S. Bureau of the Census, *Current Population Reports, Statistical Abstract of the United States, 2001.*

10. P. Sahasporn, E. E. York-Crowe, D. A. Williamson, D. H. Ryan, and G. A. Bray, "Americans on Diet: Results from the 1994–1996 Continuing Survey of Food Intakes by Individuals," *Journal of the American Dietetic Association* 102 (2002): 1247–1251.

11. L. R. Young, "The Contribution of Expanding Portion Sizes to the U.S. Obesity Epidemic," *American Journal of Public Health* 92 (2002): 246–249.

12. The United Nations Economic Commission, *Trends in Europe and North*

America: The Statistical Yearbook of the Economic Commission for Europe, 2003, Chapter 2, "Families and Households."

13. D. A. Leon and V. Shkolnikov, "Social Stress and the Russian Mortality Crisis," *Journal of the American Medical Association* 279 (1998): 790–791.

14. M. Wines, "An Ailing Russia Lives a Tough Life That's Getting Shorter," Freedom Toll: Why Russians Are Dying Younger (series), *New York Times,* December 3, 2000.

15. J. Luo and F. B. Hu, "Time Trends of Childhood Obesity in China from 1989 to 1997," Takemi Program, Harvard School of Public Health, Boston; Information Center of Public Health, Chinese Academy of Preventive Medicine, Beijing; Department of Nutrition, Harvard School of Public Health, Boston.

Commentary by Marc Lippman, Fes, Morocco, "Letters," *Newsweek* (international ed.), New York, September 9, 2002, 8.

"Social and Cultural Trends—Obesity in China: Tracking Nutrition in Transition" (Department of Epidemiology, University of Pittsburgh, 2004).

16. A. C. Bell, K. Ge, and B. M. Popkin, "The Road to Obesity or the Path to Prevention: Motorized Transportation and Obesity in China," *Obesity Research* 10 (2002): 277–283.

17. T. M. Nephew, G. D. Williams, F. S. Stinson, et al., "Surveillance Report No. 55: Apparent per Capita Alcohol Consumption: National, State, and Regional Trends, 1977–1998" (Bethesda, MD: National Institute on Alcohol Abuse and Alcoholism [NIAAA], 2000).

18. "Cigarette Consumption, United States, 1900–2002," *Tobacco Outlook Report,* update, Economic Research Service, U.S. Department of Agriculture, Office of National Drug Control Policy, White House.

19. Office of National Drug Control Policy, White House Update, 2003.

20. K. M. Flegal, M. D. Carroll, R. J. Kuczmarski, and C. L. Johnson, "Overweight and Obesity in the United States: Prevalence and Trends, 1960–1994," *International Journal of Obesity and Related Metabolic Disorders* 22 (1998): 39–47.

21. Budget of the United States Government: Economic Report of the President, 2003. Statistical table, "Consumer Credit Outstanding, 1952–2002."

22. S. M. Foote and L. Etheredge, "Increasing Use of New Prescription Drugs: A Case Study," *Health Affairs* 19, no. 4 (July–August 2000): 165–170.

9. The Toxic Spiral of Weight Gain

1. G. P. Chrousos and P. W. Gold, "Stress and Stress Disorders," *Journal of the American Medical Association* 267 (1992): 1244–1251.

R. A. Ruden, *The Craving Brain* (New York: HarperCollins, 1997).

R. M. Sapolsky, *Why Zebras Don't Get Ulcers: An Updated Guide to Stress, Stress-related Disorders and Coping* (New York: W. H. Freeman, 1998).

M. M. Woolsey, "Eating Disorders: A Clinical Guide to Counseling and Treatment," American Dietetic Association, 2002.

T. Lewis, F. Amini, and R. Lannon, *A General Theory of Love* (New York: Random House, 2000).

D. S. Charney, "Psychobiological Mechanisms of Resilience and Vulnerability: Implications for Successful Adaptation to Extreme Stress," *American Journal of Psychiatry* 161 (2004): 195–216.

A. S. Karlamangla, B. H. Singer, B. S. McEwen, J. W. Rowe, and T. E. Seeman, "Allostatic Load as a Predictor of Functional Decline: MacArthur Studies of Successful Aging," *Journal of Clinical Epidemiology* 55 (2002): 696–710.

O. M. Wolkowitz, E. S. Epel, and V. I. Reus, "Stress Hormone–Related Psychopathology: Pathophysiological and Treatment Implications," *World Journal of Biological Psychiatry* 2 (2001): 115–143.

A. Peters, U. Schweiger, L. Pellerin, C. Hubold, K. M. Altmanns, M. Conrad, B. Schultes, J. Born, H. L. Feling, "The Selfish Brain: Competition for Energy Resources," *Neurosciences and Biobehavioral Reviews* 28 (2004): 143–180.

R. Thayer, *Calm Energy: How People Regulate Mood with Food and Exercise* (New York: Oxford Universtiy Press, 2001).

N. E. Adler, A. C. Snibbe, "The Role of Psychosocial Processes in Explaining the Gradient Between Socioeconomic Status and Health," *Current Directions in Psychological Science* 12 (2003): 119–123.

G. F. Koob, "Alcoholism: Allostasis and Beyond," *Alcoholism: Clinical and Experimental Research* 27 (2003): 232–243.

10. Spinning Out of Control

1. E. Epel, R. Lapidus, B. McEwen, and K. Brownell, "Stress May Add Bite to Appetites in Women: A Laboratory Study of Stress-Induced Cortisol and Eating Behavior," *Psychoneuroendocrinology* 26 (2000): 37–49.

2. D. S. Ludwig, J. A. Majzoub, A. Al-Zahrani, G. E. Dallal, I. Blanco, and S. B. Roberts, "High Glycemic Index Foods, Overeating, and Obesity," *Pediatrics* 103 (1999): E26.

3. E. Somer, *Food and Mood: The Complete Guide to Eating Well and Feeling Your Best* (New York: Owl Books, 1999).

4. G. J. Wang, N. D. Volkow, F. Telang, M. Jayne, J. Ma, W. Zhu, C. T. Wong, N. R. Pappas, A. Geliebter, and J. S. Fowler, "Exposure to Appetitive Food Stimuli Markedly Activates the Human Brain," *Neuroimage* 21 (2004): 1790–1797.

5. L. B. Siorensen, P. Moller, A. Flint, M. Marents, and A. Raben, "Effect of Sensory Perception of Foods on Appetite and Food Intake: A Review of Studies on Humans," *International Journal of Obesity and Related Metabolic Disorders* 17 (2003): 1152–1166.

R. J. Wurtman and J. J. Wurtman, "Brain Serotonin, Carbohydrate-Craving, Obesity and Depression," *Obesity Research* 3 (November 1995), suppl. no. 4: 477S–480S.

6. D. P. Burkitt, A. R. Walker, and N. S. Painter, "Dietary Fiber and Disease," *Journal of the American Medical Association* 229 (1974): 1068–1074.

7. M. C. Howarth, E. Saltzman, and S. B. Roberts, "Dietary Fiber and Weight Regulation," *Nutrition Reviews* 59 (2001): 129–139.

8. S. Stanley, K. Wynne, and S. Bloom, "Gastrointestinal Satiety Signals III: Glucagon-like Peptide 1, Oxyntomodulin, Peptide YY, and Pancreaticpolypeptide," *American Journal of Physiology—Gastrointestinal and Liver Physiology* 286 (2004): G693–G697.

9. E. Naslund, N. King, S. Mansten, N. Adner, J. J. Holst, M. Gutniak, and P. M. Hellstrom, "Prandial Subcutaneous Injections of Glucagon-like Peptide-1 Cause Weight Loss in Obese Human Subjects," *British Journal of Nutrition* 91 (2004): 439–446.

10. M. I. McBurney, "The Gut: Central Organ in Nutrient Requirements and Metabolism," *Canadian Journal of Physiological Pharmacology* 72 (1994): 260–265.

D. Attaix, E. Arousseau, A. Manghbati, and M. Arnal, "Contribution of Liver, Skin, and Skeletal Muscle to Whole-Body Protein Synthesis in the Young Lamb," *British Journal of Nutrition* 60 (1988): 77–84.

11. E. Epel, R. Lapidus, B. McEwen, and K. Brownell, "Stress May Add Bite to Appetites in Women: A Laboratory Study of Stress-Induced Cortisol and Eating Behavior," *Psychoneuroendocrinology* 26 (2000): 37–49.

12. G. M. Reaven and A. Laws, eds., *Insulin Resistance: The Metabolic Syndrome X* (Totowa, NJ: Humana Press, 1999).

13. I. Mattiasson and F. Lindgarde, "The Effect of Psychosocial Stress and Risk Factors for Ischaemic Heart Disease on the Plasma Fibrinogen Concentration," *Journal of Internal Medicine* 234 (1993): 45–51.

14. R. L. Weinsier, "Etiology of Obesity: Methodological Examination of the Set-Point Theory," *Journal of Parenteral and Enteral Nutrition* 25, no. 3 (May–June 2001): 103–110.

A. E. Macias, "Experimental Demonstration of Human Weight Homeostasis: Implications for Understanding Obesity," *British Journal of Nutrition* 91, no. 3 (March 2004): 479–484.

15. C. J. Small and S. R. Bloom, "Gut Hormones and the Control of Appetites," *Trends in Endocrinology and Metabolism* 15 (2004): 259–263.

16. Y. Shi and P. Burn, "Lipid Metabolic Enzymes: Emerging Drug Targets for the Treatment of Obesity," *National Review of Drug Discoveries* 3 (2004): 695–710.

17. R. Cancello, A. Tounian, C. Poitou, and K. Clement, "Adiposity Signals, Genetic and Body Weight Regulation in Humans," *Diabetes Metabolism* 3 (2004): 215–227.

18. M. F. Dallman, S. F. Akana, A. M. Strack, K. S. Scribner, N. Pecoraro, S. E. La

Fleur, H. Houshyar, and H. Gomez, "Chronic Stress–Induced Effects of Corticosterone on Brain: Direct and Indirect," *Annals of the New York Academy of Sciences* 1018 (2004): 141–150.

A. M. Lemieux and C. L. Coe, "Abuse-Related Posttraumatic Stress Disorder: Evidence for Chronic Neuroendocrine Activation in Women," *Psychosomatic Medicine* 57 (1995): 105–115.

19. M. L. Pelchat, "Of Human Bondage: Food, Craving, Obsession, Compulsion and Addiction," *Physiological Behavior* 76 (2002): 347–352.

Wurtman and Wurtman, "Brain Serotonin, Carbohydrate-Craving, Obesity and Depression," *Advances in Experimental Medicine and Biology* 398 (1996): 35–41.

P. J. Rogers and H. J. Smit, "Food Craving and Food 'Addiction': A Critical Review of the Evidence from a Biopsychosocial Perspective," *Pharmacology and Biochemistry of Behavior* 66 (2000): 3–14.

A. C. Toomvliet, H. Pijl, E. Hopman, B. M. Elte-de Wever, and A. E. Meinders, "Serotoninergic Drug-Induced Weight Loss in Carbohydrate Craving Obese Subjects," *International Journal of Obesity and Related Metabolic Disorders* 20 (1996): 917–920.

E. S. Epel, B. McEwen, T. Seeman, K. Matthews, G. Castellazzo, K. D. Brownell, J. Bell, and J. R. Ickovics, "Stress and Body Shape: Stress-Induced Cortisol Secretion Is Consistently Greater among Women with Central Fat," *Psychosomatic Medicine* 62 (2000): 623–632.

E. E. Epel, A. E. Moyer, C. D. Martin, S. Macary, N. Cummings, J. Rodin, and M. Rebuffe-Scrive, "Stress-Induced Cortisol, Mood, and Fat Distribution in Men," *Obesity Research* 7 (1999): 9–15.

H. Steiger, M. Istreal, L. Gauvin, N. M. Ng Ying Kin, and S. N. Young, "Implications of Compulsive and Impulsive Traits for Serotonin Status in Women with Bulimia Nervosa," *Psychiatry Research* 120 (2003): 219–229.

S. Pinaquy, H. Chabrol, C. Simon, J. P. Louvet, and P. Barbe, "Emotional Eating, Alexithymia, and Binge-Eating Disorder in Obese Women," *Obesity Research* 11 (2003): 195–201.

20. G.-J. Wang, N. D. Volkow, J. Logan, N. R. Pappas, et al., "Brain Dopamine and Obesity," *Lancet* 357 (2001): 354–357.

21. D. E. Comings and K. Blum, "Reward Deficiency Syndrome: Genetic Aspects of Behavioral Disorders," *Progress in Brain Research* 126 (2000): 325–341.

T. Hampton, "Genes Harbor Clues to Addiction, Recovery," *Journal of the American Medical Association* 292 (2004): 321–322.

22. E. T. Hsiao and R. E. Thayer, "Exercising for Mood Regulation: The Importance of Experience," *Personality and Individual Differences* 24 (1998): 829–836.

23. D. Scully, J. Kremer, M. Meade, R. Graham, and K. Dudgeon, "Physical Exercise and Psychological Well-being: A Critical Review," *British Journal of Sports Medicine* 32 (1998): 111–120.

24. A. N. Vgontzas, C. Tsigos, E. O. Bixler, C. A. Stratakis, K. Zachman, A. Kales, A. Vela-Bueno, and G. P. Chrousos, "Chronic Insomnia and Activity of the Stress System: A Preliminary Study," *Journal of Psychosomatic Research* 45 (1998): 21–31.

25. J. Kaukua, T. Pekkarinen, T. Sane, and P. Mustajoki, "Sex Hormones and Sexual Function in Obese Men Losing Weight," *Obesity Research* 11 (2003): 689–694.

26. H. Bruch, *Eating Disorders: Obesity, Anorexia Nervosa, and the Person Within* (New York: Basic Books, 1973).

27. K. D. Carr and V. Papadouka, "The Role of Multiple Opiod Receptors in the Potentiation of Reward by Food Restriction," *Brain Research* 639 (1994): 253–260.

28. W. Schultz, P. Sayan, and P. R. Montague, "A Neural Substrate of Prediction and Reward," *Science* 275 (1997): 1593–1599.

29. K. A. Bruinsma and D. L. Taren, "Dieting, Essential Fatty Acid Intake, and Depression," *Nutrition Reviews* 58 (2000): 98–108.

30. M. B. Zemel and S. L. Miller, "Dietary Calcium and Dairy Modulation of Adiposity and Obesity Risk," *Nutrition Reviews* 62 (2004): 125–131.

31. S. J. Solomon, M. S. Kurzer, and D. H. Calloway, "Menstrual Cycle and Basal Metabolic Rate in Women," *American Journal of Clinical Nutrition* 36 (1982): 611–616.

Glossary

Above the Line In a state of emotional balance, relationship intimacy, and spiritual connection in which the drives to go to excess fade and we have clarity, connection, and vibrancy.

Allostatic Load The cumulative negative impacts, the wear and tear and neurobiological changes due to repeated cycles of allostasis and inefficiencies of the body in responding to environmental stress and psychosocial disadvantage or recovery from it.

Balance A state of emotional equilibrium, instead of feeling way high, way low, or numb or having thoughts but no feelings; feeling sad, not depressed; angry, not hostile; afraid, not panicked; and guilty, not ashamed. The state in which emotional appetites fade. One of the six developmental rewards of retraining the feeling brain.

Below the Line In a state of emotional imbalance; relationship merging, distancing, or control struggles; and spiritual disconnection in which the drives to go to excess increase and we experience confusion, disconnection, and despair.

Checking In Shifting our focus from outside or from thoughts to inside and feelings, becoming aware of how we feel and what we need. One of the three Solution Skills included in the 3-Day Solution.

Community Connection In Solution training, participants have Solution buddies with whom they practice the skills. When participants are below the line, they contact buddies on their Community Connection list until they find someone who has time to listen to them do a cycle. The buddy listens without interrupting. When the person is done with his or her cycle and is above the line, the buddy makes a supportive statement, that is, gives the person a tender morsel. The retraining of the feeling brain is enhanced when cycles are done in the loving presence of another.

Distancing   Being emotionally very separate from another, aware of how we feel and what we need but not aware of how the other feels and what he or she needs. Associated with lack of empathy for others and persecuting others.

Doing Cycles   Asking ourselves the questions of the nurturing and limits cycles when we are below the line, which results in our moving above the line. One of the three Solution Skills included in the 3-Day Solution.

Earned Rewards   "What are the earned rewards?" is the last question in the limits cycle. It is the payoff, the benefit, the lesson learned that we receive when we follow through with our reasonable expectations. We feel the earned rewards after we face the essential pain and it motivates and energizes us to take action.

Emotional Housecleaning   Involves completing the sentence "I feel _____ that . . ." for eight basic feelings: angry, sad, afraid, guilty, grateful, happy, secure, and proud. Moves us above the line when we are on our way below the line. Not as effective as doing cycles in moving us above the line when we are way below. One of the three Solution Skills included in the 3-Day Solution.

Emotional Trash   Unhealed hurts from the past that make it more difficult to stay above the line when faced with present stresses. We do cycles to feel the pain of the past, heal that pain, and learn from it. When we heal these hurts, we feel emotionally lighter and have more energy.

Essential Pain   "What is the essential pain?" is part of the limits cycle. It is the unavoidable reality of the human condition or the situation we must face, feel, and accept in order to follow through with our reasonable expectation. When we face the essential pain, we pop above the line and feel secure and energized so we can follow through with our expectation with relative ease.

External Solution   What we do when we cannot soothe and comfort ourselves from within. We reach outside ourselves to soothe and comfort ourselves with an external gratifier. Because we have disconnected from ourselves, and because in that state our neurotransmitters are unbalanced, we are likely to go to excess.

Feeling Brain   The limbic system, one of our three brains (the other two being the neocortex, or thinking brain, and the reptilian brain, or brain stem). The feeling brain is the seat of emotional balance, relationship intimacy, spiritual connection, and the drives to go to excess. Retraining the feeling brain enables and promotes changes that can be sustained.

Integration   Self-accepting, feeling whole and authentic. Not feeling all good or all bad but complete. One of the six developmental rewards of retraining the feeling brain.

Intimacy   Closeness with another person, the skill of being close without distancing from or merging with the other person. Having an awareness both of how we feel and what we need and of how the other person feels and what he or she needs. One of the six developmental rewards of retraining the feeling brain.

Lifestyle Surgery   Standing back from our life and identifying and making substantial changes in aspects of life that are neglectful or abusive. Makes it easier to use Solution Skills and achieve success with Mastery Living.

The Limits Cycle   One of the two cycles that form the foundation for The Solution Method. This cycle mirrors responsive self-parenting and creates power and safety. It includes the following questions: Are my expectations reasonable? Is my thinking positive and powerful? What is the essential pain? What is the earned reward?

Mastery Living   Focusing on the moment and making each day complete and vibrant, including balanced eating, physical activity, meaningful pursuits, and time to restore physically, emotionally, intellectually, and spiritually.

Meaningful Pursuits   Activities that give beyond ourselves and require us to consider others, the community, and the greater good. Time to restore gives to us, and meaningful pursuits give to others. These activities increase our sense of fulfillment and mattering.

Merging   Not intimate. Being overly close to another emotionally, aware of how the other person feels and what he or she needs but not aware of how we feel and what we need. Associated with people-pleasing and rescuing others.

Neurotransmitters   Chemicals (primarily dopamine, serotonin, and the endorphins) that transport electricity across the synapse from one nerve cell to another in our brain and affect our energy and mood and drive to go to excess.

The Nurturing Cycle   One of the two cycles that form the foundation for The Solution Method. This cycle mirrors responsive self-parenting, increases authenticity, and accesses intuition and emotional memory. It includes the following questions: How do I feel? What do I need? Do I need support?

Popping Above the Line   The experience during the moment when doing a cycle triggers a change in the feeling brain that moves us to a state of clarity, connection, and vibrancy. The flash of experience when we move from below the line to above the line.

Reasonable Expectations   The first part of the limits cycle, identifying expectations that are reasonable, not harsh or easy. These expectations begin the process of creating safety and power from within.

Sanctuary   An abiding sense of security, a sense that there is a safe place within that sees us for who we are—light side, dark side, and all. A nurturing, not indulging or depriving, inner voice. Not feeling lost or abandoned. One of the six developmental rewards of retraining the feeling brain.

A Solution   Having retrained the feeling brain to the point that we have emotional balance, relationship intimacy, spiritual connection, and, within the limits of genetics and circumstance, freedom from the whole range of common excesses.

The Solution Method   A method of retraining the feeling brain so that we stay above the line spontaneously more of the time and naturally process daily life in such a way as to minimize the unnecessary pain we cause ourselves and maximize health and happiness. Also called developmental skills training, mastering the skills that give us emotional intelligence and enable us to evolve.

The Solution 1-2-3 Eating   A system of choosing foods based on selecting at least one food from each of three groups: The Fiber Group, Healthy Fats, and The Protein Group. All foods in these groups support having a diet that is nutritionally adequate, prevents degenerative diseases, and promotes weight loss and maintenance. We consume foods from the fourth group, White Stuff, when we really need to, and we do so with complete enjoyment and no guilt. It is not a diet but an emotionally intelligent way to determine what and how much to eat.

Solution Skills   The tools to create a nurturing inner voice, stay balanced in response to current stresses, heal hurts from the past, and follow through with lifestyle changes. Three of the basic skills are used in the 3-Day Solution Plan.

Solution Training   The longer-term use of The Solution Method, with skills and practices in addition to the introductory ones included in the 3-Day Solution

Plan. Requires the completion of six Solution Kits and support such as Solution groups, the Solution Internet community, or self-help Solution circles.

Spirituality   The experience of feeling connected to the divine, God, or the spiritual as we define it. This aspect of Solution training is shaped to be consistent with each participant's religion, traditions, or beliefs. A deepening of spirituality is one of the six rewards of retraining the feeling brain, which is the seat of the soul, the part of us that experiences transcendence.

Stepping Out of the Toxic Spiral   Using Solution Skills and Mastery Living to trigger the cascade of changes in mind, body, and behavior that create weight loss without rigid diets.

Tender Morsel   A supportive, nurturing, and honest statement made to someone who has just done a cycle by the individual who has listened to that cycle in a group setting or during a Community Connection. The statement starts with the word *I* and reflects how it was for the listener to listen to the cycle; for example, "I learned so much from listening" or "I appreciate how much courage it took to do that cycle." Tender morsels enhance the intimacy and safety of Community Connections.

Thinking Brain   The neocortex. It processes knowledge, insight, analysis, planning, and deciding. Most interventions for weight loss are processed primarily by the thinking brain. There is no significant relationship between what is processed by the thinking brain and the most primitive human drives, such as overeating.

The 3-Day Solution Plan   An introduction to The Solution Method in which we use three basic Solution Skills and Mastery Living to live life above the line for three days.

Time to Restore   Activities in which we give to ourselves and meet our needs so that we have the balance and vibrancy to give to others and to fulfill our purpose in life. Taking time to restore ourselves physically, emotionally, intellectually, and spiritually.

Toxic Spiral of Weight Gain   The many small but important changes in mind, body, and behavior that synergistically create the shift into gaining weight or the continuation of weight gain.

Vibrancy   The personal vitality, spirit, and radiance that is associated with life above the line.

Acknowledgments

Many people have contributed generously to this method over the now 25 years of its development. There would be no Solution Method without the support and stimulation of colleagues and participants at the University of California–San Francisco, especially early on from Marion Nestle, Ph.D., M.P.H.; Charles E. Irwin Jr., M.D.; Jonathan E. Rodnick, M.D.; Mary S. Croughan, Ph.D.; and Larry L. Dickey, M.D., M.S.W., M.P.H. I am deeply grateful for the wisdom and courage of Jim Billings, Ph.D., M.Div., and the many ways that his presence has guided the evolution of this work. Igor Mitrovic, M.D., has been a tremendous support in reflecting on the neurobiology of the method.

Members of UCSF's Center for Obesity Assessment, Study and Training (COAST), whose contributions and research have enriched this work. Elissa S. Epel, Ph.D., whose groundbreaking research on stress and obesity and her many discussions of the issues have been so important to this work. Also, I am most grateful to Robert B. Baron, M.D., M.S.; Nancy Adler, Ph.D.; Alka M. Kanaya, M.D.; Andrea Garber, Ph.D., R.D.; and Robert H. Lustig, M.D., and Amy Levine and Quita Keller were generous with their support.

Other colleagues have given generously of their knowledge and support, including John Foreyt, Ph.D.; William Shore, M.D.; George Saba, Ph.D.; Carl Greenberg, M.S.; Velia Frost, M.F.T.; Mary Crittenden, Ph.D.; Marna Cohen, M.S.W.; Susan Johnson, M.D.; Lisa Frost, R.N., P.H.P.; Dennis Styne, M.D.; Lee Lipsenthal, M.D.; Ruth Marlen, M.D.; Ken Goodrick, Ph.D.; and Michael I. McBurney, Ph.D., F.A.C.N. The work of Robert E. Thayer, Ph.D.; Ronald A. Ruden, M.S., Ph.D.; Virginia S. Satir, M.D.; Erik H. Erikson; John F. Schumaker, Ph.D.; Joe Dispenza, Ph.D.; Fari Amini, M.D.; Richard Lannon, M.D.; Thomas Lewis, M.D.; and Dean Ornish, M.D., has informed the method in im-portant ways. I'm very grateful to John Gray, Ph.D., whose work inspired the feeding activity on the second day of the plan and who has contributed to the method throughout the years.

The staff of the Institute for Health Solutions, the nonprofit organization that disseminates professional and individual training in the method, has shouldered many responsibilities with kindness and good cheer during the writing of this book. I am deeply grateful to Kelly McGrath, director of operations; Sabrina Geshay, director of provider relations; Sean Maher, coordinator of customer service and information technology; Lynne LoPresto, coordinator of the Solution Maximizing Success program for those with extreme obesity; Michele Gorman, director of client relations; Meaghan Maher, graphics coordinator and administrator for the recipes and plan testing; and Brandon McGrath, customer services coordinator.

Earlier, Bernadette Payne spearheaded the development of our client services department, and Barbara Krohn responded to the needs of high-medical-risk participants. Consultation and support from Nora Farnsworth, David Bott, and Bryant Young have been invaluable. I am deeply grateful for the talent of Teka Luttrell, our graphic designer, who created the design of our Solution Kits and shared his wisdom and spacious thoughts with me on numerous occasions. Dave Radlauer generously shared his talents in producing our CDs for the Solution Kits; Nina Hill, Jill Johnson, and Kit and Warren Weagant of Command Productions shaped the sound for our Solution CDs and Alan Syiek has been a gracious and skilled webmaster for the Solution Internet community. Keith Parker's information technology advice and generous support have been tremendously valuable to our daily activities at the institute.

Many providers have made special contributions to this work. Deanne Hamilton, M.S., R.D., our director of lifestyle training, dealt with many clinical and professional training issues in my absence, all while planning her wedding. Judy Zehr, M.A., M.H.R.M., gave generously of her time despite pressing personal demands; Peggy Ernster, R.N., L.M.H.C., continues to be a source of enthusiasm in applying the method; and Jackie Placidi, M.S.W., has been consistently generous in sharing her insights and encouragement and care in this work. C. Anne Brown, Ph.D., has been such a joy and privilege to work with. And the many insights of Susan Stordahl, L.C.S.W., continue to broaden my view of the work. Barbara McCarty, R.D., has given so much to the method, including in the early days when our needs were the greatest. I'm grateful for the gentle persistence and depth of spirit of Mary Killian, R.D., L.D.N., and the honesty and laugh of Bonnie Hoag, M.F.T. I am deeply grateful to so many Solution providers and providers-in-training who shared their enthusiasm and their knowledge as this work was developed, including Gigi Acker, R.D.; Donna Acosta, R.D.; Merilee Amos, M.S., R.D.; Robin Anderson, R.D.; Neala Ausmus, R.D.; Mary Bergman, M.P.H., R.D.; Mari Bickford, R.N.; Gretchen Brickson, L.C.S.W.; Barbara Brown, M.S., L.P.C.; Sandy Buchanan, R.D.; JoAnn Campbell,

L.M.H.C.; Saoirse Charis-Graves, M.S.; Kristi Colbert, R.N.; Gale Cox, R.D.; Sylvia Cramer, Ph.D.; Roxanne Crocco, M.S.W., L.S.W.; Candy Cumming, R.D.; Tammy DuPerron, R.N.; Sonia Elkes, R.D.; Judy J. Fitzgibbons, M.S., R.D., L.D.; Misa Garbacz, R.D.; Ellen Good, M.S.W.; Donna Hemmingway, R.D., L.D.; Patsy Hollingbery, R.D., Ph.D.; Denise Holmes, R.D.; David A. Ingebritsen, Ph.D., L.P.C.P.; Vicky Jackson, M.F.T.; Annika Kahm, B.S.; Sandi Kaplan, M.S., R.D.; Denice Keepin, M.A., L.M.H.C.; Jeanette Lamb, R.D.; Elizabeth Larkin, L.C.S.W.; Diane C. Lesley, M.A., L.L.P.; Luise Levy, M.S.W.; Paula Lickteig, R.D.; Nancy Logue, Ph.D.; Eve Lowry, R.D.; Cheryl C. Marshall, R.D.; Sandra Martin, R.N.; Joanne Mason, M.F.T.; Anne S. Nuss, L.M.H.C.; Robin O'Hearn, Ph.D.; Cynthia Payne, M.S., R.D.; Carol Quartana, R.D.; Carra Richling-Knox, R.D.; Vicki Rowe-Currence, L.C.S.W.; Greg Sawyer, M.D.; Tina Sawyer, M.F.T.; Sarah Schuyler, Ph.D.; Jill Shaffer, R.D.; Madeline Simpson, R.N.; Paula Staffeldt, L.P.C.; Joy Staley, L.M.H.C.; Lynn Sterba, L.C.S.W.; Shirley Swartz, M.S., R.D.; Darcy Trego, R.D., C.D.E.; Colleen Verbeke, M.A., L.L.P.; Maribeth Webber, C.R.T.; Andrea Wenger-Hess, R.D., C.D.E.; and Alia Witt, R.D., M.F.T.

I am particularly grateful to our nutrition team, the certified Solution providers who worked tirelessly on the menu plans, testing the recipes submitted by participants, calculating the nutritional contributions of each menu and recipe, and coming to consensus about interpreting science that is often not clear. They are Jill Shaffer, R.D.; Carra Richling-Knox, R.D.; Donna Acosta, R.D.; and Sylvia Cramer, Ph.D., Alia Witt, R.D., M.F.T., and Eve Lowry, R.D., contributed to the recipes in this book.

Jill Shaffer lives in a house surrounded by woods in Pennington, New Jersey, with her husband, Brian; their three children; and their chocolate lab. She has been a Solution provider for seven years and specializes in obesity and eating disorders in her private practice. Jill is a Solution trainer, who coaches health professionals in the method and participates as a provider at our Solution retreats. I have always seen her as a sensitive clinician but enjoyed knowing the side of her that loves to cook! Jill brought her clarity, sense of style, and taste for good food to her work with our team.

Carra Richling-Knox has been a provider for five years and recently moved to Boulder, Colorado, from the Bay Area. She lives with her husband, Tod, and their new baby son, Jacob. Carra did all the nutritional analyses for the menus and recipes in this book, making the adjustments in the meals' recipes, and lists that would create precisely the balance of nutrients we recommend—all while taking time for yoga, conducting Solution groups, maintaining a nutrition private practice, and mothering an infant. She brought calmness and steady persistence to her work with our team.

Donna Acosta is a new Solution provider, who lives with her two small children and husband in Las Vegas. She participated in our first Solution retreat, and I so appreciate her passion, frankness, and strong opinions about nutrition and cooking. Donna is an experienced developer of cookbooks and cooking courses and brought to our team her sharp editor's eye and her love of good food. She also kept us on track to make these menus appealing to more people, often saying, "We can't include that recipe. You can't get *that* ingredient in Las Vegas!" Donna compiled and edited the final menus and recipes for this book.

Sylvia Cramer has been a Solution provider for eight years and specializes in Solution training for participants with high medical risk. She has a Solution practice in Lite-Weighs, an obesity clinic in Redlands, California. She drew upon her joy of traveling internationally with her husband, Giovanni, and daughter, Alessandra, in testing these recipes, which reflected the regional foods of the world.

The strength of this team is formidable. Its members are all professionals with scientific training in foods and nutrition and have a Solution in their own lives and are committed to bringing these skills to others. Working with these women on this project was a most rewarding experience. The opportunity to engage in creative work with people who shared the same scientific training, were above the line, and had a common heartfelt purpose was exciting and nourishing. I am deeply grateful to each member of our nutrition team for their many hours and late nights of service, as well as to their groups and families who participated in the testing and refining of these recipes. Special thanks to Meaghan Maher for all the administrative activities involved in this process.

So many program participants tested our three-day plan and submitted favorite recipes. I am grateful to each and every one of them. There were many times when I posted questions and surveys on our website. The formidable response was wonderful, with literally hundreds of participants sharing ideas and offering insights. Najwa Jardali's prizewinning recipe, Salata with Grilled Chicken, is featured on day 6 of the plan. Others who made formidable contributions to this work include John D. Galbraith, Kieran Bahn, Chris Hegge, Greg Cooper, Liz Rodgers-Ponce, Barb Roberts, Trisha Delp, Aeron Hicks, Mike Bell, and the inspiration and memory of Mike Bell Jr. I am grateful for the generosity and spirit of Hawley Riffenburg, Lisa Reyes, Pat Cherry, Mary Lane, Diane Merlino, and Dawn Galbo.

Kris Salvatore read the entire manuscript, offering editorial comments despite formidable obstacles. Christina Amini, the daughter of the late Fari Amini, M.D., whose writings on understanding the limbic system informed this work, and Audrey Webb offered editorial suggestions. Melissa Ayres, a graduate student at New York University, was tireless in locating and reviewing scientific articles for this work. Sean Maher was good-spirited and very effective in locating research articles for this work.

I am particularly grateful to Caroline Sutton, my editor at Random House, who has offered to this project her keen eye for concept and has carefully edited the words on these pages, improving my writing considerably. Caroline's involvement has been a true gift to the method. I appreciate Christina Duffy's attention to detail and meticulous care in guiding this work through production, and Susan J. Cohan's thorough copyediting. My agent, Jimmy Vines, has made the writing of this book so much less stressful. His enthusiasm has been contagious, and his advice has been extremely helpful. I have no idea how this book could have been written without the support of these very special people.

During the writing of this book, my parents, Rosie and Jack McClure, offered encouragement and ideas, day by day, helping with everything from fixing my sprinkler system to offering opinions on possible titles. My children—Haley, Joe, and John—each gave very different kinds of support as well, all of which changed the work in important ways. I'm so very grateful for the wise words and ongoing care of my brother, Steve McClure, and the support of Vivian McClure and Sarah, Lisa, and Michael.

I'm particularly grateful to Andrea, Daniel, Sophie, and Sarah Sharp; Dede Taylor; Kathleen Flickinger; Emily Kearney; Jock Begg; Jena and Brett Walter; Laura Doyle; Donna Fletcher; Colleen Mauro; Ann Squires; Kathy McHenry; Stephanie Moriarty; Janice and Ralph Echenique; Lou Thoelecke; Mike Mooney; Betsy and Bryant Young; Lisa Reyes; Kela and Carlos Cabrales; Kate and Yaz Krehbiel; Gail Aultschuler; Tom Morrison; Suzanne Danielson; Andrea Liguori; Louise Malandre; Ben LaMort; Sister Marina Ioki; Brian Inciardi, Lisa Wilkins and their daughters, Heidi and Hailey; and Dan Rosenthal.

My first publisher, Bob Mellin, spearheaded the application of this method to childhood and adolescent obesity, The Shapedown Program, and without his support over the years, there would be no Solution Method. Also, Sharon Nielsen has given of herself to this work for many years.

Finally, I feel a deep gratitude to all the providers, staff, and participants who have made our Solution community and Solution retreats possible. At our first retreat, a diverse group of people came together for three days. We had expected them to have a restoring, productive, and fun time, but soon realized that something of a different dimension was occurring. Perhaps due to the power of collective resonance coupled with the focused intensive use of these skills. Most participants felt transformed by the experience—which is what inspired the creation of this three-day plan. I am very grateful to each person who participated in our first 3-Day Solution Plan.

ABOUT THE AUTHOR

Laurel Mellin, M.A., R.D., is the *New York Times* bestselling author of *The Pathway*. She is an associate clinical professor of family and community medicine and pediatrics at the University of California, San Francisco's School of Medicine, and the director of The Institute for Health Solutions, a non-profit organization.

Her research and writing have received awards from the American Medical Association, the American Bariatric Society, and the U.S. Department of Consumer Education, and have been featured in *Fortune, U.S. News & World Report,* and *Time,* and on *Oprah, Good Morning America, Today,* and *The Early Show.* She has three children and lives in Marin County, California.

The mission of her non-profit organization, The Institute for Health Solutions, is to design, evaluate, and disseminate the method described in this book, developmental skills training, for the prevention and treatment of common problems and the promotion of health and happiness.

Visit the Institute's website at www.thepathway.org for information about joining a Solution Group or Circle, becoming part of The Solution Internet Community and obtaining your first Solution Kit. If you are a licensed health professional who is interested in inquiring about professional training to become a Certified Solution Provider, visit her website or e-mail health@thepathway.org. To contact the Institute for Health Solutions directly, call (415)457-3331 or e-mail 3daysolution@thepathway.org. For information regarding the application of the method to childhood and adolescent obesity, the Shapedown Program, visit the program's website at www.childobesity.com.

ABOUT THE TYPE

This book was set in Walbaum, a typeface designed in 1810 by German punch cutter J. E. Walbaum. Walbaum's type is more French than German in appearance. Like Bodoni, it is a classical typeface, yet its openness and slight irregularities give it a human, romantic quality.